"THE THING INSIDE MY HEAD"

A FAMILY'S JOURNEY THROUGH MENTAL ILLNESS

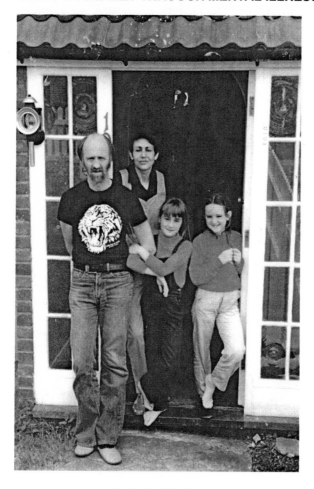

By Lois Chaber

'One million people commit suicide every year'
The World Health Organization

Lois Chaber

Published by
Chipmunkapublishing
PO Box 6872
Brentwood
Essex CM13 1ZT
United Kingdom

http://www.chipmunkapublishing.com

Copyright © Lois Chaber 2007

Edited by Lucy Dow and Mary Dow

In this book, many persons' names, especially those of medical personnel and patients, have been changed or kept anonymous to protect confidentiality and privacy. Furthermore, the content of the book represents the personal views and interpretations of our family—Sybil, Molly and Neil Macindoe and myself, Lois Chaber—whether of events that occurred in medical, educational, or legal institutions or of persons involved in any way in our daughter's care. The book mainly concerns events between 1978 and 1999, and as the primary author I declare that I have no information on or opinions about the current policies or personnel of any of these institutions.

"THE THING INSIDE MY HEAD"

Foreword

Human life is suffering but Sybil Macindoe suffered more than others with a severe and complex mental health problem, known as Obsessive Compulsive Disorder (OCD) and Anorexia Nervosa. It was an extremely distressing and handicapping condition for both her and family that ultimately led to her tragic death.

This book provides some insight into both the experience of Sybil as well as that of her carers and professionals. We can all learn from her narrative and from the different perspectives of her family and carers. I felt moved by her experience and was left wishing that she could have taken advantage of the newer developments in treating OCD.

The impact of OCD on the family is often hidden. Her family's observations and narrative are extremely balanced and provide a cautionary tale for sufferers, carers and professionals alike. There is lots of information and self help material about OCD but this book is a valuable addition to our knowledge about OCD and Anorexia Nervosa and its impact on others.

David Veale
Consultant Psychiatrist in Cognitive Behaviour Therapy,
South London and Maudsley Trust and the Priory Hospital
North London.

Lois Chaber

"THE THING INSIDE MY HEAD"

Acknowledgments

The resource that matters the most is people.

(Marjorie Wallace, on what is really needed in NHS mental health services, in "Broken Promises," by Minette Marrin, in *The Sunday Times Magazine,* July 8, 2007, pp. 40-49.)

People, many of them friends, were invaluable to me in the course of putting together this work over the past eight years. My first timid request for someone other than my husband to vet the earliest versions of chapters was met by an old US friend, Susan Teich, now a retired attorney. Her constructive comments and encouragement over an extended period of time gave me the momentum to carry on churning out the pages slowly but steadily. Oddly enough, the second volunteer to carefully review the early manuscript was also a retired US lawyer, a newer friend, Judson Levin, who also helped greatly with formatting it. At a critical juncture, I was given professional advice by the UK freelance author, Rebecca Loncraine, on sharpening and editing my too-voluminous manuscript. The second version was given a judicious overall reading by another US friend and academic colleague, Michael Rosenblum, who also reminded me that my friend Dolores Rosenblum had acquired special expertise in medical narratives. Dolores diligently presided over a third round of revisions and fed back a steady stream of inspired criticism. Finally, my oldest American friend, Barbara Phillips, a licensed clinical social worker, intensely critiqued the opening chapters during my search for a publisher. Thank heavens for email, which made possible this in-depth scrutiny by my former compatriots.

Many of my English friends also provided encouragement and various kinds of helpful feedback, having read all or parts of the manuscript at various stages. Grateful thanks go to Lesley Hill, Merita Banda, Mary Waldron, Michelle Soliatis and Pat Mountney. I am also

Lois Chaber

grateful to Tessa Baradon of the Anna Freud Centre Parent-Infant Project for reading the opening chapters and provoking me to further insights about my relationship with my daughter.

I am extremely indebted to those people whom I interviewed for this work, some of whom are given pseudonyms herein, whose willingness to talk about their interactions with Sybil made it possible to write a multi-vocal narrative: Family members who participated were my husband, his cousin Edna Keylock, and my daughter Molly; local friends included Sybil's former classmate and neighbour, 'Asha'; Sybil's adult pen-pal, June Keyte; Sybil's dancing teacher, Lesley Hand, and Sybil's temporary foster mother; from the Bethlem Royal Adolescent Unit, a senior nurse and a school teacher talked to me; the former Admissions and Marketing Officer from Jacques Hall, Jane Lee, was extremely helpful; and, in Clacton, two of Sybil's keyworkers from Granta Housing, Diane and Michael, and the chaplain for Clacton Hospital, Reverend Richard Smith, also granted me long interviews. Sybil's sister, Molly Macindoe, deserves special thanks not only for drawing upon difficult memories but also for providing the book's cover image and enhancing the photos within, distressing as these tasks were. Thanks also to Sue Patch, Theresa Coyne and June Keyte for allowing me to use personal letters, to Carole Fabricant for sending us the moving Pavese poem, and to Sarah Henderson for updates about the Coroners Bill.

I am very grateful for the advice and services of my publisher, Chipmunka—not least for the welcoming answer by CEO Jason Pegler to my initial, tentative inquiries: "You have come to the right place." I have been lucky to have two very conscientious and generous support workers, Mary Dow and Lucy Dow, to do the final formatting and editing of my text. Andrew Latchford's pragmatic legal advice has also been very helpful and his patient stewardship of the paperback edition is much-appreciated.

"THE THING INSIDE MY HEAD"

It has become a cliché to bestow all-out gratitude on one's spouse at the end of authorial debt lists, but it is a gesture I cannot avoid. Without the unmitigated support (technical, financial, and emotional) of Neil Macindoe, my husband—not to mention his own narrative contributions—this book could never have been written, and without his detailed scrutiny of various versions of every chapter, my prose style, such as it is, would be clumsier and more inaccurate.

Formal acknowledgement must be paid to the following organisations for the permission to reproduce substantial parts of works held in copyright or unpublished material:

A line from "Daughter" by Ellen Bryant Voigt, in *The Forces of Plenty:* With the kind permission of WW Norton & Company, Inc.

Stanzas from "Nocturne" by Cesar Pavese, translated by William Arrowsmith, in *Hard Labour:* With the kind permission of the Johns Hopkins University Press.

Extracts from *Up and Down the Worry Hill: a Children's Book about Obsessive-Compulsive Disorder,* by Aureen Pinto Wagner: With the kind permission of Lighthouse Press, Inc.

Extracts from Radio 4's 'You and Yours' programme of February 13, 2003: With the kind permission of the BBC.

Extracts from '*One in Ten*': *A Report by the National Schizophrenia Fellowship into Unnatural Deaths of People with Schizophrenia-April 1991 to January 1999*: With the kind permission of Rethink (Formerly the National Schizophrenia Fellowship).

Extracts from Crown Copyright material, *Certifying and Investigating Deaths in England, Wales and Northern Ireland: An Invitation for Views, August 2002* and *Death*

Lois Chaber

Certification and Investigation in England, Wales and Northern Ireland: The Report of a Fundamental Review 2003: With the kind permission of the Controller of HMSO and the Queen's Printer for Scotland.

Extracts from Sybil Macindoe's Medical Notes from the Bethlem Royal Adolescent Unit: With the kind permission of the South London and Maudsley NHS Trust; extracts from Hill End's consultant's letter of 26 November 1992: With the kind permission of the Hertfordshire Partnership NHS Trust; extracts from letter to the Coroner of 27 May 1999, by the former Director of Acute Services: With his own kind permission and that of the North Essex Mental Health Partnership NHS Trust.

"THE THING INSIDE MY HEAD"

Prologue: Why?

*When I first went to the Bethlem, Mrs. Wells, who I had been living with in foster care, drove my mum and I down to the Bethlem. I wasn't eating; I had an ng [nasogastric] tube up my nose. I wasn't talking. I had my head right back as if I was looking up at the ceiling and my eyes rolled right back. I kept my eyes and head like this all the time except for when lying down in bed. I didn't communicate at all except for a sort of smile, which meant agreement or 'yes'. On the second day there my key worker Jane was on shift. That was when I started communicating with ticks, crosses and question marks. Jane suggested it **and the thing inside my head which I thought was God said I could do it**.*

> *From Sybil's 1997 Memoir of her two years at the Bethlem Royal Adolescent Unit*

From Medical Assessment of Sybil for admission purposes, Bethlem Royal Adolescent Unit, December 27, 1992.

[Sybil's] Patient Profile:

Physical: Small, thin (said to be 36 kg.) girl obviously malnutritioned. Peripherally blue, postural oedema [swelling, inflammation], noisy breathing, standing with arms rigid and head extended backwards. No solids since 09/11/92. n/g [nasogastric] feed tube in situ, incontinent of urine. Immobile.

Emotional: Appeared sad, did cry when being told how we assumed she must be very sad.

Social: No social contact at all—isolates herself, total gaze avoidance.

Lois Chaber

Language: Mute since admission [to Hill End Unit; Nov. 1992].

Family: Mother has history of depression.

Summary: Sybil is a 14-year-old girl with an extremely disabling and risky mental health problem. She has withdrawn and regressed to a point where she now receives care appropriate for an infant. This it would appear protects Sybil from other psychic constructs and brings her parents together where otherwise the family would fragment.

From an interview with Sybil's former
Associate Nurse at the Bethlem Royal
Adolescent Unit:

There was some feeling before that there had been a major trauma, and this was the result of it. I suppose I just didn't really believe that. I think it was a case of a combination of things that had happened. Sybil would often say quite shocking things, like, "Do you think my father sexually abused me?" And I'd say, "No, I think what has actually happened and why you find it so hard to talk about it, is that it all seems like nothing". And one of the things was the family being in Qatar and unable to leave because Neil's passport had been taken away... And it was by her bringing up things like that, that gradually she realised we weren't expecting one big disclosure.

"THE THING INSIDE MY HEAD"

Oh why did it go wrong? Why?
I must be strong.
Sometimes I want to write out my whole story,
But I don't have the patience to achieve that
glory.
Everything is like an instant in my mind,
An explosion where you can see everything, all
my troubles
Going up in the air for one second
Then it falls and becomes muck and rubble.
I have so much I'm carrying inside me,
But I fumble in the dark
For the door to let it out.
I feel like turning all those pains,
Those memories into a single scream or shout.
Where will I go when I am finished writing?
I am living, putting on a show, for the rest of my
life.

Poem by Sybil, Nov. 21st, 1996.

* * *

My daughter Sybil suffered from obsessive-compulsive disorder, mutism, extreme anorexia, and severe depression in the course of her brief history. She died a suicide, in 1999, after many dark days of illness mingled with bright flashes of her engagement with life. Her poem above, discovered by us after her death, moved me to write this memoir, in which I attempt to answer her anguished question, *"Why?"* The 'answer' is not simple:

Sybil's "*whole story*" is intimately bound up with my own psychic struggle and with the trials of our family members, both individually and collectively, in five different countries. Articulating the connections between our family difficulties and Sybil's illness helped us, in some measure, to come to terms with her tragedy. Our hope is that other families can resonate with the story of our decisions and indecisions and our quests for help.

As time went by, Sybil's fate was also profoundly affected by the strengths and the shortcomings of the successive counsellors and institutions that tried to help her. In this respect, *"her story"*—accounts of her treatments that unfold throughout the latter two thirds of this book—may possibly help bring about changes in how mentally ill young persons like her are treated by the National Health Service and other relevant bodies.

My complicity in Sybil's tragedy, however debatable its degree, has led me in writing this memoir to draw on the voices of other participants in Sybil's life, with their complementary information and countervailing views, with the aim of composing a fairer "*story*". Not the least of these voices is Sybil's, taken from her many diaries and other writings. Her own views of events, sometimes confused, sometimes searingly insightful, always illuminate.

"The thing inside my head" still haunts those who loved Sybil best, and we are confident she would have wanted sufferers, families and carers, among many others, to learn and benefit from this cautionary tale. Sybil's express desire in her poem "*to achieve that glory*" meant, I believe, that she wanted to touch people's hearts not only with her sufferings but also with her brave struggles against them. We dearly hope this book goes some way towards her reaching that goal.

"THE THING INSIDE MY HEAD"

PART I

Lois Chaber

"THE THING INSIDE MY HEAD"

Chapter 1: Mothering

> The mother-child relationship is the essential human relationship.

> (Adrienne Rich, *Of Woman Born: Motherhood as Experience and Institution*, WW Norton and Company, 1976, p. 127.)

Pinned precariously to the edge of one of the many bookshelves in my over-crammed study in our North London home in 2007, is a faded, coffee-stained pencil sketch of my face, lovingly drawn by my mother over sixty years ago when we were waiting for my father to come home from World War II. My face is in profile, my brunette hair held back over my ear with a hairclip, my chubby cheeks and full lips emphasised, my eyes with their thick, brush-like eyelashes cast demurely down. My mother, Sylvia Garfinkel, a highly intelligent amateur artist and a would-be art teacher, jettisoned her college degree just one term from completion to marry my father, Bernie. In this affectionate if hasty sketch she has captured a serious but sensuous child of about two and three-quarters, out with her mother for one of many intimate walks together through the stony outlying grounds of Fort Tilden and the adjacent Rockaway Naval Air Station (now Jacob Riis Park) on a peninsula jutting out from the southernmost part of the New York City Borough of Queens. Some of the fort's barracks are being used to house wives and families of GIs fighting overseas. We live upstairs in of one of these very basic two-storey wooden units with our cat—my first ever—Tabby, whose long white whiskers I one day cut off just as a whimsical experiment, despite my affection for him. What I remember from the day of the sketch is a large, flint-grey rock, on which my mother may have been sitting, the soft pleats of a light-coloured skirt she was wearing, and the hazy view of a bridge—probably the Marine Parkway Bridge—in the distance.

Lois Chaber

Roughly two years later: My father has come safely home from the war about a year earlier. We are still living in the cramped quarters of the Fort Tilden GI housing because my dad's relations, owners of a prosperous dairy corporation, are taking their time to mull over a possible position in the company for him. But tonight I am settled snugly into one of the two double beds in the dingy, one-bedroom, inner city Brooklyn apartment of my Grandma Minnie and my Grandpa Ben, my mother's parents, who are baby-sitting me while my own only recently reunited parents dine out with good friends, celebrating a special occasion, perhaps their anniversary. I am awakened from deep sleep around midnight when harsh yellow lights are suddenly switched on in the bedroom. As I focus sleepily on the two framed prints by Gainsborough on the opposite wall—prints I then know only as "Blue Boy" and "Pink Girl", with their satiny costumes—I become conscious of people scurrying around the apartment, and I can hear my mother's heavy sobs, my grandmother's high-pitched wailing. Confused and frightened, I learn only in subsequent days—from whom, I am not sure—that my father is dead at twenty-nine, having fatally choked on a chicken bone, with bystanders too ignorant to help, as he lay sprawled on the restaurant floor. For the rest of our life together, my mother never utters a syllable about that night.

1950: My mother has recently remarried—a well-educated electrical engineer, Richard—surly, thickset, and swarthy as *I* see him—and we are ensconced in a modest three bedroom brick house in Queens, New York, just on the margins of upwardly mobile Long Island. Unable to form any kind of amicable relationship with my stepfather, also widowed, who has brought his own three-year-old son and baby girl into the marriage, I am closer than ever to my mother at eight years old. Bedtimes are special. We are a Jewish family but not religiously observant, and my main connection with faith is the little universal prayer my mother has taught me to fervently repeat by my bedside each night: "Now I lay me down to sleep/I pray the Lord my soul to keep/

16

"THE THING INSIDE MY HEAD"

If I should die before I wake/ I pray the Lord my soul to take."
After this, my mother comes up to 'tuck me in', and the
climax of her visit is the goodnight kiss: I hurl my arms
around her, greedily drinking in her reassuring warmth,
squeezing her tightly in a passionate hug and implanting a
sloppy kiss on her lips in an attempt to imitate the romantic
movies I have watched on early US television. If she forgets
to come up or I have been naughty and she holds off, I am in
anguish; I long for that climactic embrace, sobbing quietly,
unable to sleep until I hear her slow footsteps on the stairs
telling me she has relented and is coming up for a belated
goodnight.

It is early autumn 1953, and I am an introverted,
studious, chubby eleven-year old sitting with my mother in
the waiting room of a child psychiatrist. Here on sufferance,
I glumly occupy myself by staring at a huge glass tank with
goldfish flitting back and forth, only surmising that my
presence here has something to do with my frequent
sullenness and periods of total withdrawal at home as well
as my ongoing hostility to my stepfather, who frequently
delivers stinging smacks and snide insults. In the inner
sanctum of the psychiatrist, a somewhat patronising middle-
aged woman with glasses and frizzy mouse-coloured hair, I
hesitantly reveal my last night's dream at her insistence: I
am a promenading queen surrounded by admirers, but
something sinister lurks around the corner, which has filled
me with dread. This shadowy menace is what concerns me,
but the doctor dismisses my dream lightly, telling me it's just
an echo of the English queen's glamorous coronation I have
watched on TV a few months ago. This is my single
memory of visits to this psychiatrist, which soon end as
mysteriously as they have begun, possibly because funds
have run out (my paternal grandmother is paying) and 'they'
don't feel I am benefiting. My depression is not addressed
again in childhood, nor am I minded later, as a young adult,
to obtain help.

Lois Chaber

In the early spring of 1955, I am in bed after yet another upsetting confrontation with my stepfather, listening to him and my mother quarrelling heatedly in their bedroom below. Since the early days of the marriage, she has been coming between him and me, shielding me, deploring his occasional verbal and physical violence to me—at the expense of her own marital peace. Now I hear her telling him she is leaving with me for good, and she starts packing a suitcase. I break out into a sweat, panic-stricken. I hate "the ape" (my bratty name for Richard), but I am in horror at the thought of leaving my own cosy, cheerful bedroom, our respectable, comfortable middle-class suburban life, my sleek, newly-built junior high school, all my material comforts and neighbourhood friends; I cannot bear the thought of returning to the dowdy Brooklyn apartment of my too-often-quarrelling grandparents, I cannot face living in near poverty while my mother, as before, earns a meagre salary as a department store sales assistant and my grandmother digs second-hand Marvel comic books out of the building's incinerator for me to read. I sneak down, face tear-stained, to find my mother and clasp her round: "Mummy, I don't want to go; please let's stay here." She is surprised, disconcerted, but gives in to my pleading, unpacking the suitcase. Even at twelve and a half, I am sickeningly aware that I have sold out my mother and myself.

From that day, my mother gradually withdraws from her role as my valiant defender and we move apart like two orbs in an expanding galaxy. When the family moves further out on Long Island to an even more attractive split-level home in thriving Hicksville, she throws herself into the social activities of the 'Sisterhood' of a local Jewish Centre that the family has recently joined in a new onset of religious respectability. Meanwhile, I grow away all together from any kind of faith, 'converted' by my avid reading of George Eliot's novels and other agnostic fiction in my teens. Coming to sexual awareness, I retreat from my mother into a shell of proud adolescent secrecy. Behind a façade of indifference, I am nevertheless bitterly pained when she studies my

"THE THING INSIDE MY HEAD"

excellent report card, only to remark: "How come you went down from a 96 to a 90 in English this term?" or when I strain in my bedroom to hear the half-joking, half complaining anecdotes about my latest blunders in the kitchen or my failures in the high school social scene, with which she regales her Wednesday night mah-jong ladies down in the wood-panelled 'finished basement'.

In the summer of 1962, I leave my home and my college studies against the wishes of my mother and stepfather to marry passionate but unstable Frank, a fellow sophomore student at Ithaca College in upstate New York, where I have changed my major from music to English. I walk out the door with no regrets after a noisy, angry family quarrel, as my mother stands watching, tears streaming down her face, and the neighbours stare from their windows. A week later, I return when the house is empty to collect some clothes and belongings; on my dresser, my mother has left her wedding ring from my father, a thin gold band, with a note bearing a single Shakespearean quotation that pierces my heart: "How sharper than the serpent's tooth it is to have a thankless child."

In 1965 I am sitting in a small, packed classroom at UCLA, the University of California at Los Angeles, concentrating worshipfully on the analysis of "The Beggar's Opera" issuing from the lips of my deliciously cynical professor, Maximillian Novak, who will win me over to eighteenth-century studies. Frank and I have made our way across the continent and after a dismaying, poverty-stricken year of office jobs in downtown Los Angeles, have resumed our university studies. Suddenly, I happen to glance up at the half-window in the door of the classroom and there, standing outside and peering in hopefully, is my mother, with her carefully coifed auburn-died hair and her black-rimmed spectacles; she has the largest, most beaming smile I have ever seen on her face as she meets my shocked and embarrassed gaze. Here on a business trip with Richard, she has searched me out after three and a half years of our

Lois Chaber

total non-communication, and, a much-mellowed middle-age now, reconciles with Frank and me later in a hotel room. Mady, my younger stepsister, now an attractive sixteen-year old who has been a companion to my mother on many excursions, stands by her side.

Charlottesville, University of Virginia, 1969: As a PhD. student working on Samuel Richardson, the so-called eighteenth-century "father of the novel", author of prolix but psychologically complex woman-centred novels, I am living in a cheap student flat with my second husband, Edward, a slim, red-haired, flirtatious fellow graduate student. My marriage to Frank collapsed in 1967 early in my Virginia days, a result of his egregious gropings after sixties-style sexual freedom—a classic fate for an immature marriage. Embarrassed and proud, I once again broke off communication with my mother, dreading her "I told you so." Out of the blue, I now receive a letter from Mady (once again my relatives have ferreted out my whereabouts—like the "Hound of Heaven" chasing hidden sinners "down the arches of the years"): my mother has had a severe heart attack and is in hospital; don't I want to come and see her? Edward and I make a post-haste car journey up the East Coast to Long Island, my first trip back to my old haunts since my elopement. With great anticipation I enter her hospital room. I am nubile, tanned, sporting two flowing pigtails that make me look ten years younger than twenty-seven and wearing a psychedelic chartreuse mini-skirted sun-dress—my late sixties look. Timidly, hopefully, I greet my mother—our first reunion since California—but the first thing she says to me, in her extremely nasal New York accent, smiling weakly, is, "You look just like Mady!"

Three and a half years of lukewarm interchanges between my mother and me pass by—we are both shy, and I am always "too busy" completing my dissertation during my first year of teaching at the State University of New York at Albany. In autumn 1973, in the middle of the night, a telephone call from Mady informs me that my mother, only

20

"THE THING INSIDE MY HEAD"

fifty-four, has died in the aftermath of open-heart surgery. Still unable to deal with my hated stepfather, I boycott the funeral. Yet, the words "my mother is dead" become an obsessive mantra for me, to this day, in the shower when hot pelting water releases my emotions, at bedtime when my insomnia kicks in, and whenever my chronic anxiety has me in its vice.

Late 1975: Albany, the capital of New York State, is throbbing with the activities of 'The Movement', 1970s radical feminism. This evening I am about to tell the other members of my consciousness-raising group—teaching colleagues and friends from the State University, all of us in our thirties and forties, three 'political lesbians' and three (including me) 'straight' women—that I intend to marry and start a family with Neil Macindoe, a thirty-two year old New Zealander teaching architecture at Rensselaer Polytechnic Institute in a neighbouring city, whose craggy masculinity and air of self-sufficiency I find very sexy, despite his thinning red hair. My marriage to Edward exploded in scandal two years ago when he 'came out' as a homosexual—a chic move in the 70s. I try to explain that Neil is the quietly mature, stable, professionally dedicated man I have always really needed—a stark contrast to my two previous half-Italian, impetuous and unreliable partners—and that he fully supports my career and independence, but my friends are horrified and dismayed that after two arrant failures I am willing to subject myself to marital constraints again. Am I betraying The Movement in which I have been so actively involved—speaking, marching, writing—since coming to Albany in 1972? But I am thirty-four and my biological clock is ticking ominously, like Captain Hook's crocodile. My lesbian colleague and friend Nadia, who has two adorable girls from a previous marriage, tries to clear the air with a wisecrack: "What's so great about having children? It's just like a bowel movement—push, push!" and she laughs knowingly.

Lois Chaber

To be sure, this second wave of feminism that I have lived through in Albany as a member of our large local umbrella group, Capital District Women, has inadvertently promoted somewhat contradictory myths about motherhood, leaving me confused, though I *think* I want a child—if only for Neil's sake. One popular rallying cry of the times has been, to be blunt, "Motherhood Sucks"—a deliberate frontal assault on the centuries-long propaganda for women about the maternal ideal, the platitude that "biology is destiny". Along with my friends and students, I have read and admired 1970s spokeswomen like Germaine Greer and Shulameth Firestone, who have denigrated motherhood in favour of women's self-liberation and self-fulfilment. The weekly message coming from my consciousness-raising group has been the need for self-assertion; traditionally, motherhood has called for self-denial, even self-sacrifice.

However, The Movement has offered a second myth that in its own way underestimates mothering: "Doing it All"—the assumption that by sheer force of will the new woman can have her cake and eat it, be a "Supermom" and a career woman as well, without compromising either. If I have unconsciously absorbed the early feminist hostility towards motherhood, I presently subscribe openly to this latter myth; it suits the self-image I have constructed in my successful university years: a determined Amazon who can do anything she sets her mind to. Even before leaving the University of Virginia, in my final days as one of their most promising graduate students, I had been drawn to this new zeitgeist. Looking at me wryly one day, the eminent scholar Irvin Ehrenpreis, one of my mentors in the English department, commented with obvious male satisfaction, "You'll find that you have to compromise your professional goals once you get married and have a family." I retorted that this would by no means be the case. "What will happen if you can't get a position near your husband?" he needled. "I'll just commute," I answered, with the confidence of the naïve and inexperienced. Here in Albany now, I have absolutely no doubts that when I marry Neil I will be able to

22

"THE THING INSIDE MY HEAD"

successfully combine teaching and mothering, even though my obsessive perfectionism has already made it difficult even to combine teaching and scholarship in my current assistant professor position.

Autumn 1977, Tehran: I have not only married Neil but have followed him to the Middle East so that he can take up architectural practice again in the only part of the world where the construction industry is booming in the aftermath of the Western oil crisis and recession. We have been trying for several months to get me pregnant—without success—but now the signs have been promising and I am waiting my turn at a rickety public telephone booth, hoping to hear the results of a pregnancy test. I am accompanied by Debbie and Sarah, two of my new friends and colleagues from Damavand College for Women, where I have been teaching since September. Unlike Pars College, the small coeducational Iranian institution of tertiary education with its sullen students and sinister, labyrinthine administration, where I'd taught for one term after arriving in Tehran in January 1977, Damavand is a bastion of order, regularity and enthusiasm. Formerly a Presbyterian missionary college, Damavand, under a special dispensation from the Iranians, is administered and staffed primarily by Americans and semi-independent from government control. The college has a very limited curriculum—no science or math, only humanities subjects—but I have been delighted with its moderately feminist agenda, including the annual celebration, with great fanfare, of the two important national commemorative days for Iranian women: the abolition of mandatory veiling and the more recent granting of suffrage.

My Damavand colleagues and I are plunk in the middle of downtown Tehran, with horns tooting aggressively all around us and the nauseating stink of petrol fumes permeating the polluted air. We have rendezvoused here in order to accommodate Sarah, a rangy American hippie type, fluent in Farsi, who lives nearby and is going to translate the pregnancy test results from the Iranian clinic. Sarah dials

23

the number, and Debbie and I wait tensely, as several grubby-looking, swarthy Iranian men in the telephone queue look on with bemused curiosity. A broad grin breaks out on Sarah's face as she screams out the results—striving to make her voice heard above the clamour of downtown traffic—so that not only Debbie and I hear the news about my intimate biological condition but also the very embarrassed and disapproving Iranian men waiting nearby. All three of us hoot and jump around, like silly schoolgirls, celebrating my first pregnancy.

"THE THING INSIDE MY HEAD"

Chapter 2: Iran: Born into Trauma

Babies, who are born prematurely with very low birth
weights, may have social and emotional problems
because they are 'shell-shocked' by a world they
have entered too early.

> (Dr. Elizabeth Hoy, developmental psychologist, quoted
> in Sarah Boseley, "Premature babies are socially
> damaged," in *The Guardian*, "Home News", April 10,
> 1999, p. 16.)

There is wealth of research which reveals a great
deal about the experiences of babies living with
mothers who feel depressed or angry, almost
always because they are insufficiently supported

> (Sue Gerhardt, *Why Love Matters: How Affection
> Shapes a Baby's Brain,* Brunner-Routledge, 2004, p.
> 57.)

"Dokhdar darid!" —"You have a daughter." A busy
Iranian nurse in blue and white uniform pauses fleetingly and
with a smile delivers these words to me, my first introduction
to my newborn daughter, nowhere in sight. "Where is she?"
My befuddled mind is just swimming into consciousness as I
wake from a gas-induced sleep, lying on a stretcher in a
deserted, blank corridor reeking of antiseptic, somewhere in
the Tehran Clinic on May 18th, 1978. But I am soon flooded
with euphoria: I have so wanted a girl child! My ardent New
York feminism has predisposed me to anything female. I
silently vow to raise one of the new women of the twentieth
century—*my* daughter will show them all what women can
achieve! And I vow to compensate for the distance my
mother and I both put between us in my teen years. My
newborn Sybil—whose name, in the Jewish tradition, I have

25

chosen in honour of the deceased *Sylvia*—will redeem that unfulfilled relationship. With all my heart, I'll strive to share her hopes and fears, tears and laughter, in a close and warm companionship.

As these thoughts of a disembodied 'Sybil' float through my mind, Neil enters the corridor, munching a sandwich, cheerful and reassuring, his usual sanguine self. "Sybil," he tells me, "is in an incubator." Born seven weeks premature and weighing less than two kilos, she is alive and wriggling, but has been whisked away from us because she has jaundice and her lungs are not one hundred per cent ready to face the world. He has witnessed Sybil's fraught entry into the world even if I haven't and has seen her tiny legs poking out of my cervix in a breech birth. As soon as she started to emerge, he explains, my Iranian obstetrician, Dr. Farhat, concerned to avoid any hysteria should this very premature baby be stillborn, ordered his assistant to unceremoniously knock me out with gas—no matter that we had opted for natural childbirth! His fears of a distressing scene have deprived Sybil and me of that primitive maternal bonding, that immediate reposing of the infant on the mother's heaving chest. This disappointment adds to the day's trauma.

Earlier this morning, I had awoken suddenly, awash in liquid, horrified and humiliated. "Have I peed in the bed?" Only gradually did Neil and I, first-time parents, realise that my amniotic waters had erupted and something was terribly wrong. With me stretched out on the back seat of our Volkswagen camper van, Neil raced westward through Tehran's demented traffic to the clinic, where they told us I was about to give birth. It was almost two months before my due date! Having attended only the first two sessions of a Lamaze antenatal course, we had snatched up the course manual to bring along to the clinic, where I was then hooked up to a drip. But my child labour was so accelerated that Neil couldn't turn the pages fast enough to keep pace with the successive stages my body whistled through—an eerily painless, almost slapstick process. Before we knew what was happening, I was wheeled down to the delivery room and Dr. Farhat was there, looming over me. Now, the birthing over, I am lying here, a mother, but with no *physical* sense of my baby—happy, but disoriented. What can little half-formed Sybil be feeling?

The policies of the impressively modern clinic I deliberately chose add to our mutual ordeal. This Tehran Clinic, priding itself on its scientific superiority in a still only partly-modernised country, has modelled itself, I now realise, on the coldly clinical and aseptic practices of Western birth technology. But it is already about a decade behind current Western medical thinking, influenced by the counter culture of the sixties and the feminism of the seventies that have promoted more natural and humane birthing practices. My friend Carole, whom I am to meet several months later, gave birth in a California hospital to a critically-ill baby, who remained in intensive care for months; nevertheless, she was encouraged to come every day to her daughter's ward and, with mask, gown and gloves, to sit by the incubator and touch and talk to her infant to promote salutary maternal bonding. I, here at the Tehran Clinic, am soon begging just to *see* my child. Neil and I are permitted only a quick peek from the corridor into the intensive baby care ward, where one of several metal incubators holds our newborn Sybil, whose tiny pink button of a face and waving limbs we can just barely make out. The obstetrician assures us mechanically that her medical needs will be met, and I am guided upstairs to a private room where I am to stay overnight and recuperate from my episiotomy. Having no experience and little knowledge of birthing norms and hospital procedures, we meekly defer to authority.

Anyway, I am absorbed with difficulties of my own in hospital. While I am lucky that the birth has taken place just the day before Dr Farhat is due to go on leave for two weeks, I am now left in the care of his partner, a brusque Iranian doctor totally uninterested in me because I'm not his regular patient. For the most part, my contact is only with young Filipino nurses, who slip in and out of the room, offering strange pills to me that they are unable to explain in their extremely limited English, pointing to basins of hot water and trying hard to communicate through gestures. Nor can I really relax and indulge in the 'fun' reading I had thrown into my bag, thanks to professional responsibilities nagging at me. Nearly as soon as the grogginess wears off, I begin to prepare for the two Sophomore Communication and the two Western Literature classes that I teach at Damavand College. Sybil's birth, conveniently due a week after the close of the term, has actually come three days before the end of classes and the start of final examinations, creating a host of practical difficulties. There is no provision for maternity leave at Damavand.

I am already in a delicate position vis á vis my Iranian students. The teaching schedule at Damavand was much more time-consuming than what I was used to in my tenure-track position in New York, but I had managed to meet the intensive demands of the first term and enjoyed warm relationships with the young women. The second term, with my advancing pregnancy, proved much harder. Each day I was bone-weary by the time I zigzagged home through afternoon traffic in our van and struggled up the stairs with my heavy tote-bag. I had always been what students call a "demanding teacher", but the recent hormonal changes had heightened my obsessive perfectionism. I assigned the students difficult texts to read and insisted on their "thinking for themselves", determined to wean them from the system of rote learning they'd been brought up on in Iran. My spiralling demands having alienated many students, I was already in danger of compromising my fine teaching reputation when Sybil burst in upon my life so inconveniently. Now, propped up here in my hospital bed, depleted but anxious, I am doggedly composing final exams and correcting earlier tests Neil has brought from the flat.

"THE THING INSIDE MY HEAD"

When the substitute obstetrician finally gets around to signing me out (a day late), Neil escorts me home to our airy, modern flat in Bombast Zuo, a cul-de-sac in suburban North Tehran, the two of us leaving behind a baby we have only been allowed to glimpse once.

* * *

"Unreal" is the best description of the next few days. With Sybil secreted away in a hospital incubator, I continue to mark student work—multiplied by the recent final exams and term papers that Neil has collected for me, do the housework and shopping, and regularly sit down at the kitchen table to express the milk in my swollen breasts by hand (no breast pumps available at that time in Iran!) into little plastic bags for freezing, hoping to maintain my supply for the absent baby. I am totally spaced out, however. Have I really given birth, or have I imagined the whole experience? "My daughter" remains an abstraction for me.

After a week, the powers that be in the paediatric ward consent to let me come in at last to see, touch and feed Sybil since she is now well enough to be removed from the incubator. The paediatrician and the obstetrician have wanted to bind my breasts and dehydrate them because of Sybil's indefinite stay in hospital, but the support of the local La Leche League, an American group that militantly promotes breastfeeding, has given me the audacity to defy the doctors.

On the ward, Sybil is put in my arms for the first time. Here she is—tightly swaddled in a sheet, all head and penny-coloured hair; her tiny face a miniature of Neil's. Her weight has fallen to three and two thirds pounds, and when I pick her up gingerly it is like holding a tiny porcelain doll. Terrified but eager, I put her to my breast. To my dismay, she is totally uninterested. Later I learn that premature babies have little appetite and their suckling instinct is low or undeveloped. Moreover, the nurses have already been bottle-feeding her for several days. With time, patience and determination, it *is* possible to get a 'preemie' to breastfeed, but here in the clinic the nurse on duty refuses to allow me more than three or four minutes to try and the nursing staff never gives me a second chance. They are worried, they tell me, that Sybil will miss a feed and thus lose even more weight. A couple of days later, when one of the nurses changes her in my presence and unwinds her swaddling, I see for myself her scrawny arms and legs—and I am frightened!

This visit and the ones that follow—my very first days with Sybil—turn into a nightmare. I have been told that though doctors in Iran are well-trained (usually abroad), the nursing situation is deplorable. Because of the Islamic belief in the separation of the sexes, nurses are seen by many in Iran as akin to prostitutes, and there is no tradition of professional nursing. It is hard to recruit nurses, even from other developing countries, and they are in short supply. Here in the paediatric ward's intensive care room there is only a single nurse per shift to care for nine to twelve babies at a time. One particular nurse never changes Sybil's nappy once during my five hour visit; my baby arrives home eventually with an angry-looking diaper rash.

They staff agree to let me express milk into a bottle and then feed that to Sybil each day, but no one shows me how to hold the bottle or burp her, and they regularly supply me with bottles that have clogged-up nipples. Too insensitive to allow me to use a ward bedroom for which I am not paying, the nurses in charge have put me into the cramped nursery office. There I sit squeezing milk from my breasts and then trying to give Sybil the bottle, with janitors, visitors, and staff parading past all the while. She does not feed well. "It's hopeless," I moan inwardly, frustration smothering the fragile joy of being with my baby at last.

I am grudgingly allowed to administer two feeds a day. In-between, I sit in the overly air-conditioned waiting room downstairs, marking papers and eating my brown bag lunch. The two day-nurses whose shifts overlap with mine are moody and unpredictable—one day chatty, the next cross—and annoyed by the whole arrangement. Because my participation in Sybil's care, minimal as it is, is completely dependent upon their compliance, I play the sycophant and keep smiling regardless of what happens. In reality, I am seething inwardly with aggravation and anger. About midweek, one nurse abruptly tells me I am upsetting their schedule and causing Sybil to lose weight. I burst into tears. This frightens the nurse and she becomes a bit more helpful for a time.

The enforced week-long separation from me that my baby has already endured, in addition to our present strained and intermittent contact—what consequences will they have for Sybil? Sue Gerhardt, in *Why Love Matters,* warns that the high levels of cortisol (the stress hormone) produced in human infants by early separation from the mother have been linked to mental health problems later in life. My own early physical estrangement from my baby coupled with the bizarre sensation of being a mother *yet not a mother*—how will these emotional mishaps affect my ability to relate to Sybil?

* * *

Dr. Farhat, at last back from his holiday, is frank about the below par nursing standards at the hospital and very pessimistic about Sybil gaining weight there. Preemies usually have to be at least five pounds before they are released from hospital. Sybil at two weeks is still less than four pounds, but under the circumstances he will let us take her home, advising us to hire a private nurse. With the help of the highly-organised American Women's Club of Tehran, we are quickly able to hire a registered nurse, whom we use off and on for two weeks. Neither the nursing nor the hospital bills are covered by any insurance, and as neither Neil nor I have the usual generous expatriate contract and

Lois Chaber

we pay our oil-boom Tehran rent out of our own pockets, our finances are now quite strained.

The nurse, Claire, a grey-haired, kindly, middle-aged American woman, has previously worked in a premature baby centre in Seattle and is a genuine expert. She is the only person close to a mothering relative on the scene here for me. My good friends Debbie and Sarah are childless and inexperienced. Claire cheerfully demonstrates all the essentials to us, diapering, bathing, burping Sybil and so on, and sews some miniscule cloth nappies for our exquisite infant, too tiny for commercial baby wear. She provides some cheer and encouragement at an otherwise very difficult time for us, taking up a broom to briskly sweep my neglected kitchen as soon as she enters the flat each day. The only other helpful figure around is my Damavand student Shahla, a married woman back in college to better her job prospects and one of the few pupils *not* alienated from me. Shahla visits our flat twice, bearing aromatic Iranian chicken soup for me and some teeny, hand-sewn paisley nightgowns for Sybil.

These are the bright spots in Sybil's new life and my early motherhood, otherwise a time of emotional and physical stress for all of us. Neil is scurrying around to buy supplies for Sybil and doing the grocery shopping, on top of a demanding new job. Disappointed by the incompetence and constant jockeying for power of his Iranian colleagues in his initial position with Educational Building Industries, a government firm, Neil quit at the time of his work permit renewal and joined a related firm, Padeco, where he now works in a more professional situation on a project to design an industrial park for an area near Isfahan. But with the birth of Sybil, and the consequent disruption in our lives, even his new expatriate colleagues are not terribly sympathetic when he comes to work late after a night of broken sleep or has to nip out for urgent baby needs. So Neil is also exhausted and under pressure, but he is borne up by an intuitive and powerful devotion to Sybil. Yet, as the mother, now at home all day with Sybil, I bear the largest burden of responsibility for her emotional environment.

To be sure, the post-partum upheaval of body and mind that I am experiencing is natural to all new mothers, but this is intensified by my clinical status as an "elderly primagravida"—the unflattering term for an older first-time mother. At thirty-five and a half, I have less energy and resilience than a younger mother, and am more set in my ways as a self-focused career woman. My formative years in the radical feminist movement in New York, absorbing that movement's flagrant reversal of traditional values, moreover, have left me dimly resentful of the heavy demands of maternal care, and this has fed into my personal history of neurosis: Tendencies to depression and anxiety that have dogged me since childhood, aggravated by personal losses, are now triggered by the stress of caring for a fragile infant. Sybil's dangerously low weight and her failure to gain pounds in hospital (she is so tiny we have to use a small plastic salad bowl to bathe her) are terrifying to me, an inexperienced mother isolated in a developing country. Motherhood is more a source of anxiety than pleasure. Gnawing at my insides is my internal 'needy baby', which will prove a giant obstacle to becoming a mature and giving mother.

During those early weeks at home with Sybil, I fall into the tempting habit of allowing the more stoic and stable Neil to take over the mothering at difficult moments, justifying this to myself with the feminist slogan of 'shared parenting'. When Sybil inevitably wakes in the night crying with hunger, I am overwhelmed. My ongoing exhaustion coupled with my underdeveloped faculty of self-denial virtually binds me to my bed in helplessness, like a Gulliver tied down in Lilliput by tiny but unyielding ropes. More often than not, the cord that should link my heart and my breasts to Sybil's piercing cries is severed, as if by a merciless intruder. It is almost always the half-awake Neil who gives

Lois Chaber

Sybil her midnight feed and walks her tenderly around the room to soothe her back to sleep.

Although I spend most of my day with Sybil, Neil's contributions to her care are nearly always to be more selfless, more gracious. Yet, the British feminist Melissa Benn, pondering what role "nature" ultimately plays in parenting (*Madonna and Child: Towards a New Politics of Motherhood*) has asked, "How much does a young child need its mother more than its father? How much deeper does the once-fibrous connection of mother and child go, and how long does it last?" These are questions with which 1970s radical feminism was not overly concerned.

Despite my unacknowledged resistance to maternity, on another level of my perfectionist psyche I still obstinately and naively cling to the alternative myth of the feminist 'Supermom', who copes effortlessly with both domestic and professional demands. But the confidence born of ideology soon suffers a humiliating crash to ground, Icarus-like, amidst the material realities of our daily life.

Having to use tiny cloth nappies has meant several washes a day—all hung out by hand on an outdoor terrace clothes line as we have no dryer. Housecleaning is crucial in highly polluted Tehran. A fine black dust settles daily over everything in the house, and gritty sand from the surrounding desert also accumulates stealthily on furniture and floors. We cannot afford Claire beyond the initial two weeks to help with Sybil because of our pinched finances, we have no family here, and we don't seem able to hire domestic workers at this very difficult time. The attractive young Iranian cleaning woman who came to us weekly for several months had borrowed from us a considerable sum of money and said she was going on a short holiday just before Sybil's birth. She never came back. Over the last few weeks, we have interviewed five or six different individuals who smile and nod in response to our limited Farsi and

"THE THING INSIDE MY HEAD"

promise to show up for work, but then disappear into the Tehran fog.

I have persisted in trying to breast feed Sybil, working at reverse-weaning to get her off the bottle. Every hour-long feeding session is a labour of love—or is it just obsessiveness? I spend about fifteen minutes offering Sybil my breast, in all possible positions, longing to feel her tiny lips clutch at my nipple, to no avail. Then I spend another fifteen minutes resignedly squeezing my milk into a bottle, followed by the actual feed, a tedious process as she has a minimal appetite and does not suck vigorously, and finally I go through my semi-competent burping routine, awkwardly positioning this passive infant on my shoulder.

I rise each morning grimly determined to reach the gold standard of motherhood, only to feel my energy ebbing from the first hour and to succumb guiltily to the temptations of an afternoon nap. In-between housework, feeding sessions and nap, my slog through the quagmire of unmarked student work drags on. My common sense struggles to assert itself: "Dammmit, Lois, Why can't you just breeze through these essays and assign estimated grades?" But up to now I have prided myself on my professional dedication, egged on by the internalised ghost of my demanding mother, and any threat to this self-image adds to my sense of wearied defeat. Melissa Benn speaks of a "particular quality" to the fatigue of a working mother that comes from "conflict, from attempting to dwell within two worlds that are governed by quite different values".

This difference in values I soon discover in my dealings with Damavand College. On June ninth I receive a call from the irate Iranian assistant to the Dean, asking where my final grades are, without so much as a single polite enquiry as to how Sybil and I are doing. When I try to explain why it will be at least a week before I can submit them, she launches into a near-hysterical tirade. I ask to speak to the Dean herself, hoping to get a more sympathetic hearing from this elderly American woman, a former missionary and an enthusiast for women's rights. Already deeply humiliated, I receive the Dean's call. When I launch into the difficulties of caring for a very premature baby, with no domestic help, she cuts me short, inquiring tartly, "What would we say to one of our students if they came to us with such an excuse?" Slapped in the face, as it were, I cannot think of a retort, and the Dean continues to harangue me. When I am reduced to pleading for help with the marking, she insists I should find and pay someone myself.

The birth of my baby has created a crisis for me, a loss of my primary sense of identity as a competent academic. And to my consternation, my milk, already waning in flow, dries up completely. I am now a failure both as a teacher *and* as a mother.

* * *

This private turmoil is taking place in a context of public trauma. We have been aware of unrest in Iran since the autumn and winter of 1977, when there were demonstrations and disturbances by radical university students protesting against the Shah's repressive regime. Now during 1978, our second year in Iran, the economic and political discontent that has been bubbling under the surface is coming to a head. This past January, everyone had been shocked by the news of right-wing violence against the secularised state in the Holy City of Qom, the centre of Iranian Shiite Muslim conservatism, soon followed in February by left-wing violence in the western city of Tabriz: attacks on cinemas, liquor stores and other symbols of Westernisation. Damavand College had nearly cancelled its annual programme celebrating Iranian women's suffrage, but finally just told everyone to keep a low profile. Female voting and the banning of the chador (the traditional head and body covering) in schools and universities, keystones of the Pahlavi dynasty's modernisation programme, are anathema to conservative Shiites. By March, violence and

"THE THING INSIDE MY HEAD"

sabotage had spread to Tehran and other major cities, and on our road trip to Afghanistan for the Persian New Year holiday, Now Ruz, late in that month, we witnessed government tanks ominously surrounding the magnificent shrines in the eastern Iranian city of Mashhad, another key holy site.

Indeed, the whole region seemed to be destabilizing. Less than a month after our trip to Afghanistan, a Marxist coup erupted there, ousting the ruling strongman Daoud, whose face we had seen plastered over every public wall. In Sybil's birth month, May, there was further rioting in Qom and at Tehran University, with the unrest increasing in June. We obtain all this disturbing news through the expatriate grapevine, dependent on anonymous Iranian sources and the BBC World Service. We now hear that the exiled religious leader Khomeini has started to demand an Islamic state, but Neil and I, at this point, do not think it will really climax in a revolution; the Iranians, we believe, are too indecisive, too fond of individual intrigue, to unite under one banner and overthrow the government. Nevertheless, the situation is contributing to our sense of upheaval and is part of the inauspicious environment in which Sybil spends her early life.

Outwardly, however, by late June, Sybil, except for her weight and size (improved since hospital days but still way below par for her age), seems like a contented baby in her cot, blinking her bright blue eyes at us. At times she fusses and wails, but we have learned to resort to a pacifier, or dummy, to quiet her down, and she takes to this easy way out with perhaps too much alacrity. (In later years, we will have a devil of a time getting her to relinquish her beloved "chew-chew".) Having done my baby-book homework during this time—both the American Dr. Spock *and* the English Dr. Jolly—I make the decision to feed her on a schedule rather than on demand, partly because she doesn't *have* very much demand but also because I crave a modicum of order and regularity amidst all the other internal and external turbulence.

The paper-marking ordeal, with the help of an assistant I hire, finally comes to an end, and, happily, we have been invited to housesit in July for some German friends going on holiday. This means living for six weeks in a spacious house equipped with a reasonable-sized swimming pool, a lovely garden and patio and a once-a-week housemaid, all of which will offer great relief to us after our two months of fraught parenthood. But alone in this large and empty house every day, I am going round the bend during Sybil's long feeding sessions, her appetite still very weak. I borrow from one of our American friends a guitar book that contains the melodies and lyrics of famous folk-songs such as "Green Sleeves" and "My Darling Clementine", and I devote these six weeks to memorising the tuneful stanzas in order to sing to Sybil during these tedious bottle feedings. The vivid lyrics ease me into mothering and pleasure us both. Words, especially literary words, will always be a bridge to Sybil for me, and the ritual of daily singing to my child/children becomes one of the few happy legacies of those dark days in Iran.

In late August, we return to our flat amidst the country's furore over the Rex Cinema incident in the city of Abadan—the burning alive of innocent Iranians because they are enjoying a 'corrupt' Western recreation. With sporadic violence continuing throughout the country, we cancel our plans to have a last-minute holiday down in Shiraz; it is just too dangerous to travel now. We have finally been able to arrange some domestic help. An extremely impoverished Iranian woman with her salt and pepper hair tied back in a green kerchief, the widow of a humble shoe-shine man, who has endured many hardships and is struggling valiantly to raise two pre-teen girls on her own, is going to work for us daily, her previous foreign employers having left Iran. She conveys to us, in her limited English vocabulary, that she has refused to work for well-off

"THE THING INSIDE MY HEAD"

Iranians in recent years because they are arrogant and overbearing. Our heart immediately goes out to Leyla, who is simple, open, warm-hearted, and takes well to Sybil. She is forty, only a few years older than I, but with her corrugated face, missing teeth and sagging body, the consequence of a life of hard physical labour in a country without health care provision for the poor and uneducated, she looks at least twenty years older.

* * *

For me, the summer over, the biggest decision concerns my upcoming year of teaching, and I spend a week agonising over this. On the one hand, all my feminist principles dictate that I maintain my career while being a mother; countless times during the past year I have protested that I would have no trouble teaching and taking care of my (as yet unborn) baby; I have even offered myself as a candidate for Head of the English Department at Damavand since the current Head, another (childless) woman friend of mine, is departing. "For sure I can handle it," I have proclaimed to the administration. Now, however, I am totally deflated after the marking fiasco. Although we have Leyla, our previous unhappy experiences getting and keeping domestic help make me wary of wholly counting on her. Bad vibrations about Damavand from the insensitive treatment I received during the summer also colour my reasoning.

The final blow to my self-esteem is delivered by the new Head of English, a young man chosen over me. He informs me by phone, with acute embarrassment, that they have to break their promise to let me teach the junior year students (on a three-day-a-week contract) because my old sophomore students, now juniors, have balked at having me again: "Dr. Lois is *too* hard." This means I would be back to teaching the (new) sophomore English majors *four* times a week. My efforts to make my ex-students 'think for themselves' have completely backfired. Sadder and wiser

Lois Chaber

now, I know deep in my gut that I can't manage fragile little Sybil and still propel myself into college four full days a week. Despite Neil's supportive urgings on behalf of my career, I decide, finally, to quit my Damavand position. For the present, I will be that most shameful of creatures, a stay-at-home mother.

At least this will allow me to put in some time on unfinished scholarly articles begun during my assistant professorship in New York but never completed, thanks to my obsessional tendencies. I am eager to pick up the threads of my feminist defence of Daniel Defoe's famous adventuress, Moll Flanders, who has been almost universally condemned by literary critics for her maternal abandonment of her numerous children and for her account book mentality. *I* will argue for her as a heroine of female survival—at whatever cost—and celebrate her relationships with the mother figures in her own life.

I might have been able to have the proverbial cake and eat it could I have foreseen that not long after the term commences in September, Damavand College suspends classes "temporarily". This is supposedly a voluntary gesture of solidarity with the increasingly radicalised students at other Iranian universities who are striking in protest against the Shah's regime, forcing their institutions to close down. In fact, our own normally submissive young women have risen up against us, like the Greek heroine Antigone they read about in our Western Literature course. A large number of them, mostly the more religious students from the provinces, have been disrupting classes and performing small acts of sabotage in support of the Revolution. They see Damavand, with its quasi-feminist policies, as colluding with the Shah's regime and insulting religious tradition. My former Damavand expatriate colleagues, including my good friends Sarah and Debbie, leave Iran provisionally to wait out the results of the unrest in nearby countries.

"THE THING INSIDE MY HEAD"

Events bode ill. On September fourth the streets of Tehran are filled with a massive Anti-Shah, anti-American demonstration, which Neil witnesses and photographs while driving across town. The army is called out, but protestors stick flowers in the soldiers' rifle barrels, and the English-language newspapers translate their street cries as, "Soldiers, you are our brothers. Why do you kill people?" I am touched by this and cut out this headline to use in a colourful collage I am constructing to commemorate Sybil's birth in Tehran: disparate paper fragments depicting all phases of majestic Iranian history as well as the destructive events—from earthquakes to civil unrest—swirling around us. A huge general strike follows next, orchestrated from Iraq by Khomeini, and martial law is subsequently declared. But on September eighth, boisterous protestors in Jaleh Square in Tehran defy the ban on demonstrations and are massacred by panicky soldiers, becoming martyrs to inflame the Revolutionary cause.

Despite the snowballing violence, our little family is enjoying the uninterrupted heaven-sent autumn weather of Tehran: crisp, clear, sunny and moderately warm during the day, comfortably cool at night. The many pot plants on our little first-floor terrace are blooming apace and we dine out there in the evenings, Sybil resting quietly in her cot, Neil and I often cooking lamb kebabs on our little hibachi barbeque and contemplating our Armenian landlord's formal rose-garden below. We have settled into an amicable routine, one that makes life, at long last, relatively manageable. Sybil is fed twice a day by me, once by the affectionate Leyla, and once in the evening by Neil. But she invariably has a long cranky, colicky period in the late afternoon—a mood Leyla describes with sibilant aptness as *asabani*—and I depend heavily on the squeaky little rubber dummy and my repertoire of songs to get me through these dragging hours. Almost as soon as Neil walks through the door, I thrust Sybil into his arms, panting with relief like a weary climber shedding her backpack on the last phase of the mountainous ascent. Neil baths her with great relish

Lois Chaber

when he comes home, cooing at her softly while tenderly handling her slippery, soapy little body in the former salad bowl. Sybil is steadily gaining weight and sleeping through the night, and I am able to make progress on my *Moll Flanders* article.

In October, our focus is still on our domestic problems—Sybil's first cold and a spate of near simultaneous mechanical breakdowns in the household, including our Volkswagen van. But outside our tasteful flat, which we have decorated sparely in Modernist black and white, worsening unrest is being fomented. Khomeini, we hear, now in Paris after the Shah has manoeuvred to have him kicked out of Iraq, is calling for more general strikes in Iran, and the postal services, the oil industry and others are on hold. Graffiti saying 'Death to the Shah' appear in the streets. One day our faithful Leyla bursts into the flat, tears flowing and baggy trousers torn. She has found on the street, she tells us, a flyer saying "The Shah is poo-poo," and, angry and upset, has tried to run quickly to the nearest police station, only to fall and scrape herself badly. Leyla is an adamant supporter of the Shah because he has made it possible for girls like her own two adolescents to have a free education, which means they will be able to get skilled, higher-paying jobs, unlike herself: "They [will] no have [bad] teeth like their mummy!"

The planning for the industrial park, with Neil's significant contributions, is finished and his job with Padeco comes to an end. We now consider our options. We own no property elsewhere nor does Neil have any present employment prospects outside Iran. Yes, the political situation here is very shaky and violence is mounting, but, despite all the hassles of the last three months, we still feel strongly in favour of staying in this fascinating country where we have taken so many thrilling expeditions before Sybil's birth—to blue-tiled Isfahan, to Zoroastrian Yazd, to the lush Caspian jungles, to neighbouring Turkey with its many-domed mosques, and more. The thought of dismantling our

"THE THING INSIDE MY HEAD"

now reasonably stable household, packing up and having to completely start a new life who-knows-where with a still very small baby dismays us. Remaining here and weathering what we see as a temporary political glitch, we decide, will be the best for Sybil and for us. Neil will look for another job in Tehran.

* * *

Sybil seems to be thriving now: all the more reason not to leave. By mid-November 1978, although inhabiting the body of a two or three month-old (only about twelve pounds in weight), she has the gestures, desires, and alertness of a six month-old. If she wakes before us, she looks with quiet attention at the colourful pictures of zoo animals taped to the headboard and sides of her crib. Her face and thighs are pleasantly plump, but her torso is slim, her tiny bottom like two little crab-apples. She is all eyes, which are large, round, sky-blue, almost smothered in long black eyelashes, a contrast to her auburn eyebrows and the fine auburn down now growing back on her head; and all mouth, a wide cupid's bow with an incredible range of expressions, from tiny O's of wonder, curled pouts, raucous open guffaws, to glowing wide grins of delight. These last two months she has distracted us from the political nightmare unfolding around us by her change from a squalling, colicky sleeping-eating machine into a good-natured responsive little elf.

And we still find opportunities for pleasure outside our cosy flat. Around the time of Neil's birthday in early November, along with a pleasantly eccentric English couple, we drive about forty minutes outside Tehran into the surrounding Alborz Mountains, to a small village, for a hike up a mountain valley trail that seems to wind into infinity, passing autumnal foliage, ghostly poplar trees and friendly villagers who hail us with "Salaam Aleikum". In our down ski jackets (the weather having finally turned cold), Sybil bundled up and fast asleep in a canvas sling worn by Neil,

Lois Chaber

we walk for two hours, light snow gently falling on us at times, and stop for a trailside lunch of bread, cheese, homemade chutney and leftover birthday cake.

But meanwhile, around the same time in November, there has been a convulsive surge of violence in Tehran: massive student demonstrations, street riots, killings and the burning and pillaging of banks, ministry buildings and the British embassy. On my birthday, November 6th, the current prime minister steps down, a military government is installed, and the martial law curfew is rolled back from midnight to nine o'clock. Tehran is progressively becoming a black hole: all foreign newspapers and magazines banned, all cinemas and cultural centres "temporarily" closed and daily rumours of electricity and water shutdowns. Town-wide panic occurs after a one-day petrol supply strike. I wait four hours in our camper van, part of a massive queue that winds up a hill and around corners, and manage to finish two books before being served. There have been deliberate government electricity blackouts at night to deter Khomeini's followers from broadcasting from the rooftops his speeches taped in France, but we still hear angry cries of "Allah Akbar" and periodic rifle shots piercing the night air. Becoming inured to this menacing clamour, we burn brass kerosene lamps and sometimes diaper Sybil clumsily by candlelight.

Neil lands a new job. However, by now virulent anti-foreigner sentiment is spreading, forcing the government to appease the populace with measures to constrain expatriates. There is now a ban on new or renewed work permits for expatriates, making it impossible for Neil to take up this new position. Most foreigners are leaving anyway, but we are undeterred. Neil will try to find work under the aegis of the Iranian government, which does not require a work permit. Claire, Sybil's former nurse, gets her husband to recommend Neil for a position with the building division of Boeing International, which works for the Ministry of Defence. On the weekend we step gingerly through the broken, glassless doors of our bank, withdraw our remaining money and go to another bank to convert it into traveller's cheques, just in case, but we really want to 'hang in'.

Yes, despite our liberal politics, Neil and I do not have a lot of sympathy for the current Revolutionary movement. In fact, Neil is even willing to put himself forward for a job with Boeing that indirectly aids the Shah's government—and this is more than just blinkered self-interest on our part. We most certainly find the repression and corruption of the present regime repugnant, and we know there is a contingent of Marxist-Leftist protestors (including students) in the anti-government coalition with whom we *can* identify. However, we are also aware that the largest, most powerful group in this coalition is constituted by the conservative Islamists who want to turn Iran into a hard-core theocracy, which makes us shudder. Already Shiite leaders are calling for non-Shiites—Armenian Christians, Iranian Jews, Sunni Muslim tribal members, Protestants, and members of the Baha'i sect—to be purged from the government and civil-service.

As a feminist, I am especially incensed that these Shiite 'revolutionaries' are also itching to turn back the clock for Iranian women, despite their vague public disclaimers. This autumn, to appease the opposition, the Ministry for Women's affairs has been eliminated from the Cabinet and a bill *reversing* the only recently reformed 'Family Protection Law' (giving women almost equal rights in divorce), has been put before the Majlis (Iranian parliament) because, as the newspapers declare, the reforms "take away the rights of men and violate Islamic law". The much-touted Women's Organisation of Iran, a government-supported group that lobbied for women's rights and benefits, has vanished from view, as if by the twitch of a malevolent fairy's wand. All of this makes us profoundly uneasy about the revolutionaries' future intentions, and, like Leyla, pragmatic supporters of the Shah's government as the lesser of two evils.

Lois Chaber

Meanwhile, I am managing to juggle caring for Sybil—which I view as part of a household rota—with my academic endeavours, putting the finishing touches on my *Moll Flanders* arguments and tackling another half-finished article on the eighteenth-century novel. Despite Sybil's advances and my own, I am still moody, quite often 'down' for no reason I can fathom; I do not think much about the implications of having given up teaching. Neil is finding it hard to cope with intermittent sulks and explosions on my part, and perhaps even little Sybil senses when my head and body are buzzing with irritation as I diaper or feed her. Motivated by the fact that I have run out of the Valium prescriptions that were forged by a good friend of mine in the States, I seek help from a local Iranian physician; however, this general practitioner offers me only platitudes and pills—some not very effective tranquillisers as well as more of the highly addictive Valium. My depression remains essentially untreated.

Right up to Christmas Day we are still determined to stay here, looking forward to giving Leyla a raise and buying her a pair of spectacles when Neil starts a new job. Sybil, fortunately, appears to be oblivious to the dismal situation around us, consuming jars of cereal, pureed banana and applesauce, learning to drink a little from a cup, and making gradual headway in sitting up. She responds with muted delight when I sometimes play 'this little piggy' with her toes while changing her nappy. But my happiest moments are when Neil and I, putting aside any antagonism the day may have brought forth, together avidly check Sybil's progress against a little American manual that sets out what the baby should be doing each week of her new life. As we inspect and analyse Sybil's every gesture, every bowel movement, every incipient smile, I feel intimately and lovingly connected—to my husband.

In the very last days of December, we learn that the Boeing manager has been ordered to put a freeze on hiring. Soon the company leaves Iran all together, thus ending

"THE THING INSIDE MY HEAD"

Neil's attempts to circumvent the new anti-foreigner laws. Our money is running out. We have been living on our meagre savings since Neil's job ended in October, and a large portion of our funds are tied up in a mandatory Iranian customs guarantee for our camper van, untouchable until we and it leave the country. Iran itself, thanks to strikes and disruption, is on the verge of total economic collapse and the many recent mass demonstrations have become increasingly fundamentalist in nature. Damavand College officially dismisses all its foreign employees, and virtually all of our other friends have decamped. We now finally abandon our hopes of staying here, but we do not know where to go next. Neil starts writing job enquiry letters to just about every country in the world except Saudi Arabia. Meanwhile, we are slowly freezing in the flat as the landlord, unable to obtain supplies of heating oil, has lowered the temperature to the absolute minimum.

In early January the Shah attempts to conciliate the opposition by appointing the liberal Shahpur Bakhtiar as prime minister to replace the military governor, but this does not deter the revolutionaries. Neil jumps at the chance when he hears that an American planning company, William Pereira Associates, is looking for an architect in the Arabian Gulf country of Qatar, a short distance away. A telephone interview goes well, but they need to see him in person before making a decision—not so easy with Iran Air on strike and no other airlines coming into Tehran. We are stranded and broke.

But word gets around that the airport is re-opening and Pan American Airlines is tentatively scheduling a few flights from Tehran to the US. We purchase a ticket on our credit card for the 15th of January for a flight stopping in Istanbul, where we will change airlines and fly to Qatar via Beirut, the only way to reach the Gulf at this point. Our household items and the Volkswagen van we leave indefinitely with an Iranian agent since all commercial shipping is on hold due to strikes. On the 15th, Neil's Iranian

47

Lois Chaber

friend Saeed speeds from his house the moment the official curfew lifts at 6:00 am, collects us and drives manically to the airport so that we can make our 9:00 flight. At the airport there is a grand mêlée of all those foolish people like ourselves who have not had the sense to leave Iran earlier. We wait anxiously in an enormous queue with our fourteen pieces of luggage, including Sybil in her carrycot and two cats in a kennel, plus numerous coats we are wearing on our backs in the overheated and overcrowded terminal. Eventually we embark on the circuitous route to Qatar, discovering in Istanbul that the Shah himself has departed Iran one day after us.

* * *

When we finally reach Doha, the capital of Qatar, Neil is properly interviewed and awarded the job, but we ask to have a week's holiday before he takes up the position, explaining that we badly need a break after our Iranian ordeal. We have previously arranged to visit a good American friend of mine recently married to a Frenchman and living in Nantes. My friend Suzette, a pleasingly plump ex-student from the State University at Albany with face like an angel and long, hippie-straight hair, is ten years younger than I, but very mature for her years. Our mutual idealism and moral earnestness had formerly brought us together, despite my faculty and her student status.

Not long after our arrival in their modest flat in Nantes in the beginning of February 1979, Suzette and her husband Jean-Marc suggest a motoring tour around some nearby picturesque seaside towns. It seems like an ideal scenario for two war-weary virtual refugees from the Middle East. However, the abrupt re-immersion into Western civilization, the suddenly very normal environment, the release from tension, danger and uncertainty, as well as the re-connection with an old friend, all have the effect of culture shock upon me, overturning my initial relief and joy and setting the stage for the claim my recent traumas have made

"THE THING INSIDE MY HEAD"

on me. My conflicted feelings about motherhood well up strongly within me, like dark lava rising to the surface of a volcano. Each time we have to stop and attend to Sybil's needs—a change of nappy, a feed, a settling and comforting—I find myself instigating whiny quarrels with Neil as to whose turn it is to take care of the baby, much to Neil's embarrassment and Suzette's dismay. Sybil, disoriented by the various changes of scene, becomes more so with the tension mounting between Neil and me. There in the baby carrier that is resting on a makeshift seat, I see, not my little daughter in the adorable yellow-striped woollen jumpsuit that Suzette has bestowed on her, squirming in discomfort—but only a distasteful chore, a small smelly body that will inevitably be smeared with shit.

Back at Suzette's flat that night, all I want to do is sleep in order to soothe my inner needy child. Gradually coming to consciousness quite late the next morning, head heavy with guilt, I sleepily overhear Neil and Suzette talking. They are both already up, dressed and caring for Sybil. I hear Suzette, who has always looked up to me, telling Neil how shocked she is at my behaviour: "I never thought Lois would be such a bad mother." Neil mutters his concurrence. Hot waves of mingled shame and anger sweep through me, and I can only think to escape into more sleep. I cannot face them. I reach stealthily for my Valium tablets and drug myself back into a stupor.

After a while, Neil tries to wake me up, shaking my shoulders, but I am too far-gone—in more ways than one. I have crossed over the line from acceptable, if not admirable behaviour, to unacceptable, openly outrageous behaviour. Where will it lead? Through a fog of drugs, I hear their remonstrating voices, but I keep sneaking more Valium to prolong my semi-oblivion, blotting out the knowledge that I will have to get up sometime. When Neil confiscates my pills, I manage to pick the lock of his briefcase and retrieve them. I lose all track of the time, the day. . .

Lois Chaber

All of a sudden, in true nightmare fashion, men in white coats are entering Suzette's flat and forcibly removing me from bed and into an ambulance. I awake to find myself in a French mental ward. Everything is hazy, terrifying. I am sitting at a long dinner table with other patients, struggling to muster the remnants of my college French with my brain in a stranglehold of distress: *Je . . m'appelle. . Lois . . . .*

This shameful episode is another damaging separation for mother and daughter, but *this* time, I chide myself, I have voluntarily abandoned Sybil, leaving her entirely in Neil's care. It has been a time of crisis for him, too:

> *We needed medical help. I asked Suzette to call her GP, who came to the flat; after examining Lois, he recommended she be admitted to hospital. After calls to the US Embassy and American Hospital in Paris to see if they had an option and being told they needed Lois to be taken to Paris, I had the doctor provide a prescription for an ambulance to the Central Hospital, University of Nantes.*
>
> *When in Iran there had been difficulties. We had had situations similar to what was happening in France. I had managed to keep going through them all, but when Lois became distraught in Nantes and not able to deal with any of us around her, me, Sybil and her good friend Suzette, I could not go on imagining that I could handle this state of affairs or that it would fade away. It seemed to be becoming a habit in our relationship. In Tehran I had accepted working through each such event in the interests of keeping things stable, especially for Sybil, but in France I became sharply aware*

"THE THING INSIDE MY HEAD"

how abnormal such events were and needed to take drastic action. I was afraid my own personality was being eroded, but mostly I was afraid of the effects on Sybil. I decided to deal uncompromisingly with this crisis, first by deciding to have Lois admitted to hospital and then by getting my family's support so that I could present Lois with both the medical and the interpersonal necessity of achieving a long-term solution. My first intent was to have Sybil taken to New Zealand while having Lois commit herself to working through her problems, either by herself in the US or with me in Doha.

With Lois asleep in the flat, knocked out with pills, and Suzette and her husband at work, I shouldered Sybil in her back pack and trudged a lonely day through cold snowy streets in Nantes to the telegraph office from where I called my family in New Zealand to tell them what had happened, explain my desperate need and get their assurances of help. While my mother Edna and sister-in-law Denyse were arranging their passports and flights from New Zealand to France, I went the next day to the hospital, where the specialist described Lois as a "habitual neurotic" and was prepared to discharge her once I had made arrangements. I then confronted Lois with my plan for Sybil and the option of whether she, Lois, would go to the US or Qatar. I know that my decision to take Sybil away, even if only temporarily, was done with only partial medical advice and certainly without legal advice, but I was close to desperation.

Lois Chaber

Neil finally comes to see me in the hospital, carrying Sybil in his arms. My remorse so strong it is a visceral stab in my chest, I reach out longingly to take her and hold her, but she shrinks from me, clinging to Neil. This is the worst punishment I can receive, even more hurtful than Neil's ensuing words. He tells me he has arranged for Sybil to be taken to New Zealand and raised by his relatives, as I am not fit to do it. Panic-stricken, I plead with him, tearfully: "Please don't send my baby away!" Only after I make many promises to seek professional help for myself in Qatar does he at last agree that we will go there as a family. Somehow I manage to pull myself together enough to be discharged. I am never to see Suzette again. We leave for Paris together, and then on to Doha, all of us bearing invisible wounds on our way to yet another foreign country.

"THE THING INSIDE MY HEAD"

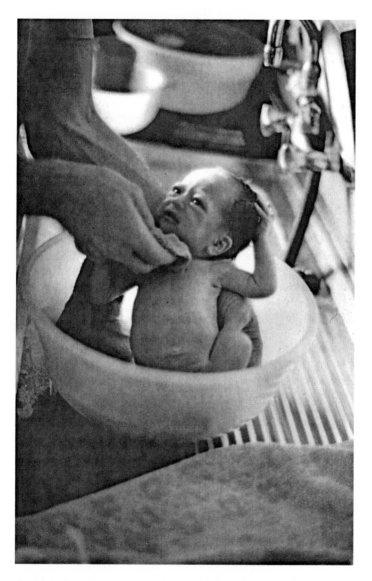

Bathing Sybil in our salad bowl, Tehran, 1978

Lois Chaber

Chapter 3: Qatar—A Family Album

> Language is by nature, fictional; the attempt to
> render language un-fictional requires an enormous
> apparatus of measurements . . . but the Photograph
> is indifferent to all intermediaries: it does not invent;
> it is authentification itself.
>
> > (Roland Barthes, *Camera Lucida: Reflections on
> > Photography*, trans. Richard Howard, Vintage; 2000, p.
> > 87.)

A photo of Sybil's first time on a beach in Qatar,
taken not long after we arrive in late winter, 1979, is
enshrined in our first family album, one of many. With his
trustworthy camera, a manual Nikon he takes everywhere,
Neil has captured her running headlong down the clean
sandy beach, with only a hint of civilization visible, the
bottom of a dark blue car in the upper left-hand corner. Sybil
is stark naked—a *seeming* tabula rasa or blank slate—with
an absolutely confident and gleeful expression on her
disproportionately large, sand-smudged face, framed by
short, coppery hair. Her thin legs look as if they will only
precariously support her small lean torso. She has just
barely learned to walk. Will the family's new expatriate
sojourn be a fresh start for the happy child of that photo or
will Sybil's emerging personality be shadowed by the
traumas of Iran?

* * *

By late February, 1979, shortly after we have read
with dismay that Khomeini and his followers have finally
trumped the Shah's rump of a government in Tehran, our
little family is settled comfortably in a spacious one-story
house or 'villa', which is filled with expensive golden teak
furniture and carpeted wall to wall in warm, muted colours.
This luxury villa and its exorbitant rent, paid by Neil's new

"THE THING INSIDE MY HEAD"

company, William Pereira Associates, as part of his employment 'package', are typical of the inflated life style that characterises this small Arab state.

Qatar is situated on a peninsula protruding into the Persian Gulf, adjacent to Saudi Arabia and the United Arab Emirates. Before its petroleum-producing days, it was a barren peninsula roamed by nomadic tribes, its sparse population surviving on camel herding in the interior and fishing and pearl diving along the coast. Eventually, it became one of the "trucial states" extending from Iraq to Oman and linked to Britain as protectorates by a series of treaties negotiated over a hundred-year period starting in 1819. After the Second World War, Britain, for political and financial reasons, ceded independence to these protectorates one by one, starting with Bahrain and Qatar in 1971. British interests and personnel still dominate in Qatar, unlike in Iran, where there had been a strong American presence prior to the Revolution.

Petroleum was discovered in the Gulf in the 1930s but not fully exploited until after World War II. From the 1960s onward, Qatar, like the other Gulf States, was transformed by the oil revenues pouring into the money-chests of the ruling Al-Thani family. Its members have used a large part of their wealth to establish a relatively modern infrastructure and a welfare state in which housing, utilities, and education are free for Qatari citizens, basic commodities are subsidised, and taxes are non-existent except for a small levy to support the PLO.

This accelerated development, similar to that in Iran only more so, has resulted in the build-up of a large expatriate presence that comprises eighty per cent of Qatar's population in 1979. Seemingly a colourful potpourri of Eastern and Western peoples, the foreign community is in fact as openly hierarchical as an ancient caste system. At the top are the Western administrators, businessmen, and technocrats, pocketing their comfortable expatriate salaries

Lois Chaber

and living in oversized villas like ours, along with some select non-Qatari Arabs, mostly Egyptians and Palestinians, who are also employed as elite administrators. Descending rungs on the ladder are occupied by large numbers of Easterners—the remaining foreign Arabs as well as Indians, Iranians, Pakistanis, Filipinos, Koreans and so on—working a range of jobs from skilled tradesmen, shopkeepers and sales personnel to waiters, 'houseboys' and nannies. At the bottom, perhaps, are the be-turbaned, pyjama-suited Baluchi tribesmen from Pakistan, pushing garbage barrows, watering lawns, breaking up stones along the roadside—employment that no present-day Qatari would even consider. The Qataris themselves, a small minority, range from the fabulously wealthy Al-Thani royals and their offspring, highly prosperous traditional merchant families, various tiers of civil servants and administrators, to ex-Bedouins settled into free housing in purpose-built new towns.

This variegated humanity of Qatar lends itself well to Neil's avid photo-taking, often with the exotic wares of the Doha souk (bazaar) in the background—delicately-flowered Persian carpets and red, yellow or brown spices spilling out of large hempen bags—an aesthetic oasis in this otherwise arid land. We acquire many friends, colleagues and helpers of all nationalities from the entire range of Qatar's social strata. Even our gentle, bearded Baluchi gardener, Mahmood, becomes a true friend when he sits day after day with Neil in the mid-1980s, patiently holding our cat Lucy while Neil scrapes off her ringworm sores, a consequence of diseased camel dung fertilising our lawn, formerly the site of a camel market. Sybil's developing personality also benefits from this multi-cultural environment. If anything, she becomes decidedly partial to making friends with girls of other ethnic and racial origins, perhaps finding them easier to get along with as they are lower in the school pecking order, which mirrors the larger community in many ways, and gentle Sybil is vulnerable to bullying from the 'white' English girls who rule the roost.

56

"THE THING INSIDE MY HEAD"

Despite the population's diversity, Qatar's native ruling class remains firmly committed to the mores of the Wahhabi sect, a fundamentalist branch of Sunni Islam originating in the eighteenth century, making Qatar in 1979 the strictest, most puritanical of the Arabian Gulf countries next to Saudi Arabia, also Wahhabi. During our stay, Qatar is a 'dry' country like Saudi, with no commercial sale or public consumption of liquor, but, here, unlike in its rigid neighbour, Western expatriates can purchase liquor to drink at home through outlets controlled jointly by the Qatari government and British officials. Similarly, as in Saudi Arabia, the native women are extremely restricted—they cannot drive cars or go out of doors unveiled, for example. The difference is that in Qatar expatriate women like me are allowed to drive and to dress Western style (within reason). Without these ameliorations for Westerners, life in Qatar would be far less tolerable for us.

* * *

Not long after our arrival, I go for an "assessment" with a senior government psychiatrist, a stern, elderly Arab. I explain that I am still quite depressed, but able to do intellectual work, like writing. He immediately deflates me, chiding, "You'll have to be able to do more than that," meaning, of course, my domestic duties; yet this doctor, not prepared to help me with these conflicts, offers me exactly five minutes of his time and a new prescription. The government medical system—including the psychiatric department—is a free but no frills service during our time here in Qatar. Psychotherapy, which I badly need and have promised Neil to obtain, is not available. I am to see a series of junior psychiatrists from here on in, all of them pressured to get through as many patients in a day as possible and disposed only to offer one medication after another.

Fortuitously, I come across for the first time a brief explanation of post-natal depression (PND), which affects

57

Lois Chaber

about ten per cent of new mothers and causes them to experience tension, irritability, lack of energy, and a general inability to deal with the demands of the baby—not to mention the accompanying guilt! This discovery prompts me to try re-connecting with Suzette in Nantes by sending an apologetic letter, but her reply is minimal, and the renewed correspondence eventually peters out, my good friend lost forever. I am still unaware at this time that "maternal depression", as defined by Tracey Thompson in *The Ghost in the House,* is something even more sinister: a condition extending its tentacles beyond PND, aggravated by the ongoing stresses of mothering and transmitted from mother to child, sometimes over generations, by learned behaviour as well as genetics. My underlying problems, with all their implications for Sybil, remain unresolved.

As a consequence, the first few months in Qatar witness some very unpleasant conflicts between Neil and me, often triggered by incredibly trivial issues—should we not invest in a compartmentalised baby food plate? Neil adamantly decrees 'No!' —and some of these escalating confrontations leave me in hysterics. In the absence of a family therapist, Neil's way of coping with these tumults is by literally dragging me into the car and off to the government hospital, where I am forcibly sedated by thuggish male assistants and then dismissed, returning home to sulk in stony silence for days. Gradually, however, these incidents ebb in amount and intensity, and we settle into a reasonably stable domestic routine.

The Qatar office of Neil's new American employer consists of a small team of architects, planners, and engineers working to plan various aspects of the 'New District of Doha'—an eastward extension of the city on reclaimed land. When Neil leaves for Pereira's office early in the morning, I settle myself and Sybil on the floor of the little hallway between the kitchen and my large study, gather round me Sybil's steadily accruing pile of toys and nursery rhyme books and devote myself—for a stipulated period of

"THE THING INSIDE MY HEAD"

time—to creative play with this rewardingly bright and responsive baby. As long as I can be both verbal and didactic, baby care is endurable. We are employing an Indian woman part-time to relieve me later in the day so that I can retreat to my golden desk and work on my academic projects. Sybil and I get to see Neil for a mid-day dinner since companies in Qatar work on a traditional Arab schedule: employees get a three hour siesta break and then work until around seven in the evening every day except Thursday, when work ends around lunchtime, and Friday, the Muslim Sabbath, the one completely free day.

The strict division of my time between Sybil and the household on the one hand and my scholarly work on the other, works well for me, but possibly helps to promote, along with her still-regulated feeding schedule, Sybil's growing need for well-defined structure. To be sure, regular schedules have been often recommended for babies (depending on the latest paediatric fashions), and with some flexibility need not be detrimental, but I cling rigidly to this routine, looking to each upcoming 'relief' period as to a distant gleaming shore whose promise enables me to get through the messy business of baby care each day. The obstacles to bonding in Iran plus my own troubled personality have put a damper on my maternal generosity. Once, when Sybil is cranky and resists being handed over to her baby-sitter, clinging to me and crying piteously, I make a decision I later regret deeply: I steel myself against her sobs, thrust her into the nanny's arms and walk into my study, shutting out the noise of her distress.

Nevertheless, Sybil appears to be thriving. At first intimidated, this lithe little baby now practically gallops around our large house on all fours and exploits everything in it, including the brass keys protruding from the kitchen cabinets, to gracefully raise herself up. We are so pleased with her 'normal' progress that by spring 1979 we decide to try for a second child. Despite the only recently-ended turmoil in our lives and my difficulties with motherhood, I am

Lois Chaber

amenable to this idea—perhaps for all the wrong reasons: Neil greatly desires another child and I want to please him. It will be psychologically healthier for Sybil to have a sibling, the sands of my biological clock are running out (I am going on thirty-seven), and, very persuasive with me, domestic help is affordable with Neil's oil-boom salary–if difficult to obtain, due to immigration restrictions on single women.

At the end of May, when Neil is chugged across the Gulf from the southern Iranian port of Bushire by a motorised wooden dhow, returning from a risky but necessary trip back to Iran to oversee and accompany the shipping here of our remaining personal effects and the camping van, I joyfully announce my second pregnancy. But shortly afterwards, our Indian nanny suddenly tells us that 'her sheikh', who is her legal sponsor, has recalled her to work for him, and she has no choice if she does not wish to be summarily deported. Neil has been trying to recruit another nanny/housemaid, but in vain. With another baby coming, in yet another foreign country, stressed by the hormonal uproar of the first trimester, heavily engaged in revising my *Moll Flanders* article for publication and clearly unable to turn to the brusque Islamic psychiatrists I have been seeing briefly at intervals, I panic: "I just can't bear returning to the turmoil of Iran!" Overdosing with my current (not very effective) anti-depressants, I once again leave Neil to pick up the pieces and to care for Sybil, oblivious as well to the welfare of my unborn baby.

I awake to find myself in the old, shabby Rumaillah General Hospital, forcibly held down in a cramped iron bed by six terribly young but oxen-strong Asian nurses who refuse to even let me up to pee. The only good that emerges from this deplorable incident is that a new psychiatrist, the pleasantly plump, forty-something Egyptian with an elegant goatee, Dr. Shirbini, the most humane and idealistic clinician who deals with me in Qatar, takes me under his wing and promises to counsel me outside the high-pressure assembly line of psychiatric appointments.

"THE THING INSIDE MY HEAD"

Neil, who is surprisingly unreproachful to me, sorts out our domestic arrangements by finally coming up with a full-time Indian nanny. This woman, 'Maria', corpulent but solid, cocoa-coloured, gap-toothed and jovial, is older and more independent than our previous help. She lives with her second husband, Babu, a genial office clerk, in a tiny stucco cottage right across the road from us, where she will often take our children for Indian sweets and Disney cartoons on her video (we haven't invested in this new technology yet!). Like other nannies we employ before and after, Maria is a fundamentalist Catholic from Portuguese-influenced Southern India, and is to surreptitiously 'share' her religious beliefs with little Sybil. Also behind our back, she regularly nicks money and liquor from us until we catch her at it and gradually deduct repayment from her (generous) salary. Nevertheless, we keep her on because she is otherwise so reliable and Sybil has become extremely attached to her.

In late July 1979, for Neil's first company leave, we make a trip back to Albany, New York, the first since we left in 1976, partly so that I, as a thirty-seven year old, can have an amniocentesis. To our great relief, besides the negative result for Down's syndrome, the radiologist assures me the foetus has not been affected by my overdose. For Sybil, the US trip is a stimulant, reinforcing new developments; shortly before departure she had suddenly pointed at our cat Pippy, beamed, and enunciated 'kgat'(as in the beginning of 'Qatar') her first word other than 'da-da'. Here, in a more pet-friendly environment, she makes a second, generalising leap and identifies cats everywhere, in the flesh, on the walls and in the media, soon moving on to 'oogie' for 'doggie', the beginning of her life-long adoration of animals. We are thrilled with the keen intelligence that Sybil, at one and a bit, increasingly displays, and I, especially, welcome her entry into language.

At home during the next month, Sybil's vocabulary expands in leaps and bounds and she becomes absolutely hooked on books—another development that makes

61

mothering more pleasurable. As soon as she spies a propitious moment, she will run up to one of us, with pleading eyes, book in hand. When we consent to read and settle somewhere on the floor, where we have laid out huge multi-striped cushions, she literally hurls herself into one of our laps, sometimes landing a foot away, so eager is she, not just for the sentences she mostly doesn't understand, but for the sense of ritual and loving togetherness that reading evokes for our family. Sybil's wonderful sense of humour also emerges; she loves a good joke, even if it's on herself. When she whines or frets, I sometimes imitate her and she immediately recognises her silliness, stops, and laughs heartily at me and at herself. One day on the beach, when she insists on drinking from the grownup's water bottle and cold water then runs all the way down her shirt front, she guffaws heartily at her own sloppiness.

Neil is simply crazy about Sybil. I take a black and white photo of him with his 1970s look: longish hair and beard, in an art nouveau T-shirt and short shorts, sitting on our terrazzo patio, with his strong, large hands securely gripping and almost meeting across the slim torso of sixteen-month-old Sybil, who is seated, with great delight, on his bare knee. Both of their faces are identically lit up with broad, happy grins; she is a pint-sized copy of him. Neil's eyes are creased with happiness.

* * *

Autumn 1979: It is getting closer to my due date. Having rejected an initial plan to give birth in New Zealand, amidst Neil's family but without him, I am now resigned to bearing my second child in the only maternity facility in Qatar, the dingy, dilapidated, and overcrowded 'Women's Hospital', a relic of less affluent times. Conditions here are summarised in a nutshell when Mrs. Hunter, the English head midwife, confides to me: "As far as I can see, women are lower than camels in this country." Indeed, this maternity hospital is the opposite of the Tehran clinic—very

"THE THING INSIDE MY HEAD"

primitive: one has to bring one's own linens, swaddling for the baby, and all mundane supplies, including toilet paper and cutlery, since the hospital caters to Qatari domestic customs.

Around this time also, in November 1979, the US Embassy hostage crisis in Iran explodes and ripples throughout the Gulf. Panic is provoking many Americans to leave voluntarily, especially wives and children, and some US companies, as well as the US Embassy, are coercing their personnel, or at least their dependents, into evacuation, which unfortunately affects my best friend Carole McCreary, the wife of the American vice-consul, and her little daughter Katy, Sybil's first friend. Having already lived through the more immediate menaces of revolutionary Iran, Neil and I don't feel personally threatened. But the exodus of many friends and the curtailment of social activities have left us isolated and bored. And despite assurances by the Qatari government to American businesses, community tensions are growing. A local Arabic newspaper displays in its centrefold pictures of American short-wave radios and other 'suspicious' paraphernalia 'discovered' at the US Embassy in Tehran, with the aggressive comment (as translated): "The Iranians have done what we don't dare to do." Things are reaching a peak by December 2nd, the date of the Iranian constitutional referendum, when the Qatari government makes an obvious show of guarding (or is it constraining?) the Iranian Embassy and setting up roadblocks in all directions. Throughout the day impassive Iranians, nondescript in their drab, quasi-Western dress, walk past the gates of Pereira's nearby American office-villa, determined to cast their votes, as Neil's nervous colleagues watch from the windows.

In these ominous circumstances, I give birth prematurely on December 16th to my second daughter, Molly, in conditions that nearly replicate Sybil's traumatic birth in Tehran, even to the extent that my doctor, an Indian woman and the best obstetrician in Qatar, is due to go on

Lois Chaber

holiday in three days. Once again, my waters have broken suddenly, and at the hospital, my labour and delivery are over in less than two hours. Neil has to shuttle back and forth frantically, bringing more and more basic items for me and the baby, to facilitate our two-day stay here in this under-equipped facility. Unlike Sybil, however, Molly, only four or five weeks premature, weighs nearly six pounds and does not need an incubator—none of which are currently working, anyway! There is no nursery in this hospital, so this time my baby is not only lodged right next to me in a cot, but I am on my own in caring for her. This immediate intimacy makes all the difference to my relationship with Molly. But, like Sybil, she is not interested in suckling, and again the Asian nurses are at best indifferent, at worst hostile, to my desire to breast-feed. Desperate by morning, as Molly has had no nourishment at all, I am 'rescued' by a helpful Scottish nurse who walks in cheerily, swaddles Molly helpfully, and reassuringly shows me a technique for getting Molly to feed.

I persist in breastfeeding Molly, but again the apathy of a preemie and lingering jaundice, as well as my own propensity for tension, prevent vigorous suckling. Only by my putting her on the breast for two hours at a time can she can come close to draining my somewhat meagre supply of milk, which has to be supplemented with a bottle. Molly catches a cold from Sybil, and her illness and consequent sleepless nights are made worse by the ignorant prescription of a strong antibiotic by a government paediatrician. Molly's severe illness, her interminable feedings, plus constant diarrhoea and diaper rash, mean that Neil and Maria virtually have to take over Sybil's care, isolating me from her for the first several weeks of Molly's life—not a good way to mitigate sibling rivalry!

As in Iran, political unrest and baby problems are accompanied by professional difficulties for Neil. There is uncertainty in William Pereira's office as to whether the firm wants to stay (given the turbulent regional politics), whether

"THE THING INSIDE MY HEAD"

the Qatari government will renew their contract in any case, and, with regard to Neil, whether his own contract with the company will be renewed. Despite the long, productive hours he has put into the project, he does not get on well with either the office manager or Pereira's partner, who regularly commutes from the Los Angeles office to Doha. This multiple insecurity drags on into February, creating anxieties that inevitably decrease my already less-than-free-flowing milk and permeate the daily life of the children. Neil's insistence on sending out his résumé in this time of uncertainty leads to a final showdown with his bosses, and he is sacked.

Dodgy and insecure job situations are to dog Neil for many years, with serious repercussions for the whole family, and I am puzzled as to why, given that he is such a hard-working, talented and conscientious professional. I can only speculate: Neil was born with a cleft palate and hare lip, largely remedied in New Zealand through a series of difficult operations, but his disability and his medical ordeals inspired his very loving and supportive mother to instil in him a strong sense of stubborn self-pride and self-sufficiency. As a result, he doesn't suffer fools gladly, regardless of rank, and he is not prone to ingratiating himself with his superiors. At the very least, this attitude does not endear him to them.

Fortunately, in this particular crisis, Neil soon receives an enthusiastic offer of work from a project management company, McKee Associates, which has been working with Pereira's on the New District of Doha project. He is given the management position of 'Executive Architect' with responsibility to oversee the designing and building of homes for the Qatari 'senior staff', upper echelon civil servants. The downside is that we have to leave our attractive, comfortable house and our half-grown vegetable garden with cabbages, cauliflowers, and tomatoes literally ripening on the vine, because in these expatriate situations the house goes with the job. Since we have to move house,

Lois Chaber

we decide to take our first trip to see Neil's family in New Zealand with the children before Neil's new duties begin.

This flight to and from New Zealand in March, 1980, is the first of many Antipodean travel ordeals to come, due to the inordinate length of the flight there, the several mandatory plane changes, the generally unsympathetic flight attendants on Cathay Pacific Airlines, and the awkwardness of flying with very young children (both in nappies and Molly with chronic diarrhoea on this journey). The holiday begins inauspiciously, with us embarking from the old house while the movers are working all around us, thanks to the pressures put on us to vacate the house quickly, and in the confusion we leave behind Sybil's two favourite teddy bears, miss our flight from Doha Airport, and eventually lose yet another teddy bear that we have stopped off to buy. By the time we finally get to a hotel in Australia, the journey still incomplete, Sybil, totally disoriented and too young at less than two years to take in explanations of what a long air flight entails, is throwing extreme tantrums, rejecting food, balking at hotel doors and refusing to go into rooms. We are taken aback by this first glimpse of the super-sensitive, hyper-excitable side of her personality.

Fortunately for her, when we finally arrive in Wellington, the benefits of meeting Neil's extended family for the first time—especially her one and only grandparent, Neil's elderly mother, and Sybil's good-natured older cousins, who fuss over Sybil and vie to amuse her—outweigh the strains of the toilsome journeying. In Wellington also, I at last am able to consult a highly competent and sympathetic paediatrician, who gives me practical advice that results in a fulfilling breastfeeding relationship with my new infant—possibly a factor in Molly's laid-back and genial childhood personality. But Neil's challenging new job all too soon recalls us to Qatar and subsequent visits to this warm extended family are to be few and far between; we only dimly begin to perceive the costs to our children of this expatriate way of life.

"THE THING INSIDE MY HEAD"

* * *

During the spring and early summer of 1980, Dr. Shirbini, the kindly, liberal-minded psychiatrist I met when hospitalised, offers me the opportunity for some unofficial extended therapy. "I'm going to inject you with something that will make you relax and talk freely," he tells me soothingly, as I lie back nervously on an antiquated examining table in his cramped office (it is a few years yet before Qatar gets a new, state-of-the-art medical complex). By 'peeking', I discover the drug is called 'methadrin', presumably a variant of the heroin substitute methadone. Soon, layer after encrusted layer of my chronic anxiety unpeels, followed by a massive wave of almost orgasmic euphoria, so intensely pleasurable that from this day I am able readily to empathise with drug addiction! In our first session, he gets me to talk about my fraught relationship with my mother, opening up channels clogged with guilt and grief. His words afterward—"Don't you think she would forgive you?"—are like a priest's absolution.

In a second session that focuses on my own daughters, my anguish over the daily conflict between maternal caring and personal self-fulfilment, my resentment of the boredom and mental deterioration attendant upon full-time motherhood, all pour out uncensored with the help of the injection. When I emerge from my trance, he tries to comfort me: "They will become more interesting as they grow older. Trust me!" His final words to the wise are ones I am to hear ringing in my mind throughout my career as a mother: "Love them or reject them, but don't be ambivalent—that's the worst thing for children."

Much to my distress, these cathartic and therapeutic sessions come to an abrupt end later in the summer when Dr. Shirbini has to leave Qatar for family reasons. I am more desolate than ever when I have to return to routine appointments with the other apathetic and brusque government psychiatrists, especially as I have had a bit of a

Lois Chaber

crush on Dr. Shirbini. My resurgent depression gains impetus from the oppressive heat of the season and the summer exodus from Doha of most of our expatriate friends' wives and children; Sybil and Molly are also bored and miserable without their little friends. My depression, however, also arises from a more longstanding intellectual isolation and loss of confidence. Excluded from Doha's professional community, I feel alienated from 'real life'.

A vigorous pep talk over coffee from Ruth, the bleached-blonde, middle-aged wife of the Senior Staff Project Director and a down-to-earth New Yorker, reinforced by Neil, who realises that my depression is undermining my mothering, kick-starts me into job-hunting. By a stroke of luck, I walk into a teaching position in the English Department at the National University of Qatar that has just been unexpectedly vacated. Unfortunately, it is full-time not part-time as I had hoped for, but it is my best chance, and I plunge in, taking a deep breath and shrugging off pricklings of guilt. Sybil is at first not very pleased about my going off in the morning to 'the big school', as we call it, even though she has been happily attending a nursery, but she soon seems to adjust, and Molly is too young to protest.

Qatar University, for conservative Islamic reasons, consists of two physically separate campuses for men and women about a mile apart, and in September I start teaching the women, while also having to drive back and forth to the men's college for administrative and departmental matters. Although the salary is much better, the contact hours and the number of classes are as heavy-duty as those at Damavand College. The university has an officious rule obliging all faculty to be on campus from at least 8:30 to 12:30 pm, regardless of their class schedule, so I indulge in a bit of risk-taking by leaving the English Department common room a half hour before the contact hours have officially ended, despite the glares of other, more rule-bound faculty members. Most days I sneak out at 12:00, speed home in the Volkswagen van by 12:15, quickly breast-feed

"THE THING INSIDE MY HEAD"

Molly, hurriedly put together a lunch for Sybil, Neil and myself, aided by Neil, usually home for lunch by 12:45, and then take off precisely at 1:15 to make a 1:30 class. None of this would be possible without the help of Maria, whose affordability on Gulf wages is, in part, my rationalisation for working full time.

Nevertheless, I feel the strain of dividing myself up between needy children, demanding students, and my own cravings for privacy and ongoing scholarly stimulation (my English classes at the university—ranging from basic language instruction to one dumbed down literature section—being of a very low standard). But by gaining a professional status in the community and by making new, more educated, more like-minded friends in the English Department, I am now a happier person to live with, even though I cannot exorcise the motherly 'ambivalence' Dr. Shirbini has warned me against.

Meanwhile, during the sticky, oppressive summer of 1980, Neil outdoes himself by taking over, in addition to his responsibilities at Senior Staff Housing, the fast-track management of a previously cocked-up project to complete some pre-fabricated units for the Engineering Division of the men's university. He spends three months of back-breaking, all-consuming work, an average of twelve hours a day, six days a week, whipping contractors, foremen, engineers, and labourers into industry on the site. The long hours of both our jobs inevitably have repercussions: Our domestic life becomes even more regimented, our time with the children tightly squeezed— particularly unfortunate as at this time both of them are constantly getting bad colds and bouts of flu that incapacitate them for activities outside the home. Sybil has recently been so ill that she has had to stay out of nursery school and away from friends for two weeks, during which she becomes emotionally unstable and withdrawn. Her tendency to fall apart under stress is becoming increasingly apparent.

Lois Chaber

Sybil's rough passage through the 'terrible twos', from late 1980 through mid-1981, is the *only* period of her life when she is conventionally 'naughty' as opposed to simply stressed and quasi-hysterical. Neil and I find ourselves unthinkingly spanking her during her bouts of stubborn defiance or aggression. Both of us have been spanked and smacked in our own childhood and, despite my own unhappiness as a child, we don't question these old-fashioned disciplinary methods, applying them to Molly later as well—and for a longer time. For me especially, giving one of the little girls a sharp smack becomes a knee-jerk response in moments of intense irritability. The absence of an extended family in our immediate environment means there are no adults around intimate enough with us to comment candidly and sympathetically on our parenting or to provide alternative role models. We tell ourselves that such physical punishment as we sometimes resort to is more than 'balanced' by the lavish and open physical affection we bestow on the girls, but it is a practice we later come to regret dearly.

At this time, anyway, the toddler Molly is very good-natured and easy to manage, with a ready laugh or smile. Sybil and Molly have just started to engage in parallel play—when Sybil can restrain herself from tearing things out of Molly's hands! Neil and I have established a shared bedtime routine of individual songs and stories for each child, an extension of my earlier folk song repertoire, and these nightly rituals become a special family tradition, a time of warmth and security, which the girls can always count on—and will find very hard to give up in later years.

* * *

Early summer 1981: I have just arrived in bustling Hong Kong with the now-three-year-old Sybil. Neil and I have decided on separate holidays, splitting up the children, so that he can visit his mother, now ill with a recurrence of cancer, and I can visit friends and relatives in the US,

70

"THE THING INSIDE MY HEAD"

particularly my stepsister Madelyn, who has never met Sybil.
Due to a mistake in my hotel booking, there is just one bed,
a single, in our room. I am not concerned to alter this,
however, for it means that Sybil and I will have to snuggle
closely together, dovetailed like two spoons in a narrow
drawer, for our much-needed post-flight nap—a delicious
opportunity for intimacy as Sybil has never been one for
climbing into bed with her parents. This heightened physical
and emotional togetherness continues after our awakening
when we go for a dip in the hotel pool. We splash and play
our favourite water games together ("Mummy, let's play
rock-a-by-baby"), lapped by a mutually loving feeling.
Following upon the companionable flight with my now-
articulate little girl and our cosy nap, this makes me feel
closer to Sybil than any time up to now. But my euphoria is
abruptly deflated, like a punctured swimming tube, when I
notice some suspicious spots on her chest: "Uh-oh—
chicken pox!" I manage to quash these silent fears for the
time being, but the next morning, creeping down her chest
and back, the illness is unmistakeable, and I shift into panic
mode.

At lunchtime, sitting in a sleek ultra-modern
shopping centre, I go over the options with my Jewish-
Tunisian friend from Qatar, newly resident in Hong Kong,
while Sybil blithely cavorts in and out of the shiny plastic
tables with my friend's small son:

"The signs I saw in the airport," I tell my friend
Simone, "tell me that Hong Kong officials are on the lookout
for contagious diseases."

"How do you know?"

"They all stated that visitors must *immediately* notify
authorities about any possible indications."

"Oh, I wouldn't take it all so seriously if I were you."

Lois Chaber

"But I'm due to stay in Hong Kong two more days and then fly to Japan; her chicken pox is going to get more and more obvious. What if I'm 'caught' when boarding the plane and quarantined in a small hotel room with Sybil?"

"Is that so *very* bad?"

"YES!! Sybil is so hyper these days! She's been an angel so far, but, locked up for days without her collection of toys and books, she'll get extremely cranky, even hysterical, for sure! I won't be able to deal with it!"

Simone is sympathetic but bemused.

"On the other hand, if I dash my round-the-world trip and go home, I'll have to pay a large penalty fee, the airline has told me, plus the cost of the homeward flight. Neil will really be pissed! And I'll lose this opportunity to cement my relationship with Sybil... What should I *do*, Simone?"

My very wise Middle Eastern friend gently urges me to take a chance, continue onwards with Sybil and bear the burden of her illness, whatever happens. In the end, however, I return lamely to Doha, carrying the chicken-pox back to a susceptible Molly and thus putting back Neil's holiday plans by a month, so that when we eventually voyage to New Zealand all together, our little ones come down with severe colds from the bitter, wintry Wellington weather and they get to see little of their cousins, who are now too busy with school.

For me, however, one redeeming feature of the compromised holiday is the opportunity in Neil's home town for the extremely impressionable Sybil to have her first taste of the theatre—there is no public children's entertainment in Qatar. While Neil baby-sits Molly, I take Sybil off to a children's play, a marvellously silly Gothic concoction called "Bad Jelly the Witch." The woman playing the witch, fantastically made up to appear sinister and grotesque,

"THE THING INSIDE MY HEAD"

comes forth to present her first soliloquy: "I'm Bad Jelly the witch, the worst witch in the world, and I looove to eat little children..." Sybil bursts instantly into tears and I am hard put to convince her to stay for the rest of the performance. But I assure myself I've done the right thing since, though shaken, she emerges from the theatre excited and impressed, and at home in Doha later, she chatters endlessly about the play, remembering it in vivid detail. (Later in life, I am similarly to foist on Sybil 'edifying' books and films with dark overtones—like *Tess of the D'Urbervilles*—that stimulate but disturb her.)

Back in Qatar in the autumn of 1981, I get a scare at the university when I am summoned to see the much-dreaded Mr. Naimi, a stern, cadaverous-looking senior administrator, and told to "Bring your US passport." Friends in the department whisper to me quickly that an elderly Irish faculty member, whose advances I have recently spurned, has 'tipped off' the university on a hunch that I am Jewish. Living in an Arab state that is avowedly anti-Zionist but also unofficially anti-Semitic, has meant having to conceal this part of my ethnic background, for its revelation would mean deportation for the whole family. Mr. Naimi takes the passport from my trembling hands and riffles through it, hoping for some official statement of my religion—as is found in most Middle Eastern passports; fortunately, this is not the case with most Western passports, and I am dismissed grumpily without explanation or apology.

The English Department I teach in features a conventional curriculum of British classics in their (few) literature courses, so that I get to teach my Arab girls some works that I love, albeit at a very slow pace and at a very low level to accommodate their limited reading skills. They prove incapable of understanding Jonathan Swift's irony in *Gulliver's Travels,* but I am very successful in putting across to my women-only class how similar the restrictions and assumptions of Jane Austen's eighteenth-century world are to their own milieu. This is as far as I dare to lift up the veil

Lois Chaber

on my feminism in a state rife with political surveillance and repression.

In Neil's job, however, problems worse than mine are cropping up. McKee Associates has not been remunerated by the Qatari government for about a year, despite frequent obsequious, money-begging visits made here from New York by the company president, Jerry McKee. It is always 'bukra'—the Arabian version of 'mañana'. This is an extreme instance of the difficulties all contractors and consultants in this country have with the Qatari government, whose delayed, grudging payments are a byword in town. The only way McKee's can meet the monthly payroll is for the National Bank of Qatar, with a lot of grumbling, to extend the company's already enormous overdraft each time. Expatriate work in the Gulf continues to be extremely insecure.

* * *

It's scary! By late 1981 I am seeing in Sybil both my 'good' and my 'bad' genes emerging with a vengeance. Yes, she is intelligent, sensitive, and highly responsive to literature and language. She is also very whiney, prone to extreme mood changes and fearful, with a low threshold for physical and mental pain. At her bad moments, I see my own worst self, and shrink from it.

For the last year she has been obsessed by death, initially provoked by hearing us read about the violent demise of the mother elephant in the Babar books and reinforced by seeing photos in our family album of our deceased parents, not to mention our frequent shrill warnings against dangerous behaviour: "Sybil, don't take off your swimming tube in the middle of the Doha Club pool!" Now, she has been seeking any excuse to bring up this topic, 'death', usually by morbid questions such as, "What will happen to Molly if someone puts their hands around her throat?" She repeatedly asks us, "Mummy, are you and

74

"THE THING INSIDE MY HEAD"

Daddy going to die? Am I going to die some day?" Neil and I forego any mention of 'heaven' during these uncomfortable discussions, compelled to be honest by our shared religious scepticism—perhaps a big mistake. But at the same time, we evade telling her about the recent death from cancer of Neil's mother, formerly her only living grandparent.

Meanwhile, Molly, by early 1982, has what is perhaps Neil's only 'vice', stubbornness. Like her father, she tends to be stolid, genial and very independent. We have to coerce Sybil (who is three and three quarters) into putting on her underpants and socks in the mornings, while baby Molly comes running out of her room dragging an entire outfit she's managed to snatch out of her changing table wardrobe, screaming "I put on pants"—though she really cannot. Every afternoon, when Sybil wakes up from her mid-day nap, she sits on her bed, still under the bedclothes, whimpering, until someone comes in; Molly, as soon as she awakes, pops out of bed, opens the door of her room, walks into mine and says in a chirpy voice, "I'm a' wake up." Sybil is thin, Molly plump; Sybil is highly verbal, Molly at nineteen months is extremely well-coordinated and good with her hands. Our current photo album is replete with pictures of the two of them, standing stiffly side by side, with pudding-bowl haircuts courtesy of Maria, Sybil at this point towering over Molly, with a serious poker face, Molly usually laughing.

We increasingly perceive a 'see-saw syndrome', in which the two girls constantly play off against each other's personality traits and moods, reacting in opposite ways to events and stages in our family's life. To some extent part of the inevitable sibling rivalry in children of the same gender so close in age, it is possibly also a consequence of their lacking a single stable cultural background in their formative years: Born of two parents with different nationalities (the US, New Zealand), they are geographically exiled from both those parents' homelands and living in an alien non-Western cultural environment. They belong, in fact, to a growing twentieth-century demographic phenomenon that David O.

75

Lois Chaber

Pollock and Ruth E. Van Rekin call 'Third Culture Kids' in their book of that name. According to these authors, expatriate childhoods greatly affect the sense of self and world-view of such children. More than the norm, it seems to me, our little girls tend to use each other as points of reference in forming their identities, as Molly's memories of growing up in Qatar suggest:

> In the early years, Sybil seemed to be just as adventurous as me. We used to do the same things. I remember the time we cut off each other's hair. I have a mental picture of my parents coming into the room and us two sitting there with scissors in our hands and hair everywhere and everyone being very shocked. I don't remember whose idea it was and whose hair got cut. We cut off all the dolls' hair as well, thinking it would grow back.

> In the early days, she was the more adventurous one. We had some friends around, little boys. There was a beehive in our garden and they wanted to throw sticks at it. I refused to do it and went inside the house and closed the glass door. Sybil remained outside, perhaps not throwing sticks, but watching, and she got stung. I sort of said, "I told you so." Also, when we visited our [American diplomat] friends in Yemen the first time, during a picnic, Katy and Jo-Jo [their daughters] wanted to climb up a tree. I didn't climb with them, but Sybil did. The upshot was that Jo-Jo fell out of the tree and hurt herself.

"THE THING INSIDE MY HEAD"

At other times, I tended to follow and imitate what Sybil did. I remember when Pippy [our cat] died. My mum came into the house and found a note from dad on the bed and told Sybil and me about it. Then mum and Sybil ran crying to their bedrooms and threw themselves down on the bed, so I followed them and did the same thing, pretending to cry, even though I wasn't that upset.

Our roles reversed in later years; she became the sensible one who held back and I became more adventurous. I was the more domineering one, especially around other kids. For example, when we went to a big, big beach and lots of people came to visit, I was the one more eager to get in with the other kids, and I would rush off ahead, or, if she didn't want to do something, I'd just go and do it anyway even if she said I shouldn't. When we were together, she would be the one, when it came down to it, to take a back seat and let me be the one that went ahead and got attention and got my way more often than not.

Meanwhile, in late 1981, Neil, now promoted to Project Manager of the Senior Staff Housing Project (while poor Ruth and her husband are sent packing, alas), is spending at least eleven hours a day on the site and bringing work home. He has close to four hundred Arab senior staff clients, many of whom are continually barging onto the site to besiege him with complaints about the progress of their houses. His mental health is suffering. On top of this, as time goes by and the Qatari government continues to withhold payments, the company resorts to paying Neil's salary only every other month, adding to his aggravation and our worries. With me working full time at the university, and the needs of two little children calling for a whirlwind domestic schedule even with the help we have from Maria, tensions frequently run high in the house, Neil and I losing our tempers with each other or with the children. Once, things come to such a pass that Neil angrily absents himself from home for twenty-four hours. I am still seeing the state psychiatrists, at distant intervals, only for the sake of obtaining medication—but there has been no one to take Dr. Shirbini's place, no one I can relate to therapeutically. We try not to think about how this pressure-cooker environment is affecting the children.

* * *

Whatever the family tensions, however, these early years in Qatar are in other ways idyllic ones for our children. Perhaps because I am so deficient in spontaneity, finding it difficult to provide off-the-cuff amusement for the girls, and, I sometimes think, almost *fearing* to be alone with them lest I expose myself as the incompetent mother I secretly believe myself to be, I make extraordinary efforts throughout our time here to ensure they are entertained on a more formal basis. To be sure, children's entertainment here is *generally* formal, mimicking that of adults. With a disparate population, high concrete walls between houses, and violent, unpredictable traffic, there is virtually no casual neighbourhood play, obliging the mums to arrange a perpetual round of 'coffee mornings' with their children. Inviting over Sybil's friends' mothers, serving the requisite home-made refreshments, and being prepared to reciprocate the visits, is a totally new experience for me and eats up the little free time I have as a full-time lecturer. Often I have nothing in common with these women other than biological motherhood, and I have to turn mental somersaults not only to keep the conversations going while the children play but also to charm the mothers so they will continue to promote the children's friendships, on which my

"THE THING INSIDE MY HEAD"

eager Sybil so thrives, blissfully unaware of my discomfort—
or so I tell myself. Like Rhett Butler in *Gone with the Wind*, I
force myself, for Sybil's sake, to chat up the socialite
mothers I scorned before my daughter came along.

With no street life or children's television in English
in Doha, birthday parties acquire heightened significance.
By the time I throw my first one ever, for Sybil's third birthday
in spring 1981, I have cottoned on to the way the British give
children's parties. While I have grown up in New York in the
1950s with the traditional American fare of birthday cake,
ice-cream and some 'candy', the typical British birthday
party, I now gather, provides a proper 'birthday tea'—a
veritable feast, starting with cocktail sausages and petite
sandwiches and eventually encompassing a huge range of
finger food and sweets—as well as an overstuffed 'goodie
bag' for each departing child, often costing more than the
birthday gift that was bestowed—to my amazement.
Expatriate children's birthday parties in Qatar turn into highly
competitive extravaganzas, sometimes even catered in
exclusive clubs, partly because of the oil money floating
around, partly because of the infectious nature of
ostentatious Arab hospitality, but mostly because of Qatar's
cultural and physical barrenness.

As a 'guilty' working mother and a chronic
perfectionist, I jump all too eagerly onto this extravagant
birthday party bandwagon, while Neil unfailingly
memorializes these jubilant occasions by taking scores of
photos for our albums at each one. I get hold of a little book
of children's party games—like the 'turtle race': who can take
the longest to crawl to the finish line?—which I studiously
review before each occasion, drawing up an over-ambitious
agenda of games and stock-piling superfluous prizes. The
zenith of the Qatar party mania in our own family is captured
by Neil's photo of five-year-old Sybil in flouncey pale green
dress, perched high on a chair, bending with concentrated
looks over not one, but two gigantic, made-to-order,
marzipan-topped birthday cakes, her eyes bright, her mouth

pursed, trying to blow out the candles on both of them simultaneously, while a mass of excited young well-wishers surrounding the table look on. I have made the double order of cakes from our luxury local supermarket in order to provide for her entire primary school class of thirty, anxiously invited by me so that Sybil will not offend anyone and will also receive in turn lots of birthday invitations to sustain her social life.

Admittedly, this practice is spendthrift and leads to a calendar of peaks and troughs for the girls, especially the older Sybil; nevertheless, these very special occasions and the flattering attention they provide for the girls make 'birthdays' forever after into momentous, if sometimes anxious occasions, for the two girls and help to fix Qatar in their minds, in future times, as a paradise lost. Years later, just days before her eleventh birthday, Molly, crying bitterly on her bed, is to blurt out to me, "I wish I was five years old and back in Qatar!"

Our strenuous efforts to keep Sybil and Molly amused in this otherwise not very stimulating environment are rewarded in these early years by the obvious pleasure the two girls register when we succeed. In the first few years we spend in Qatar, there is not a single children's park in the country, so when a family park with playground finally opens, not quite finished, about forty minutes north of our house, we enthusiastically whisk the girls there and stay just as long as we can all stand the stink of the recently manured lawns and the accompanying flotillas of aggressive flies. Everything good about the girls' childhood is captured in a splendid close-up photo of Neil's taken at this Al Khor Park: Sybil, in colourful tee-shirt, and Molly, in bib-top overalls, four and two and a half respectively, are perched together (in their typical sisterly closeness) at the very top of a children's slide (itself not visible), against the background of a powder blue sky with puffs of clouds; they appear literally and figuratively 'on top of the world', their delight at having this brand new playground to themselves evident in their

"THE THING INSIDE MY HEAD"

glowing red cheeks, their eyes crinkled with merriment, and their mouths open in a cross between laughing and smiling.

Whatever harmony we have as a family is never more in evidence than during our favourite Friday (Sunday) pastime—going to the beach, as nostalgically described by Sybil herself in a class essay many years later:

Just about every Friday our family went to the beach. My parents drove for what seemed hours to us kids, but it was probably not very far. We were driving through desert country. We looked out for signs of water, and when we saw it, we bobbed up and down in the back with excitement, shouting, "I can see the sea!"

Sometimes our family went on our own and sometimes with friends, but excluding the friends, we were the only ones there as far as the eye could see, and if there were even just one other couple our group would consider it crowded! After a quick drink or a yogurt to quench our thirst and refresh us, my sister and I headed for the water. We were both good swimmers from an early age.

The water was clear with a tinge of blue and you could see your feet and the light-coloured sand on the bottom. It was beautiful. My mum and dad would join us and we would swim and splash about. Later we kids would play in the sand and my dad would go spear fishing. The sandcastles we made were complicated and sophisticated with towers and with water in moats. I

81

always remember us trying to make little bridges over the moat but we were never successful; they always caved in. Dad would come back with the angelfish he had caught and start a barbeque.

The beach wasn't at all pebbly but completely sandy. Further away from the sea grew wiry but robust grass, which camels would eat. It seems wonderful and amazing now that we actually came close to wild camels. Once, when we had laid out the blankets and were sitting upon them eating, a couple of camels came very close to us, spitting and eating our food. Sometimes we would see camels lying down, resting, their golden flanks bared to the sun. One time a camel herder and his camels were there at the beach; the herder milked one of them there and then and gave us the milk. Dad and I drank some but goodness knows how we didn't get ill from it.

As the afternoon drew on and it came close to early evening, my sister and I would badger our mum to help us make a 'mermaid sculpture' in the sand. My mum would draw the figure of a mermaid in the sand. Then we would fill it in, making a raised, three-dimensional picture, and decorate it with shells.

Then came the time for us to leave. The sand hurt my skin as I changed out of my swimsuit and put dry clothes on. I would go down to the sea once more to rinse the sand from my legs and feet and try and put my shoes on without them getting wet or me getting more sand on my feet. As you can

"THE THING INSIDE MY HEAD"

imagine, this was nigh on impossible. My sister and I hated leaving and would cry. Then in the car we would try to play and make tents in the back seat with towels. When we got home it was bath-time and then bed.

The experiences seem so far away now. Sometimes I feel the memories are from another life. I'm sure no beach will ever be the same to me as the beaches of my early childhood.

Lois Chaber

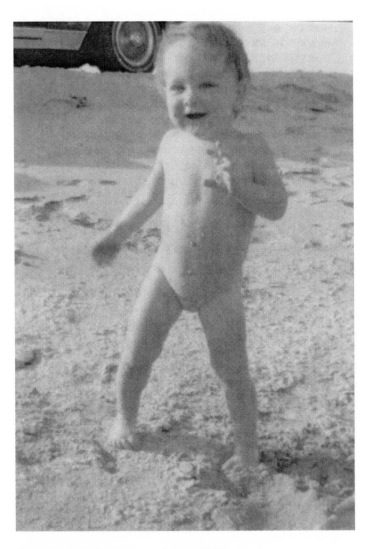

Baby Sybil on the beach, Qatar, 1979.

"THE THING INSIDE MY HEAD"

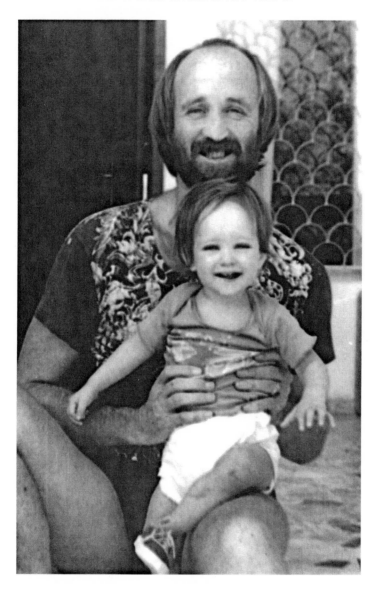

Neil and Sybil in Doha, circa 1980

Lois Chaber

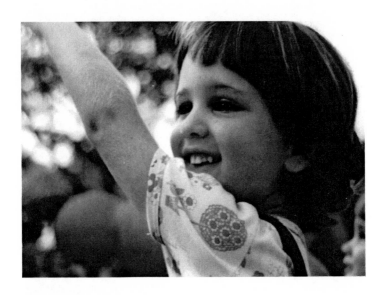

Sybil in Disneyland, 1982

"THE THING INSIDE MY HEAD"

Chapter 4: Qatar—the Picture Darkens

The [Labour Ministry] spokesman said that the
Arabisation programme is aimed at preserving the
Arab tenor of Qatari social and cultural life, and
avoiding a preponderance of any foreign nationality.

(Staff reporter, "Qatar Outlines its Manpower Policy," in
The Weekly Gulf Times, March 5, 1981.)

January 1982: Inspired by the stoic endurance of
long-drawn-out suffering by Neil's mother, who has died of
cancer this month, I resolve earnestly to foster a better self,
for my own sake and the family's. I have been coping with
life for two months without anti-depressants, only obtainable
through the government psychiatrists. My most recent one
had insisted on "massaging" my thighs—"to relax your
tension"—and, too timid to officially complain, I had just
ceased going to appointments. No visits, no pills. Proud of
my abstention, I steel myself to face upcoming hardships,
confident I can deal with my chronic anxiety and
depression—as if they can be willed away!

By late February, my spirits and resolve are slowly
being damped down by the perennial dilemma of my
motherhood again. Unlike the children's 'play dough' or
Plasticine, my time, no matter which way I twist and turn and
press it, is not infinitely flexible. Every minute I give to the
children is a minute away from my creative efforts, and every
minute given to writing is a deprivation for the children.

And Sybil's psychological life and mine are
inevitably intertwined. I continue to oversee her miniature
social life, endeavouring to recruit new supplies of friends to
replace the ones that regularly leave Qatar. In mid-March I
make a date for a 'coffee morning' with Pauline Chew, an
English woman married to a Chinese man and new to the

87

expatriate community, who has a daughter Sybil's age (nearly four). This mundane visit is to give me the first intimations of Sybil's vulnerability, and, given my tendency to overreact, is to affect my own life dramatically.

We are at Pauline's home, and her exquisite little Eurasian daughter Alison, for some unfathomable reason, does not take to Sybil, refusing to play with her or even to let Sybil use her toys. Coyly and arrogantly, Alison plays by herself, pointedly ignoring my daughter; meanwhile, Sybil, eager on her part to engage with the little girl, pleads with her and follows her around like a rejected puppy. While this is going on, we mothers try to keep up a cheerful flow of conventional chatter. I am both bored to tears and, increasingly, distraught over Sybil's pitiable plight.

Totally 'uncool', Sybil is allowing herself to be tormented by this haughty little girl, and I see myself in her. Alison's mother from time to time makes a feeble attempt to chide her daughter into playing with Sybil, but Alison is not to be moved, and the pathetic little drama goes on. Both of us mothers are very embarrassed, but we say little about what is happening, continuing to make small talk. Despite my concern for Sybil and my vicarious pain, I am too foolish, too timid, too bound by social convention simply to say, "Look, it's obvious the children are not getting along, and Sybil is quite unhappy. Why don't we just call it a day and let me take her home; we can get together by ourselves another time." Instead, I carry on, masked with a phoney smile, until finally the mid-day call to prayer booms out from the nearest mosque, and I can make excuses to leave for lunch.

I return home with my whining, tearful little Sybil, trying to comfort her, but with my face broken out and a rash on my left hand from the psychological strain of the morning's fiasco, I am probably communicating my own distress to her unwittingly. Emotional pain is ricocheting back and forth between us. That afternoon, trying to work at my desk, I feel a stress-induced, visceral belt of pain around

"THE THING INSIDE MY HEAD"

my midriff, which grows more acute as I struggle to ignore it. The new awareness of Sybil's vulnerability and a premonition of further rejections down the line fill me with helplessness and plunges me into the old familiar depression. Alternately melancholic and savage for the next few days, I am urged by Neil to see the incumbent government psychiatrist, a new man, Dr. Shawki. Abandoning my boycott of the mental health department, I make an appointment.

Dr. Shawki further punctures my self-confidence with a somewhat smug harangue. "Your 'crash' was inevitable," he tells me, categorising me as a life-long depressive and comparing my condition to diabetes: "There is no cure but there is treatment." I totally yield to this doctrine and embark on new medication, a 'cocktail' of the anti-depressant Imipramine and the anti-anxiety drug Stelazine, which I now resign myself to taking indefinitely. The depression, in time, lifts, but I continue to be, at frequent intervals, short-tempered, even shrewish with Neil and the girls; it is as if Dr. Shawki's insistence on my innate chemical deficiencies have somehow absolved me of the need for the moral striving with which I began this year.

In the early summer, I perceive more connections between my problems, my difficulties in managing my emotions, and Sybil's. She throws a tantrum during lunch at the staid Doha Club, becoming wildly frenetic over a minor frustration. "How strong I must be," I tell myself, "to help Sybil deal with her personality." That evening, I fall out with Neil over whether we should rent a video to watch that night. Before I know it, I am hysterically lashing out at him, unconsciously identifying with the emotionally volatile Sybil, while the girls look on, disturbed.

* * *

In August 1982 the family takes a highly successful round-the-world trip through the Far East and to both coasts of America for our summer holiday, but we come home to bad news. All this year, the Qatari government has been implementing 'Arabisation', a process of gradually replacing upper echelon foreign workers with recently qualified Qatari professionals insofar as possible, in all areas of work under the government. For Neil's company, McKee Associates, this has entailed the placement of a young Qatari 'trainee' with a recent American college degree to work alongside Neil on the project. Now, upon our return, we find that this very inexperienced and quite arrogant Qatari man has, by government order, summarily replaced Neil as project manager, with Neil in effect being pushed off the project. And, predictably, the project is after some weeks in a worse mess than ever.

Jerry McKee and Robert Campbell, the company bosses, to patch up their finances and salve their consciences over Neil's treatment, have decided to start up another construction company, to be called McKee International and sponsored by a local trading company, not the government, with Neil as manager. Neil is now working hard to get contracts in order to make the new company viable and staying up late at nights to meet various tender deadlines. His time is also taken up repairing things around the house and the house itself (to which our Qatari landlord is indifferent), all at our own expense, so that our family doesn't have to live in squalor. As nothing firm materialises for McKee International, Neil continues to be paid only every second month. We are depending a great deal on my teaching salary.

At the same time, the cultural climate of Qatar is darkening. The Gulf States' desire to emulate the Islamic fundamentalism of the Iranian Revolution, together with their very real fear of Iran during its war with Iraq, raging since 1980, is having an increasing effect on government policies. Despite sending their young men to the UK and the US for university education and embracing Western technology, the Qataris and other Gulf Arabs are feeling quite threatened by

"THE THING INSIDE MY HEAD"

the creeping influence of Western culture in their countries. The first indication of change this year has been a sudden blanket ban on female performers of any kind entering the country, resulting from two separate but similar 'scandalous' incidents in which hotel or club entertainment featured some scantily-dressed women. The thin flow of cultural events we have therefore been enjoying in this country now narrows to a nearly non-existent trickle, as the ban affects everything from pop stars to string quartets.

Another result of this paranoid zeal is the sudden 'banning' of Christmas in December 1982. Up to this year there has been a low key but varied succession of festivities held around Christmas time—not only expatriate group and club functions but also commercial parties and dinners promoted by local hotels and restaurants. In the middle of this month there suddenly appears in the local English language paper an announcement that there is to be no public celebration of Christmas because it is against the tenets of the Islamic religion. All previously advertised public functions are forthwith cancelled, and rumours are rife about Christmas turkeys held up at customs and vats of Christmas pudding mix confiscated from hotels. Western-style supermarkets are made to stay open on Christmas, and we foreigners at the university are required not only to teach but also to attend a general faculty meeting on that day. Needless to say, all this puts a damper on the expatriate community's private celebrations of this holiday, including our own quasi-secular but enthusiastic family gift-fest centring on the little girls. Sybil is confused and upset that "Mummy has to work on Christmas", her favourite day of the year.

In the New Year 1983 there are more untoward events that prey on her. During 1982, demand has increased to attend the new and popular but highly-regimented pre-school in which we have reluctantly enrolled Sybil after all her little pals deserted her former laid-back play-school. The owner's greed has motivated her to repeatedly enlarge the premises—to the children's disadvantage. Originally a small venue for a small group, the location was subsequently changed to a larger house; next, the playground there was appropriated to hold first one, then two port-a-cabins. Now, over the Christmas break, the school has been moved to two interconnected, quite unwelcome-looking double-storey houses with large, difficult stairs (most homes and schools in Doha being single-storey). Despite the fact that a bored four-and-a-half-year-old Sybil has been whining all through the long holiday break for the pre-school to re-open, she is traumatised by the discovery of the unfamiliar and unattractive venue on her return.

The first day she is just stunned and dazed; the next day she is crying when Neil leaves her there, and the third day, when he brings her up to her class, crying again, the teacher informs him that she cried hysterically the entire previous day. Disturbed, Neil brings her home for the day, where she plays apathetically, and she is adamant about not going to school on the following day. Fearful of this becoming a permanent impasse that might impinge on my working time, I urge Neil to take her in anyway. While Sybil's crying very gradually abates over the next week and a half, she insists that her daddy spend some time in the classroom with her each day—this from a little girl who in the past has thrived in play-school and grows restless during term breaks. She also starts to express fears of abandonment, convinced we are not going to collect her at the end of the school day: "Will we leave her somewhere? Will we disappear? Are we really going to stay at home each night?" At the end of the second week of the term, she says to me: "You know, mummy, I didn't cry today, but my feelings are still sad."

Sybil gives us no real explanation for her behaviour—the first of many times we are to be stymied by her unwillingness to talk about her feelings. We toy with the idea of seeking psychiatric help for her at this point, but dismiss the idea; comforting ourselves that the episode is within the bounds of normal school anxiety and, as usual, too caught up in our own frenetic schedules.

* * *

The big event of 1983 is a severe economic depression here in Qatar and in the Gulf States generally, primarily caused by the world-wide oil glut although there are rumours of financial mismanagement in Qatar, at least. In the spring, the government begins a drastic cost-cutting operation that involves the halting of most government projects and the refusal to pay out even for finished projects, on one excuse or another. Consequently, dozens of foreign companies have to pull out and thousands of expatriates leave, including many of our friends and more importantly, those of the girls, these periodic upheavals in the foreign community forming part of their lives as 'third culture kids'. At a time that is economically bad for our family, government subsidies on basic foodstuffs are dropped, and the price of petrol is allowed to rise. I have been promoted at the university, but my pay rise is still churning its way through the bureaucratic mills of the Ministry of Education.

Moreover, as part of its increasing vindictiveness against the original McKee Associates, the Qatari government early this year invokes a law stating that no company that works for the government can also do private work, and quashes the new company, McKee International. Neil has had the carpet pulled out from under him again, and, of course, has still not been reimbursed for losing every second month's pay over the last two years. Undaunted, however, and typically optimistic, Neil starts up his own small project management consultancy, Project Design, and a genial Egyptian friend, Bashir, arranges for Neil's little company to be sponsored by his own boss, a sheikh who is the Minister of Education and brother to the Emir. But how Neil will fare in this poor economic climate, we do not know.

Lois Chaber

The main reason we have—once again—chosen to stay on in a dubious situation is that Neil hopes, eventually, to be reimbursed for the large sum of money owed to him by Jerry McKee, the company president, who has become a good friend of ours over the years during his frequent visits to Qatar. However, relations between McKee's and the government continue to deteriorate, and the withheld government payments fail to come through. All spring, Jerry keeps promising Neil a cheque, but either he leaves one behind and it bounces, or the continually 'already sent' cheque from New York never arrives. But Neil still insists on the velvet glove approach. Things come to a climax when Jerry is twice nearly thrown into gaol at the airport for non-payment to McKee's commercial creditors, and, on a day when we are expecting him for dinner, he abruptly and secretly leaves the country, with no call to cancel the dinner, no apology, no cheque for Neil—a personal as well as a financial betrayal. And, as McKee Associates is soon unconditionally expelled from the country, Jerry never returns.

These financial strains, however, seem not to be unduly affecting Sybil. By spring '83, she has apparently recovered from her trauma at pre-school, and although she regresses at times into extreme crankiness, she has generally settled down so much that my own mothering abilities flourish for a time. Sybil, very precocious, picks up on the grown-up world with frightening alacrity. Recently, I have borrowed a friend's Siamese male cat to try, for a second time, to mate him with our new cat Lucy, saying to this friend as Sybil and I leave her home, "I hope he does the job this time." Sometime later, when this young male is indeed mounting Lucy in front of us all in our entry hall, five-year-old Sybil shouts out with glee, "He's doin' the job, he's doin' the job!" and when Molly inquires, "What is he doing?", she replies impatiently, "Something special Molly." In fact, Sybil who is really strikingly beautiful at this age, with her oval face framed by auburn hair, large long-lashed almond eyes and kewpie-doll nose and mouth, is both chasing and

"THE THING INSIDE MY HEAD"

being chased by several five or six-year-old boys in succession, and we find her regularly mooning about the house, cooing "I'm in love with David" or "I'm in love with Scott."

Sybil's application to attend the over-subscribed, quasi-official British primary school, called the English-Speaking School, is successful and she starts the infant division in September. She has just missed starting a year earlier because the school's cut-off point is April 30th and hers is a May birthday. Along with others who have narrowly missed the start date, she has been put into a special accelerated class that is supposed to condense four years' work into three so that she and her classmates will eventually catch up with their peer group. Sybil is one of the oldest, and, being so bright to begin with, soon becomes the star pupil. Her reading and writing abilities have expanded geometrically, and, one time, she is asked to read one of her miniature essays to the whole infant school at assembly. All of this has boosted her little ego, even though she is still not terribly adept at making girl friends. She makes one new friend with whom she becomes quite close, a tiny, be-spectacled, very sweet Iranian girl, also not very popular with the other pupils. Paneez is the first of a series of Asian 'best friends' she is to have.

We are pleased with the school's excellent facilities and varied activities, but we hate the hours—7:30 am to 12:30 pm (to beat the heat)—as we can never get hyper-active Sybil to bed early enough to get a good night's sleep. Thanks to her school achievements, this year Sybil overshadows her younger sister (who is to join Sybil at the infant school next September), but Molly does her utmost to compensate for this. When Sybil grasps some new skill—like swinging herself on a swing—Molly, despite her year and a half age difference, usually acquires it herself almost at once. Compounding this, Neil and I, for our own convenience, work with them in tandem on childhood activities like roller skating, bike-riding and ball playing, for there is no neighbourhood 'gang' in this Middle Eastern country where they can casually pick up such skills. Sybil's natural lead over her younger sister is thus constantly on the verge of being eroded.

* * *

Meanwhile, as the tide of Iranian-inspired fundamentalism continues to sweep through the Gulf, Arab xenophobia becomes increasingly manifest, provoked especially by the fall in oil prices. Saudi Arabia demands ever more conservative measures in the stricken Gulf States in return for its financial aid to them. The situation is made worse by an abortive coup in Qatar, which, though quashed, scares the daylights out of the government. There is a general crackdown, made most evident to us when, for the first time in Qatar, virtually all commercial video recordings are suddenly withdrawn from the shops to have their 'sex scenes' (even the most inoffensive brushing of mouths) censored by the government.

At the university, the efforts of my colleagues and myself to persuade our female English Department students to see a rare performance of a Shakespearean play (the troupe has, with great difficulty, been given a special dispensation to enter the country) meet with little response: Thirty-five female Arab students out of two hundred who are English majors attend the performance—in their own National Theatre—and only five of these are actually Qatari. Subsequently, in the local Arabic newspaper, a Qatari religious leader delivers a virulent diatribe against the University for corrupting its women students with foreign plays. In addition, preparations for the autumn meeting of the Gulf Cooperation Council here in Qatar have entailed the installation of multiple roadblocks and security checks. It is becoming increasingly difficult for expatriates to live a 'normal' life in Qatar.

"THE THING INSIDE MY HEAD"

The biggest change in our own household is that our nanny Maria departs for India indefinitely, and I just about manage to replace her with Hazel, another South Indian Catholic. These domestic turnovers are no trivial matter to a working mother, ever insecure. Unfortunately, though Hazel treats the little girls well, she is making life difficult for me, with her quarrelsome and volatile personality, ready to take offence at the drop of a hat. Several times during this autumn term, when she has threatened to quit, I have literally gone down on my knees to her and appeased her with eau de cologne and other small gifts in order to be able to carry on with my teaching. These nannies, which our family pays generously, are my lifeline to the semblance of an academic career, in the absence of other childcare provision in Doha and given the truncated school hours.

But the Indian nannies also reinforce the Christianity that the girls, especially Sybil, are absorbing from their English primary school, with its Anglican prayers and celebrations. Sybil begins periodically questioning me, "Mummy, why don't you believe in God?" It is very difficult for me to find an answer that explains the agnostic-humanist position Neil and I hold while not demeaning or crushing her own nascent beliefs, so I am evasive and vague. After all, with the general hazardousness of life on the Gulf, perhaps religion will provide some sense of security for her. Little do I know this is later to backfire.

Meanwhile, in October, at my insistence, Neil gives up on Jerry McKee and formally puts his unpaid wages case before the Qatar Labour Court, which settles employer/employee disputes. The hitch is that the Court regulations require serving a summons on the defendant and obtaining proof of this through official channels. Since Jerry is effectually hiding somewhere in the US, it seems highly unlikely that this case will ever be heard, but Neil is determined to pursue this path to reimbursement indefinitely. Hence, we are committed to staying in Qatar for the time being, despite the increasingly pervasive gloom.

Lois Chaber

1983 ends somewhat dismally, with public Christmas activities again prohibited and the expatriate community feeling muted paranoia. Over 50,000 foreigners have left this year, a large slice out of the 200,000 total population of Qatar. We learn also that Sharia Law has now, for the first time, been fully implemented in Qatar.

* * *

Abruptly in the New Year, 1984, we are ordered to vacate our house by our Qatari landlord, who is co-opting the site for his newly married son. We are devastated, having sunk large amounts of time and money into making the neglected villa more liveable for ourselves and usable as an office for Neil's small company. Sybil, moreover, has had a happy, informal relationship with our Arab landlord's granddaughter, Mai, only possible because of our proximity to the family compound. With difficulty, we find a new villa suitable for the family and for Project Design, but the move—right in the middle of my teaching term—is disruptive and stressful for all of us, especially considering our uncertain tenure in this country. I survive only by furtively gobbling enormous quantities of chocolates from an ostentatiously large, heart-shaped box bestowed on us by Arab friends and secreted in a high cupboard.

Neil badly needs work. Thus, through his Egyptian friend Bashir, he allows himself to become involved with a bungled project to construct townhouses for a company, QIDCO, owned by Neil's sponsor, the Minister of Education, along with another sheikh and a wealthy Qatari businessman. When under another company's control, it had become mired in debts and problems due to mismanagement, graft and embezzlement on the part of its English managers. In Qatar, managers of companies, not owners, are held responsible for debts and legal problems— the province of the Sharia Court—and can summarily be thrown into gaol. The cowardly flight from Qatar of the Englishmen has left the three current Qatari owners with an

"THE THING INSIDE MY HEAD"

anti-Western bias that does not bode well for Neil. Nevertheless, he convinces them to re-start the project, with him as Construction Manager, although they hold back some of the investment money he has recommended putting into it.

As a result of the owners' tightfistedness as well as the previous financial shambles, Neil has to spend most of his 'construction' time persuading striking Asian tradesmen who haven't been paid and unremunerated subcontractors to get back to work, and dealing with lack of petrol for the project's trucks, unpaid rent for the miserable shantytown slum where the workers are housed and where septic tanks and generators are constantly breaking down, and with the personal difficulties of the impoverished workers, all the time pleading for more investment. Once again, the girls and I hardly see him, and, when we do, he is consumed by his worries and hassles.

One day in the spring of 1984, the girls and I are left waiting for Neil at our family mid-day meal. "Where is Daddy?" they persist in questioning, and I can only answer, "I don't know, hunnies," trying to smile reassuringly. Neil only returns well after lunchtime, looking harassed and upset. It seems that the original creditors of the company taken over by QIDCO, having seen construction restart, thanks to Neil's efforts, are now pursuing their debt cases again, and the only person of apparent responsibility in evidence and not immune to prosecution (sheikhs cannot be tried in the Sharia Court) is, ironically, Neil. A policeman has actually hauled him off the site—in front of all his workmen—and taken him to the court, where he has been made to waste half a day trying to explain (through an interpreter who can barely speak English) why he isn't actually the man they want because he is not the general manager and does not handle the company's finances. Under Sharia law the defendant is assumed to be guilty as charged and the burden is on him or her to prove innocence.

Lois Chaber

We try to keep this disturbing turn of events from the girls, but, soon, it is happening again and again, disrupting our family routines, and it is very hard to keep "Daddy's problems" under wraps, as Neil explains: "I concealed the extreme legal hassles from the girls until I could no longer. Policemen visiting my office, the converted large garage of our house, had to be explained." The owners keep promising to take legal measures to prevent this harassment, but they take no steps. Neil, summarily dragged off to the court again and again, has to extricate himself repeatedly from a possible jail sentence, with compounded difficulty and distress as the spring and summer wear on.

Along with Neil's persecution, in the early summer of 1984 the Iran-Iraq war is starting to escalate, and the Qataris are getting very nervous, especially as they are about to start developing a large natural gas field in the north that would make a perfect target for either of the antagonists. Moreover, after would-be Iranian hijackers attempt a landing (unsuccessfully) at Qatar Airport, the entire Qatari military is put on alert. Up to now, we have not really been overly concerned about the war (we have too much else to think about!), but now the American Embassy calls a hush-hush meeting of all Americans in the country and informs us that if there should be an "incident"—like the bombing, accidental or otherwise, of the country's desalination plant—all airports, etc. would probably be closed, making it difficult to evacuate American citizens. They tell us they will have to bus us secretly to Saudi Arabia, and, to expedite this possibility, they are now establishing a telephone chain among the American community. If we were not nervous before, we are now.

Meanwhile, fundamentalism continues to seep into my own turf at the university. A few outspoken fundamentalists among the female students start complaining about my choice of English texts—"The Fox" by

"THE THING INSIDE MY HEAD"

D. H. Lawrence, with its 'phallic symbols', in particular—and I am forced into self-censorship.

By mid-summer, Neil is so tied down on the QIDCO project and so beset by Sharia Court summons that he has to forego a summer holiday. It is up to me to take the girls to New Zealand for a reunion with the extended family that they are deprived of for so much of the time. However, Sybil is taken aback when she meets up with her beloved cousins again, for they are now ten, twelve and fourteen; in her childish mind she had thought she would somehow catch up with them in age! One day, having caught her middle cousin undressing, the six-year-old Sybil exclaims to me later with great chagrin: "Mummy, she even has breasts!" Another, more serious disappointment of the trip is learning that the New Zealand economy is in bad shape, which will preclude Neil from considering a move to his homeland in the near future to escape from our precarious life in the Gulf.

Early autumn finds Neil still working frantically on the QIDCO project site and unable to persuade the owners to contribute the much-needed funds. Out of the blue, an unofficial Qatari advisor to the project who has influence with the other high-born owner disparages the project all together and poisons the sheikh's mind against Neil. Consequently, the latter stops all payments to Neil's current and past salary (well behind, as usual in Qatar). Neil, stubbornly persistent as ever, continues working anyway until, finally, the sheikh calls all construction to a halt, leaving the townhouse clients in the lurch. Neil now resigns, never to receive another penny from QIDCO; his tremendous efforts have come to nothing—neither financial gain nor professional satisfaction.

His anger and frustration is increased by a new spate of Sharia Court debt cases against QIDCO in which the plaintiffs target Neil since no general manager has ever been officially appointed, the owners are still largely invulnerable, and he is the only visible senior professional. As the court is now more adamant about the threat of prison,

Lois Chaber

Neil is extricated only by careful manoeuvring of his own (no lawyers are ever provided) to obtain temporary exculpatory letters. It is clear to us by the close of 1984 that the Qatari owners all along have been using Neil as a scapegoat and a screen to hide behind, particularly the more vulnerable ordinary businessman. Their non-payment of Neil's salary on top of this illustrates that famous paradox of Tacitus: "It is human nature to hate the man whom you have hurt." Neil is still determined to remain in Qatar and pursue his case against McKee's with the Labour Court, despite several failures already to deliver a summons.

Although the year ends with a pall over our family fortunes and increasing restrictions on life in Qatar, there have been happy moments. We have participated in some very agreeable community events such as the Family Festival at the Doha Club—a 'knockout' contest of comical sports—and the large communal celebrations of both Independence Day and Thanksgiving by the American community. Moreover, Sybil appears to be surviving the many family setbacks so far; thriving at primary school, she also wins a recorder-playing contest there and a children's painting contest in the larger community.

This is to change in 1985.

* * *

In the New Year, my sister Madelyn makes plans to visit us here in Qatar—the only relative ever to do so. Sybil and Molly, who have warm memories of their cheerful aunt from our 1982 California visit, are bubbling over with excitement, especially since our family intends to travel with her to Yemen to see our friends the McCrearys, now working for the US consulate there, and their two little girls, our daughters' oldest friends. About nine days before Madelyn's arrival, Neil tells me—very gingerly—that we may not be able to go to Yemen because the court is holding his

102

passport. The authorities fear he may flee the country to escape the still-unresolved debt cases!

Neil embarks on a series of Byzantine manoeuvres that lead him eventually to the Deputy Director of the Department of Religious Affairs (which governs the Sharia Court). To convince this official that he *really is* in no way financially responsible for QIDCO'S debts, Neil is forced to pull out his trump card for the Deputy Director, a copy of a letter to the subcontractors once written by the owners, which sets out the limits of Neil's duties, absolving him from any financial responsibilities. He has been warned never to use this letter because it implicates his friend Bashir in the company's difficulties, for he is actually the General Manager for all his employer's, the Minister's, projects and has been hiding in the shadows all this time. On the basis of this risky letter, the Director intervenes, and after much suspense and a noisy showdown at the Sharia Court, the passport is finally returned. Since this complicated intrigue has taken place over several days of gloomy uncertainty, we have had to tell the girls that "We may not be going to Yemen with Aunt Mady because Daddy's passport is being held." Under stress, we don't think to concoct a cover-up for this ominous situation. It is to affect Sybil profoundly.

Now, however, we are jubilant about the regained passport, and all our expectations for the happy trip with Madelyn, who is by now in Doha, are revived. On the day we are packing for the imminent trip (having changed the flight several times already), Neil calls me from the sheikh's office to tell me, dismally, that Bashir the Egyptian, with whose family we have dined and gone on expeditions to the beach, refuses to sign an exit visa for Neil on behalf of his boss, without which Neil cannot leave the country. "He seems to think we won't come back," are Neil's quiet words to me over the phone. Bashir trusts his friend Neil no more than the Sharia authorities, fearing that he is using the family trip to Yemen to disguise a permanent departure that would leave the owners to deal with the mountainous debt problems of QIDCO—as they rightly should be doing! Qatari signers of exit visas are responsible for any financial and legal problems that a departing foreigner might leave in his or her wake. I insist on speaking to Bashir myself over the phone, shrilly entreating him to sign the visa since our plane is supposed to take off that evening: "Bashir, I can't believe you don't trust us! We are just going on a short holiday. All our belongings are here!" The most that I can wring from him, however, is a promise to call the sheikh in Los Angeles and obtain his "blessing", not only for the trip, but also for the payment of salary owing to Neil. We change the flight booking again.

But tomorrow comes and Bashir informs us that the sheikh has refused his permission. Glumly, we decide that I should go ahead with the flight that day, for the sake of Madelyn and the little girls, but my heart isn't in it. Despite the good fun they have in Yemen with the McCreary girls, the children, especially Sybil, are obviously shaken by the roller coaster experience of the last week and their awareness that their daddy is, in effect, a prisoner in Qatar. Sybil is to remember this whole complex chain of events, including the other Sharia Court ordeals, as the "passport problem", citing it in later times as a traumatic catalyst for her illness.

We return, and I find Neil looking more disconsolate than I have ever seen him. "I'm drained of energy," he tells me. But despite all the disappointment and stress, Neil retains his positive view of our expatriate experience:

Even under duress we learned that many normal things in life go on. While in mornings at the court I saw prisoners in chains and was myself dangerously shouting at the Qadi (judges), in the afternoons I was successfully running other small projects. While I was repeatedly called to the Sharia Court, thirty-three times in all, at the same time we were organising and enjoying big barbeques in the desert in a remote area of Qatar with up to twenty carloads of families joining us for the day, or on one occasion participating with the girls in a community Christmas Carol singing by candlelight in the sand dunes, where we could not be heard by the Qataris.

Nevertheless, he now decides we must leave Qatar—but not until next year, for he is emotionally depleted and cannot bear further court confrontations that might ensue from desperate creditors of QIDCO if his intention to leave the country were officially announced (as is the law). By next year, he hopes, the company liquidation procedure will have progressed and the legal hurdles of leaving the country will be less daunting. Desperate for work now in the early spring of 1985, Neil ironically takes up a half-time job supervising the construction of mosques for the Religious Affairs Department—the same department to which the Sharia Court belongs.

While Neil is scrambling for work, I am caught up in a ludicrous educational fiasco. A new multi-million dollar national university has been under construction for over eight years and has received international publicity for its design, an attractive fusion of modernism and traditional Islamic architecture. Now, however, fundamentalist elements in the country—conservative family dynasties and religious officials—are objecting strongly to the 'progressive' design, with the men's and women's campuses built back to back on the same site, the same laboratories to be shared on different days—a design conceived before the Iranian Revolution. Hence, the momentous shifting of the women from the old, dilapidated campus to the new one, scheduled for February '85, in which we faculty are all participating, is suddenly postponed until a huge wall to separate the two sexes can be erected and separate laboratories built.

As school ends and the summer approaches, we resign ourselves to staying in Doha with no vacation, for Neil still cannot obtain an exit visa. I have committed myself to writing a paper—a study of latent anxiety in a supposedly complacent novel of Samuel Richardson's—for a literature conference at Yarmouk University in Jordan, supposedly the highest-ranked university in the Middle East, prompted by the need to rejuvenate my flagging scholarly activity. How can I keep the children happy during the looming summer without a holiday break and, more importantly, without any playmates (due to the seasonal expatriate exodus), while still being able to write my essay? I get a brain wave: I hire a bright fourteen-year-old English girl, Dawn (one of the very few young people here for the summer), to keep the girls amused and stimulated for three hours a day from Monday to Friday, while I type away in another room.

But this solution doesn't quite work out the way I had hoped. Despite Dawn's good temper and resourcefulness, the protracted summer, during which Sybil and Molly must remain cooped up indoors on account of the intense heat, deprived of friends their own age, takes its toll on them. They become quarrelsome and whiney as the novelty of the situation wears off, competing more and more fiercely for Dawn's attentions. I remain impregnable in my study-bedroom all morning, and when they try to burst in on me to have their little quarrels adjudicated or register their complaints, I allow Dawn to drag them away while I carry on typing, once again rigidly keeping to the schedule I have set up for the day, feeling guilt but not acting on it.

The summer finally comes to an end. The girls have more or less survived, it seems, and I have more or less finished my scholarly paper. The week before their classes and my classes begin, the children's friends are gradually reappearing. I eagerly go into my usual act, phoning around

"THE THING INSIDE MY HEAD"

to set up little engagements for them, my first priority being to reunite Sybil with her best friend Paneez, the little Iranian girl from her infant class, just back from the US with her wealthy parents.

On the appointed day, Paneez comes to our house, but the two girls, separated for more than two months, seem unusually quiet and shy. About forty minutes later, I hear moaning coming from Sybil, who has retreated from the girls' playroom, where Paneez is, to her bedroom, and is writhing on the floor, sobbing violently and screaming intermittently, "Mummy, I've got pains all over my body!" Paneez looks frightened and totally unsympathetic, wailing "I want to go home." Terrified, mystified, I try to soothe Sybil and find out what the problem is while attempting to placate Paneez and convince her to stay. Sybil, incoherent and inconsolable, is not really able to pinpoint her "pains" and I get nowhere with either child. I call Paneez's mother to collect her, apologising profusely for the 'incident' and trying to brush it off lightly, but in fact mother and daughter become standoffish, the relationship never recovers from this blow, and Sybil cannot seem to make a new 'best friend'. My premonitions of three years ago seem to have been fulfilled.

Sybil continues weepy and difficult over the next couple of weeks as school gets under way and reiterates her complaints about pains recurring all over her body. Neil and I, extremely concerned, bring her to the local general practitioner for a thorough check-up, but he cannot find anything wrong and dismisses her problems. After many inquiries within the expatriate community, we locate an English paediatrician who works at the newly built, very modern Hamad Hospital, who will see Sybil privately. He books her in for a CAT scan, and when the results show no signs of any physical problem, he suggests that there may be a psychological one, for young children often present bodily symptoms when they are mentally disturbed. He advises us to obtain psychiatric help for Sybil. I sense, only vaguely, that Neil's recent 'troubles' and the summer of

Lois Chaber

intense sibling rivalry and isolation have precipitated this crisis.

Meanwhile, important changes at the English-Speaking School are aggravating Sybil's state of mind. Due to the severe economic depression in Qatar and the consequent departure of so many expatriate families, the fee-paying school is struggling to survive. As part of a radical downsizing, the special class for those children like Sybil who started late because their birthdays were just beyond the cut-off point, a class that in a carefully graduated manner enabled them to do four years in three, is now abandoned. Sybil's former classmates are dispersed into regular fourth-year classes, not only separating her from her familiar peer group of two years but also abruptly plunging her and the others into more advanced work. She goes from being one of the oldest in her class to being, literally, the youngest, and from being 'top of the class', to suddenly finding herself near the bottom.

While we investigate the possibilities of psychiatric help for Sybil, the paediatrician advises us to keep a written record of her behaviour for the next couple of weeks. The following excerpts from these notes clearly indicate a disturbed child, no longer just a sensitive and 'hyper' one, but the strange symptoms have no clear meaning for us at this time:

September 23rd: Sybil comes home at midday saying she was "lonely" at school and "couldn't breathe." In the afternoon, she goes over to a friend's house to play, but insists on reading by herself when there. She can't eat supper, saying she "feels sick." At bedtime, she folds her arms and refuses to kiss us, complaining "I don't feel well".

"THE THING INSIDE MY HEAD"

Sept. 26th: Sybil wakes up cranky and doesn't want to get out of bed. She has to be forced to eat breakfast, is sullen and uncooperative. The hostess of an afternoon party tells us Sybil was "off-colour" there. She comes home complaining of pains all over. In the evening, we try to soothe her by saying, "You can be sure Mummy and Daddy love you." Sybil says: "Why?" I say, "Because you're our daughter and you're a nice girl." She replies, "I'm not."

Sept. 27th: Sybil is up and down all day, very difficult at her music lesson and while playing ping-pong with Lois (she is unable to take criticism). She complains piteously about pains in her stomach and declares, "I wish I was never born."

Sept. 28th: It is the first day of after-school activities and Sybil is very squeamish and whiney beforehand. She complains about "pains" and is very upset when she leaves. She comes back elated and over-excited. At her recorder lesson she cannot produce low C (she has always done it before), and after a few minutes complains of pains in her stomach, then pain all over. She won't let me touch her.

Over the course of the next week she also expresses bitter jealousy of her sister, drools when she is playing her recorder (later we find out it is because she won't swallow), shows a morbid interest in diseases, is concerned that she may be poisoned, and washes her hands over and over again.

Lois Chaber

Oct. 10th: Sybil has an afternoon birthday party to attend. As party-time draws near, she tenses up and complains of pains and breathing problems. She says she doesn't want to go: "Nobody ever plays with me." I have to practically force her to go, and she later returns home cranky, confirming that "nobody played with her", complaining that she feels ill, refusing to eat, and saying again, after we finally get her to start eating, "I wish I was never born."

Sybil is just over seven years old.

We are desperate to find help for her, but our inquiries into child psychiatry either in the public health system or the private network in Qatar are stymied. There is an Arab psychiatrist with the qualifications, but he does not know enough English. Finally, I bring up Sybil's acute condition in one of my sessions with my own government psychiatrist—fortunately, still the same Dr. Shawki, who in fact has a Scandinavian mother and is not only fluent in English but also savvy about Western mores and manners—and he offers to try working with our daughter as best he can, though without expertise in child psychology. He begins to have weekly sessions with Sybil at the end of the year while at the same time counselling Neil and me together to try to smooth out some of the difficulties in our own relationship. He tells us that depression in a child often manifests itself in stomach aches and similar symptoms, confirming what the paediatrician had surmised, but reveals little about any progress as time passes. We need to turn to Molly to find out something of Dr. Shawki's method with Sybil:

All I remember is Sybil going to see a doctor and a particular game they played. We played this same game together called 'Squiggle' or something. One person would

"THE THING INSIDE MY HEAD"

draw a squiggle with their eyes closed and the next person would turn it into a picture, and then the other person would carry on with a squiggle in the same way. This was the game the doctor played with her. That's all I knew. I didn't really understand anything.

* * *

Sybil seems to get over her extreme "bad patch" in the following year, 1986, and (from my point of view) becomes "manageable", probably because she is getting special attention—if nothing else—from Dr. Shawki. Much to our distress, however, he informs us in late winter that he has decided to return to Egypt because, among other things, he is "becoming brain-dead in Qatar". When, with her psychiatric sessions having come to a close, Sybil does not exhibit the extreme symptoms of last autumn, we optimistically assume she is over the worst and resign ourselves to the lack of resources for her in this country.

Meanwhile, Neil's economic prospects here are at their nadir. The construction industry is virtually at a standstill and Neil, with no future projects in sight, is just eking out his small amount of work supervising mosques. And there is no hope of us ever going on a family holiday as the exit visa dilemma has not been resolved. The region is more dangerous than ever, what with terrorist reaction to the US 'Operation Libya' and the Gulf War constantly threatening to spread outwards, not to mention the Lilliputian war going on between Qatar and Bahrain over a tiny Gulf island. It is clearly time to go.

We hope it will be possible to 'get out' now because most of the debtors have now resigned themselves to awaiting the crawling liquidation process that is handling the officially bankrupt QIDCO's affairs. With much difficulty, Neil finds a friend in the construction business that will take over the supervision of the mosque construction and leave him legally clear. We gently break the news to the girls, who are quite distressed—as Molly explains:

> One of my last memories of Doha was when you told us we were going to leave, and we were both extremely upset because it was our home and it was where our friends were; we didn't know anything else, and we had a lovely house with a big garden. It was like anything the first time you have a big change. We plotted and planned about how we could change your minds. We were determined not to leave and planned to hide behind the door when you were moving out; you wouldn't be able to find us.

We make plans to spend a year in England, where Neil has applied to study for a Diploma in Management at the London School of Economics, one of the few reputable one-year graduate business programmes available, in order to bring his credentials and skills in line with his major job experiences in the Middle East. On the way there we will treat the family to a long overdue holiday, travelling to London via stopovers in Indonesia, New Zealand and both coasts of the US. But the way is not entirely clear yet. Neil must get clearance from the Criminal Investigation Department because of the QIDCO embroilments. This turns out to be yet another Kafkaesque experience, involving two long interrogation sessions for him and me at the grim and shabby offices of the CID. They take possession of his passport once again; he will have it returned, with exit visa in it, only at the airport. Neil will have to leave Qatar without obtaining any of the money owing to him: QIDCO is officially bankrupt, and the attempts to get satisfaction at the Labour

"THE THING INSIDE MY HEAD"

Court from McKee's have come to nothing. But at this point we are just happy to go.

Sybil and Molly share the tension and discomfort of the last couple of hours in Qatar in the un-air-conditioned old Doha Airport on a sweltering July day, while we fill out forms on dirty counters flooded with perspiration, all of us waiting for the CID representative to show up with Neil's passport, without which we cannot get onto our flight. In our intense focus on this final ordeal for Neil, we give scant attention to the feelings of loss and trauma the little girls must have in leaving the only 'home' they have ever known (Sybil has no conscious memories of Tehran). The official shows up at the very last possible moment and escorts us through passport control, still retaining Neil's documents. Only when we are literally 'out of the country', in neutral space, does he hand the passport over to Neil.

On the plane flying to Bahrain, our first port of call, I am so relieved that the ordeal is finally over that I blurt out to the girls, who consider themselves conventional Christians, that I am Jewish. I have had to conceal this from them all during our sojourn in anti-Semitic Qatar lest they expose me accidentally—a fear justified by my close call with the university. With this revelation to a dumbstruck Sybil and Molly, our new life moving westward begins.

Lois Chaber

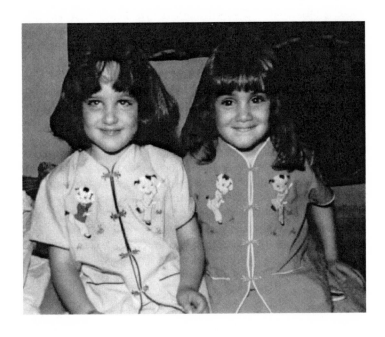

Sybil (left) and Molly (right) in Doha, circa 1983

"THE THING INSIDE MY HEAD"

Chapter 5: Sybil 'Speaks'

At least half the adults who get help for OCD already had it as children, but many of these people did not get help when they were younger. This might be because they were embarrassed about it, and did not tell anyone.

> (*Challenging OCD: Guidelines for Promoting Recovery from Obsessive Compulsive Disorder*, booklet from OCD Action [registered charity], spring 2005)

Casey's eyes filled with tears.

"Mom, I'm scared that if I don't do things perfectly, something bad will happen. Why do I have to do that? How come Jenny doesn't need to do that?"

> (Aureen Pinto Wagner, *Up and Down the Worry Hill: A Children's Book About Obsessive-Compulsive Disorder and its Treatment*, Lighthouse Press, 2000, 2004, p. 21.)

When Sybil was seventeen, one of her care-workers asked her to systematically record memories of childhood events and the feelings they had evoked. In her retrospective chart, Sybil makes several references to OCD—obsessive-compulsive disorder—a mental health problem involving intrusive thoughts of an irrational nature, usually fears of harm to the self or others, and compulsive, often ritualistic behaviour such as repetitions, hand washing and checking, meant to assuage these anxiety-producing thoughts, although in fact they just create a vicious cycle. However, neither she nor we knew anything about this disorder during the early period of her life, nor did we understand the significance of her symptoms even when we (rarely) noticed them.

Approximately one third of OCD cases emerge before the age of fifteen, according to *Obsessive-Compulsive Disorder: A Guide,* by John Geist from the Dean Foundation for Health, Research and Education in the US in 1997, and the earlier it is caught, the more likely it is to be cured. Only recently, a slew of illustrated books catering to young children with symptoms of OCD, like the one cited above, have been published to help children come to terms with the disorder and accept treatment, but during Sybil's childhood there was nothing like that available—not even general books on OCD for adults! Since 2000, on UK television alone there have been several documentaries on OCD and a full-length drama, not to mention OCD's presence in the cinema in films like *As Good As It Gets,* which have led to a crescendo of awareness about this disorder. Had Sybil been born a decade or so later and had access to the CD-ROM, *Why Me?,* developed for young people by the Maudsley Hospital, she could have been comforted by its most important message: "You are not the only person with this illness."

Sybil's memories are mostly of events in Qatar but include some from our around-the-world-journey upon leaving there and very early days in England. I have slightly rearranged some for better chronological order and have added approximate ages where none were supplied.

"THE THING INSIDE MY HEAD"

AGE	MEMORY:	FEELING:
6 or under [it was actually 2, 3 and 4]	Going to New Zealand	Happy
5 or 6	Being sent to my room till Dad came home because I threw my apple in the bin because I didn't like it and Molly told Mum.	Anger Fear
5 or 6	Pippi [the cat] ill, eaten rat-poison	Dread
[Probably about 5-6]	On our way back from our weekly visit to the beach, Molly and I would often cry. I'm not sure if it was an affected, whiney sort of crying or normal crying, but I don't think what Mum and Dad did was right whatever kind it was. Dad used to say, "Stop crying or you will get a smack! 1, 2, 3 . . ."	Angry, Alone, Scared, Humiliated.
[5]	Going to Yemen [first visit to the McCrearys] and playing with the snake cushions [large stuffed snake in their living room].	Excitement
[5-6]	Hearing or being told (perhaps asking questions about it first) that Dad had problems with his job. Mum & Dad were worried; Dad wasn't being paid most of his salary	Anxious, Angry

[5? 6? during or after Neil's mother ill with cancer]	One of my earliest memories of maybe OCD-like symptoms; a voice in my head said, "Repeat that [action] or you will get cancer." That kept on happening and I was told by something in my head not to do anything 5 times because I thought there were 5 letters in the word 'cancer'. When I found out there were 6, I questioned it in my own mind but was told by something, some-how that I couldn't do 5 or 6.	First definite memory of repeating things and OCD. Anxiety, Frustration, Fear
6	Teacher telling Dad that she wished she could have a "class full of Sybils".	Pride, Pleased
[Probably 5 and upwards]	Wetting the bed and having a chart about it.	Embarrassed, Ashamed, Guilty.
6 & 7 & 8	Finding out about (I don't know how) and believing in God. Mum and Dad gave us a Children's Illustrated Bible.	Enthusiasm Feeling left out and ashamed that Mum & Dad didn't believe in God & we weren't baptized or going to church This was very good of them.

"THE THING INSIDE MY HEAD"

5, 6 or 7	Having a snake scare. I had to avoid thoughts of snakes and had OCD symptoms watching the film 'Cobra'.	Anxious; one of my earliest/maybe 'the earliest' memories of OCD-like symptoms; scared
6	Playing with Paneez at her house.	~~Excitement,~~ Adventure
[6]	Dad looking depressed; Dad having to go to court.	Very worried, Sad, Scared, Anxious, Worried, Angry
[6]	Mum and Dad being grumpy and irritable and 'snapping' at us and Mum not giving us stickers for tidying our room anymore. I remember Molly and I talking about this and agreeing.	Angry, Frustrated, Upset.
[6]	Dad's passport taken away; we had to go on holiday that year without him [trip to Yemen with my sister].	Guilty, Anxious, Worried, Sad, Scared
7 or 8	Being told that you can wish on the 'fairy' sweets and I wished that me & my family would never die, but later thought of us all, especially Mum & Dad, growing older and older & thinner & thinner but never dying.	Fear, Panic

7	Mum finding out about the garlic beside my bed, which I sneaked from the pantry to put between my toes at night so no vampires could get me, and mum being quite angry and never asking or thinking why I did it and that I was afraid.	~~Guilt~~ Sadness, Frustration, Aloneness
7 or 8	I tried to make a sacrifice or tribute to God; I'd read about people doing that in the Bible. A voice inside my head was telling me how to do it and I had to change something and maybe repeat some things and get it right as to how the voice, which called itself God's voice, wanted it to be.	This is one of my earliest memories of the voice and maybe one of my earliest memories of OCD-like symptoms, repeating things, thoughts, having to get it right. I felt a combination of fear and peace, satisfaction and anxiety.
7 & 8	Having 'Friend Problems'	Lonely, Sad, Upset, Guilty, Angry, Frustrated

"THE THING INSIDE MY HEAD"

7 & 8	I had trouble swallowing when I played the recorder. I seemed to have lost the automatic reflex. I also kept spitting out in the sink. I can't remember this very well. Sometimes I spat on the floor. I had to, something in my head (I think it was meant to be God) told me to. I think it was for repentance or to stop bad things from happening when I did something wrong or didn't do my repeating things right. Also, for some reason, I kept thinking my saliva was poisoned. Mum and Dad couldn't understand this, got frustrated when I spat in the sink. Once the voice or intruding thought in my head told me to spit a couple of times on the carpet in my room. Then my Dad came in.	Frustrated, Confused Scared Frustrated, Confused Scared, Guilty, Frustrated, Alone
7	Getting pains in my body	Worry
7	Crying and getting attention, but when I did get attention the pains grew less.	Pleased about the attention, guilty about making a fuss; they weren't that bad. Frustration about having to feel or be guilty, which repeated the attention, because of their diminishing the more fuss I made and attention I got.
7	Going for lots of tests at hospital	Anxious but glad of the attention

7	Paediatrician saying there was nothing wrong physically, and saying it was psychosomatic and referring me to a psychiatrist.	Disappointed that there was nothing wrong physically with me, but pleased that I was still going to get attention
7	Going to psychiatrist	Anxious, a bit ashamed when I had to go during school hours and worrying that someone would know where I was going
8	Teacher saying that I've become very chatty when I should be working since I turned 8.	Shame
8	Talking about names and what they meant and Mum said 'Sybil' meant prophetess, thinking about how we hadn't had a fire drill in a long time and we got one that day, trying to read tea leaves	Powerful, Special.
8	Making up with my best friend at the time	Happy, Glad
8	On the same day as above, being told at dinner about us moving to London. Molly & I had tears streaming down our faces. London was somewhere alien to us, where our English friends went to visit their grans in the summer holiday. London was what we learnt about at school. We had nothing to do with London. I [was] thinking "but I've just made up with my best friend."	Sad, Surprised

"THE THING INSIDE MY HEAD"

8	On the day we were leaving for our halfway-around the world trip, we were all at the airport, and Dad still didn't have his passport. We were waiting for someone to bring it, but we couldn't be sure that they would. I remember praying and doing obsessional behaviour (at the time I didn't know it was obsessional), and it was agonizing, but the passport came	Agonizing.
8	We went to Australia, New Zealand, Indonesia, Tahiti and America before arriving in England. Throughout this time I still had my repeating things. Indonesia Australia New Zealand	 Enjoyed it. Didn't Mixed Feelings
8	One night [in NZ] when we stayed at Uncle Neville's, I complained of feeling dizzy, partly the truth and partly for attention & partly because of the scary repeating things. Aunt Judy, who was a nurse, said there wasn't anything wrong with me.	Angry, Guilty
8	At the park with Dad's family, I got 'funny turns' a couple of times, where everything seemed far away & distant and people's voices were distant, and I felt in a dreamlike state, but it wasn't nice; it was spooky. I got this on and off for the next few months, but this is the first time I can remember it.	I felt glad that there was definitely something wrong with me after all, but I felt scared as well.

8	In America, driving to Mum & Dad's friends, I said, "Sometimes I do something like put my shoes down and pick them up again and put them down again 'cause I think a tiger might come if I don't". I said this in a nonchalant, jokey sort of way, but I was serious. It was a bit of a cry for help and the first time I had said anything to anyone about the repeating things, and it was to be the last time for many months, even a year or more.	Disappointed, Ignored, a bit alone.
8	We stayed in a hotel [in London] for about a week. I remember having the repeating things there.	Frustration, Alone, Anxious, Scared
8	Going to visit Una [the cat we took with us from Qatar] in quarantine. She didn't seem to recognize us. She hissed and was so scared.	Shocked, Sad, Angry, Guilty
8	Going to see what school we would go to. First we went to Brunswick Park School. The first thing I remember is seeing everyone going into assembly and a girl handing out hymnbooks.	Shy, Conspicuous, Embarrassed, Awkward, Anxious
8	I can't remember very clearly, but I was really worried, after the headmaster, who was showing Molly, Mum, Dad and me around, mentioned everyone saying prayers in Assembly. I got all worried because I thought, "Well, Molly and I don't know how to say prayers." I tried to tell my parents. I wanted them to say something to the head teacher.	Worried, Ashamed, Embarrassed, Frustrated, Excluded, Upset

"THE THING INSIDE MY HEAD"

8	The first day at Brunswick Park I was in the classroom while the rest were in assembly. Term had started before we came.	Worried, Anxious, Scared, Self-conscious, Conspicuous. I was really worried about what the rest of the class would think of me.
[8?]	One day at school we were doing painting with sprays & stencils. I can't remember much about it except that for a couple of seconds something happened to me. It was a bit like the time when everything went far away and trance-like in New Zealand, but with this one when I snapped out of it and came to, I didn't know whether what I remembered of the past couple of seconds was real. It felt like I had gone into some kind of trance and dreamt or imagined something. It was really weird.	Confused, In a daze, Scared, Excited, Strange.
[8]	Our 1st Autumn Mum, Molly & I walking up Lyonsdown Rd from school & me wading through the leaves and kicking them.	Novelty, Excitement, Happiness
[8]	Our 1st Halloween in England. Went to the local library to get our faces painted, until Ricky, Mrs. Cruz's son [Mrs. Cruz was our cleaning lady] came back.	Excitement, Youthful, Happy.
[8]	Our 1st Bonfire Night. Mum & Dad bought a standard fireworks box & we did them in the garden of the flat & watched the fireworks on either side as well as ours.	Excitement, Thrilled Happy

Lois Chaber

[8]	Una came out of quarantine. At home, every time we called her she would come straight away. She was so glad to be out of that horrible place and so eager to please us.	Guilt, Sadness, Surprised, Loving. So glad to have her back.
[8 or 9?]	One day, I was doing my gymnastics or dancing practice or maybe music, I'm not sure, and I left my blue woollen jumper that Nan (Edna, Dad's mum) had knitted. Then when we went back to it, Dad found that Una had chewed a hole in it. He picked her up and held her hanging vertically in the air, & then he hit her on the head, hard, at least 2 or three times, and she couldn't even make a sound, but she stretched her paw out in the middle of the air each time he hit her.	Guilt, Anger, Horror, Pain, Anguish, Helplessness, Empathy with Una.

"THE THING INSIDE MY HEAD"

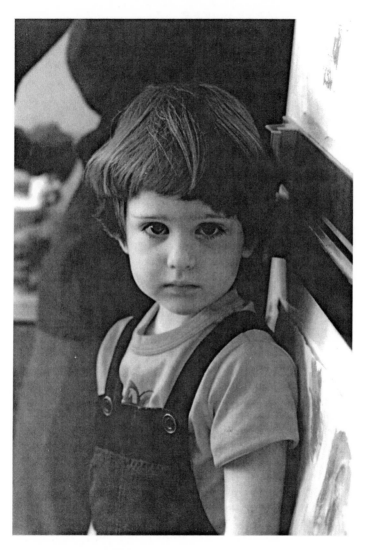

Sybil in serious mode, circa 1982

Chapter 6: Transit England

> [T]he entire cultural world they [the 'third culture kids'] live in can change overnight with a single airplane ride.
>
> (Pollock and Rekin, *Third Culture Kids.*)

"Mummy, what's a virgin?" cry out both Sybil and Molly, eight and a half and going on seven, respectively, breathlessly running into our house on Whitehouse Way in the late afternoon. They are simultaneously disturbed, embarrassed, and eager for the answer after having been teased for their ignorance by classmates from their neighbourhood primary school in North London. With my face colouring just slightly, I explain that "A virgin is a young woman who has never had sex" (having conveyed the bare essentials of 'the birds and the bees' in Qatar) and try to assuage their minor distress.

Our family has only recently arrived in an England still recovering from the bitter miners' strike of 1984-85 and riven with ideological conflict over trade union policy, unemployment, nuclear deterrence, privatisation and the governing style of Britain's first female prime minister. But Neil and I, like the children, are innocents in autumn 1986. For *us*, it is a breath of fresh air to be in a 'free country', a constitutional democracy, after our long sojourn in the repressive Middle East. We are unaware how greatly Tory policies will affect our lives.

After a couple of inconvenient months in a flat in the Borough of Barnet—an area recommended to us by expatriates in Qatar for its suburban amenities and good local schools—we are now finally dwelling in a small, quintessentially-English-middle-class house in the same borough, a brick semi-detached with drab interior, perfectly

"THE THING INSIDE MY HEAD"

adequate for the year we intend to stay here while Neil pursues a Diploma in Management at the London School of Economics. We've enrolled the girls in one of the local state schools because we do not believe in private schooling, both of us having grown up in anti-elitist countries, and, in any event, we lack the wherewithal for private fees in our current situation. But we are disappointed with the prevailing ethos of the school, which, despite the generally high quality of the teachers, is not very aspirational, and there are serious behaviour problems, especially among the boys, which was not the case in our girls' equally multicultural schools in Doha.

Our girls have been catapulted into the real world. Giggling, they blithely recite from time to time 'dirty' songs and jokes that are making the rounds of the school, but, more disturbingly, being the 'new girls', they are sometimes picked on, cruelly teased, or even ostracised by their classmates—especially Sybil, the more sensitive and timid of the two, often a target for jealousy because of her obvious intelligence and her many after-school activities. Molly gives her impressions of these early, sometimes difficult days in primary school:

I'd get very angry at school because I got told off for spelling mistakes which I didn't think were mistakes because they were different spellings, American spellings. People would ask me where I was from. I got teased sometimes. Most of the time that we were at primary school, a lot of kids didn't believe we were sisters in school or other places we went to. It was a running joke. We were very different. I spent quite a bit of time with Sybil in primary school at first. She was a lot more shy and slower at making friends. I felt it was my duty to hang around with her and bring her with me often because I didn't want her to be on her own. I know she made friends eventually, but right at the beginning we were together because we were both new to the whole thing and so we were each other's protectors.

Sybil eventually finds one good friend—once again from the ethnic minorities she feels more comfortable with—a thin, small Bangladeshi girl with spectacles and an overbite (eerily reminiscent of her former friend, Paneez), who is quite popular, but also sensitive, highly intelligent and from a family that values education highly. Asha testifies to the qualities that set Sybil apart from many of her classmates, while also pointing out her perfectly normal joy in life at this time:

I met her at Brunswick Park Primary School, and she came across as quiet, but she was friendly and she was fairly bright and intelligent and a hard worker and keen to take part in our friendship group. Sybil lived on the same street as I did just a couple of minutes' walk away, and we used to meet up at each other's houses quite frequently and we'd play lots of board games and we both enjoyed those a lot. We'd also play on the netball hoop in her garden and Sybil was very good at shooting. She was always practising hard at whatever she did.

We used to play Monopoly quite a lot and the game would go along fine, but one of my tricks was to hide my money as much as I could underneath the board so that when I had to sell my property to Sybil, she'd feel sympathetic to

"THE THING INSIDE MY HEAD"

the fact that I didn't have much money in the first place. So, to bump my amount up she'd actually pay more than she was obliged to do. Then, of course, at the end of the game I'd take out the money from under the board triumphantly. I played this trick on her quite a few times but she was always trusting and didn't seem to think it was going to happen again; it didn't seem to cross her mind. We also played a game called Coppit. It was about chasing the opponent around the board, and we'd both get excited and giggly over it. Sybil did giggle quite a lot.

She liked skate boarding and outdoor activities; she was quite adventurous. At the back of Sybil's house, there was a child's wilderness, lots of long grass, trees and a brook, and we'd often go exploring there for quite a while. I wasn't really into that kind of thing, but it's funny that although she was a quiet character, she'd be the leader in those circumstances. I think she did lots of regular things. I don't know how things went awry for her.

One thing about her was that she was a perfectionist in everything she did. I enjoyed school, and I put effort in to the things I enjoyed, but Sybil consistently put all of her effort into everything, whether it was maths or creative work or art and netball, she was very dedicated to all of them. When playing netball, if one of us other girls was goal shooter or goal attack we'd randomly throw the ball to the hoop, but Sybil as goal shooter was very precise in what she did; she actually personally followed the instructions of the teacher to raise the ball slowly towards the hoop and then concentrate *and then throw. Everything was quite controlled.*

Sybil was very good when she came to my house. My mum is very fussy about who my friends are and whether they are a good influence on me. She would always be really, really impressed by Sybil and her manners and the fact that she used to eat all of her meal while I'd still be slogging away and trying to come to terms with eating the vegetables.

Sybil was generally very quiet, so not many of the others got to know her well, but among the few people who were peripheral to us on the table, everyone knew that she was a really nice girl and that she was different in her niceness. For example, at the end of junior school we had a disco party organised by the teachers. There was a game of spin the bottle, and when the bottle pointed to you, you had to do what the slip of paper said. Sybil's task was to sing a song or remember a poem out loud. The rule was that if you performed the task, you got the sweet. Sybil was too shy to do this, but Miss Dyton insisted that she still got the sweet because she knew Sybil was shy. However, Sybil refused to take the sweet. That again was something quite alien to me because if I were offered a sweet, even if I hadn't performed a task, I still would have taken it. She had her high moral code.

Molly also bears witness to Sybil's "high moral code":

"THE THING INSIDE MY HEAD"

I remember an example of her kind and generous nature, something I've felt guilty about after I finally realised, years later, what had actually happened. When we first went to primary school we had plastic bags to bring our things in, just carrier bags. One-day mum came home with a proper leather schoolbag from a jumble sale, which she said one of us could use for school, but she only had one bag, and said, "Who would like to have it?" Sybil immediately said, "Molly can have it," and I said, without even thinking, "Oh yeah, great." I realised a year or two later, as I got older, how she probably wanted the schoolbag just as much as I did, yet she was being completely selfless, and I did not even think at the time to say, "Oh no, *you* have it."

As Asha has said, Sybil does "lots of regular things" and in many ways appears to be a happy, 'normal' child at this time, despite the 'bad' episodes in Qatar. A letter she writes at age nine, when I travel to the US during the Easter Holidays of 1987 to participate in a professional conference in Eighteenth Century Studies, reveals simply a "third culture kid" delighting in aspects of a new country that other children take for granted:

I had a great time at Anna's house. Anna [visiting from the US for a year] gave me an Easter egg and I gave her one that I had asked daddy to bring with him when he came to pick me up. We each had a small piece of cheesecake a few minutes before daddy came to pick me up but it was nowhere near as good as yours. We [went] to an adventure

133

playground and Anna and I liked a thing where there was a great big pole with a string around the top of the pole and there was a loop at the end of the rope and you had to run a little bit around the pole and then you would suddenly find yourself in the air and then as you went around the pole you would start to go down and you would land on the ground again. Anna gave me a kinder surprise (a kinder surprise is a chocolate egg with a surprise in it) the kinder surprise had some bits of a toy car in it and [a] piece of paper with instructions to make the toy car. We made the car and it runs very well. I miss you very much. Good luck with [the] confrence [sic].

On the reverse side is a crudely drawn but cheerful picture of 'Sybil' under a deep blue sky and a blazing sun, pointing to a yellow flower in the grass, with a speech bubble saying, "I'm going to pick [this] for mummy and daddy."

During 1986 and 1987 Neil is very much absorbed with re-adjusting in mid-life to the challenges of university studies at the demanding London School of Economics, while keeping the family to a parsimonious budget that will get us through the year on the modest savings we have, given the unpaid wages from McKee's and QIDCO. I am using the opportunity to write up scholarly projects I've not been able to develop while teaching full time in Qatar; it would be futile, anyway, for an American with a meagre curriculum vitae to try to find a university position in England teaching *English* Literature. And besides, I now take on all the chauffeuring of the children—not only to and from school but also to the plethora of activities I quickly and eagerly arrange for them.

"THE THING INSIDE MY HEAD"

The girls seem willing and happy to have me arrange for music (recorder) and dancing lessons and enrolment in a Brownie troop in the neighbourhood, and before long they are begging for gymnastic lessons as well. But, in addition, I rarely let a school holiday pass without searching out some extra, temporary activity for them, like the Drama Workshops at a local theatre during half term or the children's programme at a nearby sports centre during the summer. I feel convinced that these bourgeois accomplishments (most of which I was denied as a child) will fortify my girls against depression, boredom, lapses of character, and other contingencies of the soul. Even more to the point, they will protect *me* from having to deal with them in their free time. Gradually, despite my own more flexible timetable, I recreate the whirlwind of non-stop activity and rushing about that characterised our household in Qatar.

* * *

With the LSE school year finishing in the summer of '87, we decide to stay on in England temporarily' for another year; this is partly because Neil, due to illness, has an uncompleted university project, but also because we have fallen in love with London and, thanks to Neil's intense studies, have had minimal time to explore its delights or to travel to other enticing cities and towns. Neil finds a position as General Manager with a shop-fitting company, Withey's, with a promise of a future directorship if all goes well—not that we really intend to stay here. As Neil and I share a zest for touring, we embark on a series of upbeat weekend outings with the girls to all the usual tourist sights inside and outside of London. My own best side comes out at these times—including a cheerfulness I often lack otherwise. Sybil and Molly are uproariously delighted when I naively go up to an elderly gentleman dressed in black at the Tower of London and ask, "Can you tell me where the Beefeaters are?" and he answers, "You're looking at one!" It becomes a standing family joke.

Lois Chaber

I soon find in the UK a benign outlet for my feminist ideals, which have been considerably chastened by the gritty realities of motherhood and the dubious compromises of surviving in the Middle East. I join the Women's Studies Group: 1558-1837, a loose, constantly-shifting aggregate of moderate feminists, whose concern with social issues is channelled into academic scholarship. WSG is to offer me, over the next twenty years, support for my otherwise isolated research and writing and, even more importantly, many stimulating friendships.

Sybil, in contrast, continues to have trouble making and keeping friends and never attains the security of definitely "belonging" to the "friendship group" that Asha has mentioned. Moreover, as our second year in England gets under way, she lapses worryingly into periods of marked depression at times. Other people notice too, such as Edna Keylock, Neil's older cousin on his English mother's side, living with her husband Eddie in nearby Essex, who has become a kind of surrogate grandmother to the girls:

> During the school holidays Sybil and Molly used to stay with us for a few days. It was during those times when we noticed a change in Sybil; she became rather withdrawn at times, even hiding behind her hair. At that time, both girls had long hair, and she would pull it down over her face. At first we thought it was a game, but gradually we realized that, in a way, she was hiding herself.

We confide our worries to the school nurse during a routine parents' conference in the autumn of '87, and she refers us to the Vale Drive Child Guidance Centre in a neighbouring town. Neil and I are given weekly

"THE THING INSIDE MY HEAD"

appointments at the Centre with a Miss Simpson, a psychiatric social worker, starting in November. No therapy, at this point, is provided for Sybil herself because the clinic believes in "working through families"; moreover, they are short of child therapists, and we by our own admission are only temporarily residing in England.

After we fill her in on Sybil's background, Miss Simpson seems to think—as do I—that Sybil's marked insecurity (despite successes in school and activities) derives from her traumatic infantile experiences in Iran. From our descriptions of Sybil's behaviour, Miss Simpson concludes that Sybil is very repressed; in particular, she cannot outwardly express anger, aggression or any negative emotions, having moulded herself into the prototype of a sweet, well-behaved, compliant little girl for us. She advises us over and over again to "Give Sybil space"—something that I, especially, find very difficult to put into practice. My own omni-present anxiety leads me to organise *myself* rigidly, and I am a 'control freak' with the girls as well—scheduling their many activities, monitoring the related practice sessions, supervising their hygiene, and so on. Although Neil is naturally more relaxed about such things, more often than not, caught up in his new job, he acquiesces in my 'control'.

Further complications ensue when, hoping to bolster Sybil's sense of belonging and fulfil her frequently expressed religious yearnings, and I make arrangements for both girls to join a Methodist church recommended by their Brownie Leader. (My own Jewish background has been revealed too late to overcome their early indoctrination into Christianity.) To be sure, it would probably be more beneficial for us to join and worship as a family, but should Neil and I, sceptics with an aversion to organised religion and dogma, become arrant hypocrites?

The girls, particularly Sybil, are delighted with the Sunday school, run primarily by Mr. and Mrs. Wells, ardent parishioners of this Methodist Church, and with the other church activities they are invited to join, despite their chagrin that we remain politely but firmly aloof. Phyllis Wells soon begins making routine trips to our house to drop off children's Bible study pamphlets called "One to One," encouraging the girls to work through them as well as arranging to take them very occasionally to special mass prayer meetings in London. I am getting a bit worried about the intensity and scope of these religious activities, especially when I observe Sybil continually nagging the more phlegmatic Molly to finish answering the many questions in these didactic pamphlets. (Years later, Phyllis Wells is to deny any recollection of delivering these "One to One" pamphlets to our girls, answering me with a quizzical "hmmm" every time I try to jog her memory, but Molly and I remember these drop-offs vividly.)

* * *

In the school holidays of 1988, when Sybil is ten and Molly eight and a half, I enrol the girls in a summer programme at the local sports centre where they had enjoyed themselves the previous year. I am relieved to be able to amuse them constructively and also create some space for myself and my writing before we go off on our planned holiday to Scotland in August. Neil, constantly working long hours, is little affected by the girls' holidays, but, like me, has a strong sense that Sybil tends to get depressed if her days are not structured. Towards the end of the fortnight, however, things go terribly wrong. Sybil comes home one afternoon crying hysterically, and Molly tells me that some girls have been bullying her all week. She refuses to go back or talk about her experience with us and continues to screech and weep almost continuously for the next couple of days. Just on the margins of our awareness, we vaguely notice Sybil repeating some of her actions, like putting her shoes and clothes off again, on again. Although Molly has noticed covert 'repeatings' at least a year earlier, she has never spoken to us about it.

"THE THING INSIDE MY HEAD"

We are panic-stricken. Our summer holiday, a motoring trip to Scotland, is imminent and our counsellor, Miss Simpson, is away on vacation. The clinic supervisor advises us to carry on with the holiday and consult our general practitioner about Sybil. This latter doctor, at a loss, simply prescribes a children's antihistamine syrup with mild sedative properties, and so we set of with Sybil still quite distressed and dysfunctional. It does not help that, having become obsessively over-involved in the girls' music lessons—I have even occasionally resorted to smacking them if they petulantly balk at playing—I insist that they bring along their instruments (Sybil and Molly have graduated to the flute and the saxophone, respectively).

During the first few days of the holiday the full extent of Sybil's disturbed behaviour—the worst since 1985 in Qatar—now becomes apparent and persistently slows us all down. Besides her intermittent grotesque posturing and multiple 'repeatings', every trip to the toilet en route becomes a tiresome trial, with Sybil lurking in the cubicles for long periods of time, emerging only after many urgent appeals on our part. Neil and I both are shocked and frustrated, but I have less patience to cope and am often overcome with rage, once even dragging Sybil out of the toilet by force.

My occasional efforts to make the girls practice their musical instruments lead to dismal scenes of mutual distress; I soon give that up. Almost every night at bedtime, Sybil weeps pathetically, and we have to sedate her heavily with the antihistamine that our GP prescribed. But as we motor around Scotland and engage in numerous child-friendly activities like pony-trekking up a hill and picnicking on a tiny island, Sybil seems to calm down, ease off on her eccentric behaviour, and actually begin to enjoy herself by the time we are on the last leg of the two-week trip.

However, we cannot easily escape from the implications of this latest breakdown. Shortly after our return

139

Lois Chaber

to London, Sybil relapses and begins to spend inordinate amounts of time washing her hands and showering herself. When we bring our tribulations to the ear of Miss Simpson, her main advice is still "Give Sybil space", and, as much as possible, ignore her behaviour. "If she wants to stay in the shower for an hour and a half standing on one leg [her latest habit]", our counsellor enjoins, "let her". Whatever the outcome of following this advice fully, we will never know, for we find it extremely difficult just to stand by patiently during what we regard as her "antics", and Neil and I routinely quarrel over how to deal with Sybil.

By now, Sybil's strange behaviour begins to surface at primary school. According to her friend Asha, "a couple of us had noticed that sometimes Sybil stood very still, and she'd be looking at something that we couldn't see, staring into space. She would sometimes bend down and tie up her shoelaces and be over-meticulous about it, do them up very slowly and then come back and stand up again. We didn't quite know what it was about, but we let it pass." When Molly tries to ameliorate the situation, she inadvertently makes things worse:

> Sometime after the trip to Scotland, while we were still in primary school, she confided in me, trying to explain why she did certain things by saying that she would think that something terrible would happen if she didn't do them, like the devil would get her. Her friends would come up to me and say, "What's wrong with Sybil?" They wanted to know why she was being so weird. I thought I was helping by explaining to them what Sybil had said to me, but they took it the wrong way. Sybil had no idea that I had told them. I saw when they were playing netball together on the net ball team that they would stand there and would say,

"THE THING INSIDE MY HEAD"

"The devil's going to get me" and would put
their fingers on the side of their head like a
devil's horns. I don't think she noticed, but I
was so scared that she would find out, and I
was so angry with them for doing it and felt so
guilty every day. She was doing weird things—
stopping, walking at a slow pace, etc. I felt
guilty about telling them because I was always
terrified that Sybil would find out that I had told,
and I knew how upset it would make her that
they knew and were making fun of her.

Around this time, also, I first become aware of that
scourge of the 1980s, anorexia nervosa. In particular, I read
previews of a TV programme called "Catherine: Living with
Anorexia", a true account of a young girl with this terrible
eating disorder, who eventually dies, despite treatment and
her family's best efforts. I record the programme and send
away for a brochure, even though I perceive no specific
symptoms of this eating disorder in Sybil. I burst into tears
at our next session with Miss Simpson, crying out, "I just
know Sybil is going to become anorexic because of her low
self esteem." She is shocked and angry, tells me I'm
indulging in a self-fulfilling prophecy and refuses to entertain
the thought. I put the recording away on a bookshelf with
other unwatched videocassettes, for later perusal.

Having nearly forgotten about it, one day I come
home from running errands and am horrified to find Sybil
and Molly sitting on the living room sofa watching
"Catherine". Sybil looks devastated, and I snatch the video
away. They normally do not take videos to watch without my
supervision, but I have been foolish enough to leave this one
in an accessible place. Have I subconsciously wanted her to
watch it, as a kind of warning? Later that day, I find Sybil
crying, and she (for once) confides in me: "Mummy, that girl
was just like me!" That night, I force myself to watch the

whole painful recording, and I see what she means: Catherine cries a lot, has derogatory thoughts about herself, and performs other compulsive behaviours, like excessive praying, besides her food refusal.

* * *

Meanwhile, these past few months have seen Neil disillusioned with his shop-fitting company, where many less professional colleagues are pushing to retrench the business. Moreover, we have all along planned to make our permanent residence in New Zealand where, as we believe, there will be a more wholesome atmosphere, including an extended family, in which to raise the girls. Neil begins a discreet search for a position in New Zealand and, as a fall back, Australia. But Australian agencies will not consider him unless he actually emigrates there first, and, very unfortunately for our timing, the earlier recession in New Zealand is now a severe depression. Neil tries anyway, sneaking in a quick trip to Auckland in February 1989 to interview for a promising position. He comes so close to landing the job that he is utterly crushed when finally turned down, and there is nothing else on the horizon there. By default, we now resign ourselves to remaining in the UK as the least disruptive option for the family. We put the best possible face on things for the girls' sakes, but they can see that "daddy" is once again depressed over his career.

In early 1989 as well, I receive a revelatory letter from an old US friend who has read my Christmas 1988 newsletter spelling out Sybil's recent alarming conduct. She has enclosed an article discussing a so-called "obsessive-compulsive disorder" (OCD), just beginning to receive medical attention in the US, and its successful treatments with the trycyclic anti-depressant Clomipramine (Anafranil). Reading the article, we are amazed at the parallels with Sybil's behaviour—the repetitions, the excessive praying and washing—and see hope in the fact that there is a 'name' for her worrying mannerisms as well as a promising

"THE THING INSIDE MY HEAD"

treatment. Immediately, we relay our new knowledge to Miss Simpson, inquiring about the possibilities of treatment for Sybil, but she responds with muted hostility: "We don't like to give simple labels to things here," she insists, and firmly explains that the clinic does not believe in drug treatment for children. The Clinic's negative reaction discourages us from making further inquiries, and anyway, we do not even have a computer or internet know-how at this time.

However, we are soon mollified when Miss Simpson tells us that, since we have now taken up permanent residence in England, they will be assigning a psycho-therapist to see Sybil as soon as a Mrs. Greenoaks becomes available in August of this year. Inevitably, when the sessions start, the task of taxiing Sybil to and from these weekly appointments, from 4:00 to 4:50, falls on me. I find it difficult to manage since Mrs. Greenoaks will not permit me to wait in the clinic for Sybil, and there is not really enough time to return home and accomplish anything productive. I thus go to our local library, halfway between, to read and take notes. The local traffic on the high road I have to traverse is particularly fierce just before 5:00, and between this and my occasional over-absorption in work at the library, I am frequently late in collecting Sybil.

This becomes a source of friction between me and Mrs. Greenoaks, whom I find somewhat cold and impersonal, anyway. Sadly, I am not willing simply to "sacrifice" (as I see it) the two hours all together that the whole appointment and its transport takes for the sake of Sybil's mental welfare. Perhaps my poor attitude reflects my ongoing, self-centred struggle for my own psychic survival in this new country, my scramble to maintain my identity as a productive scholar.

Mrs. Greenoaks keeps her work with Sybil rigidly confidential, not involving us, her parents, at all—a policy which is to remain an issue throughout our dealings with the

Lois Chaber

NHS—and Sybil herself reveals nothing about their sessions except that they work through "play". She is quite impatient with her therapy, regularly wailing "I'm not getting better," despite our continual reassurances that this kind of treatment takes time. Only some years later is the profession to declare that psychotherapy is not the recommended treatment for OCD.

Shortly prior to the beginning of Sybil's therapy, in summer 1989, Neil's discomfort with the shop-fitting company comes to a head, particularly when they disingenuously stall over their promise to make him a company director; when he presses them, he abruptly gets the sack. But, very lucky this time, Neil succeeds in landing an excellent, highly paid position, "Development Executive", with an English property development company, Regalian—a dream come true.

Meanwhile, treatment for my own chronic problems is still minimal, despite our now residing in a developed country. I have become dependent on medication and do not complain when all that is offered me are the same type of infrequent visits, in the psychiatric department of our local hospital, with junior doctors who do little other than give their imprimatur to ongoing prescriptions for Imipramine—just as in Qatar.

* * *

During the early stages of Sybil's therapy, she begins her secondary school career at Ashmole, a comprehensive nearby. We have plumped for this instead of the all-girls state school that Sybil herself has favoured since both we and Miss Simpson believe that a coeducational environment will be more healthy and normative for Sybil, despite her vulnerability and the aggressive male behaviour we have witnessed in the primary school system. Sybil at twelve is an attractive, slim girl of medium build, with medium-length, by-now-dark-auburn hair, grey-green eyes,

144

soft, regular facial features, and a delicate complexion.
When an American friend from Qatar days visits us in
London, not having seen us for several years, and Sybil
walks into the living room, this woman gasps and exclaims:
"Wow, Neil, you will have to get a shotgun to fend off all her
suitors!" Yet, thanks mostly to her extreme shyness and
lack of confidence; she by no means enjoys the popularity,
either with boys or girls, commensurate with such good
looks.

However, Sybil by now has regained the early edge
in the schoolroom that she began with in Qatar, shining
academically at Ashmole Comprehensive and playing flute
in the school band. The downside, however, is that there is
no "streaming" for the first two years, and she complains
bitterly about the prevalence of uninterested, disruptive
students who make it difficult to work in class, and about
persistent bullying by some English girls. She is also
involved in an unstable three-way relationship with two other
girls, one of them another Bangladeshi, Purnimi, who, like
Asha, is highly intelligent, the other, Eve, an average English
schoolgirl. Molly, too, though still attending primary school,
is disturbed by Sybil's predicament and is increasingly taking
on the role of a benignly patronising older sister: "I know she
was shy and had bad times, and the people there, the girls,
were a very rough lot. There were incidents with her being
bullied by these girls and I was feeling so angry about it and
wanted to protect her, but there was nothing I could do. I
told her I'd go and shout at them if I could."

Sybil's daily return home from Ashmole—with
"Daddy" not around—is my opportunity for intimacy with her.
While Molly plays captive audience to the living room TV,
Sybil hovers listlessly in the kitchen. We both 'know' it is up
to me to elicit an account of her day and to persuade her into
a snack, otherwise she will continue to loiter and mope and
not get down to anything purposeful. I both relish and dread
this tête a tête, for if I make a wrong move, *she* may become
distraught for the rest of the day, and *I*, anguished and guilty.

Lois Chaber

"How was school today"? I prompt, and if it has been a reasonable day, I receive a somewhat compulsive rattling off of every single thing that has occurred. If it has been a bad day, there will be tears just forming in the corners of her eyes, and I will have to press the problem out of her—usually a tale of woeful injustice involving her friendship triangle ("Purnimi and Eve were *horrible*!"). I hug her tenderly—when she will let me—but my spoken attempts to brush off such incidents lightly are belied by my anxious grimace. I then urge her to have a piece of buttered toast (her favourite snack): "You know you'll feel better after you've had something to eat." But she resists, consciously denying her needs for as long as she can, like an ascetic fearing to indulge in a pleasure. Once she (finally!) makes the snack and begins to nibble, I can breathe a sigh of relief, gradually ease myself out of the kitchen and move on to other things.

We discover that Sybil's old friend Asha, bright and ambitious, has opted for a highly-reputed selective entry state grammar school, the Latymer School, further away from our neighbourhood, and we begin to feel chagrined that we did not make inquiries on behalf of Sybil. We were outsiders in the great English game of education, and automatically followed our liberal bent. In the early days, there is a nominal attempt by Asha to keep up her friendship with Sybil, but, unbeknown to us, she is increasingly put off by Sybil's strange behaviour.

When she was at Ashmole, she came round a couple of times to my house. Sybil had always been a very good eater and I had always been the poor eater; now I noticed that she was very reluctant to take her food and was even slower than I was which was unusual. When we were playing a board game afterwards, she excused herself to go the

146

"THE THING INSIDE MY HEAD"

bathroom and I waited for about ten minutes,
and I thought "What's happening; maybe she's
talking to someone upstairs," so I went upstairs
and found her still in the bathroom. I said,
"Sybil is everything OK?" and she said, "Yes,"
so I went back downstairs, waited for another
ten minutes, and then finally after another while
she came down. This happened another time
she came round. I was still sitting downstairs
and my sister said she heard Sybil retching in
the toilet. I think we must have realised
something was wrong then.

But Asha's family do not disclose their unease to us,
nor does Molly reveal anything about Sybil's growing
religious obsessions at bedtime.

* * *

During this same period, we—I especially—are
becoming aware of Sybil's adverse reaction to the onset of
puberty. Mary Pipher, an American clinical psychologist, in
her best-selling advice book, *Reviving Ophelia: Saving the
Selves of Adolescent Girls*, believes that teenage girls have
been in crisis since the late 1980s. Adolescence, at the best
of times a "hurricane" and a "crucible" for girls, has become,
in the 1990s, particularly devastating for them due to the
misogynistic, sexualised, sensationalist and media-pervaded
culture in which they come of age, avers Pipher. Alienation
from parents, eating disorders, self-mutilation, suicide
attempts, alcoholism, and drug addiction are the all-too-
prevalent consequences. Unfortunately, as Pipher points
out, bright and sensitive girls are most at risk for problems.

Sybil is a classic instance of this. But unlike those
girls caught up in the perverted spirit of the times during their
hormonal turmoil, she is repelled and alienated by the

teenage culture, replete with lurid sex and violence, which surrounds her in London. In contrast to her friends and to Molly, she is utterly indifferent at this point to pop music, though too embarrassed to admit this to people outside the family. When asked about her favourite pop star, she answers uneasily, "Kylie Minogue"—the only name she knows.

More importantly, she rejects all bodily intimations of growing up. One evening during her first term at Ashmole, as I am tucking her into bed and performing the childhood bedtime rituals that our girls have clung to all these years, I say, as casually as I can manage—and of course with unacknowledged inconsistency—"Would you like me to take you shopping for a bra?" Sybil bursts into tears at once, and turns away from me to the wall. When her first period comes, a full year and a half or so after I have given her a 'talk' and an 'educational pack', she walks slowly down the stairs of our home, with an anxious, strained face, and I am left to surmise what has happened. She becomes obsessive about concealing the fact of her menstruation whenever it occurs, insisting that I buy her the thinnest possible commercial sanitary pads and demanding constant reassurance that "Nothing is showing".

Sybil also exemplifies Piper's contention that active and dynamic pre-pubescent young girls lose their energy and their "selves" upon entering a troubled puberty. The extra-curricular activities that Sybil once revelled in now become torments for her, though she is too timid—in this family that is "too achievement-oriented," according to Miss Simpson—to come right out and ask to drop them. Her longstanding dancing teacher, Lesley Hand, comments on the change:

> When Sybil first came to dancing, she was
> a bright and bubbly eight-year-old happy child

"THE THING INSIDE MY HEAD"

with a natural sense of dance, very expressive and creative. I think she must have been about twelve when she started to change, becoming nervous and withdrawn, trying too hard, and looking frightened and scared when dancing instead of enjoying it. I would try to coax her to smile, almost begging her to be "naughty". From a technical point of view, she used to have loose limbs and could swing her legs very high. As her illness progressed, her legs became tighter and tighter and she could barely get them to ninety degrees, whereas before she could get them to eye level. She also started spending ages in the loo. Other girls would tell me she was standing in one position and not moving. I personally felt helpless and incapable of helping her; it was all so sad.

Just as painful to witness is her musical deterioration. Daily flute practice, which I still insist on, has become a devastating impasse for both of us. She refuses to practice without my "help" yet obviously resents it, and I have too much emotional investment in her musical achievements to withdraw. So we both stand there, miserable, facing the music stand, as tearful Sybil starts and stops endlessly, emitting feeble intermittent bleats on the flute. Would that I could end the music lessons like I have recently stopped her gymnastics at the urgings of her disappointed instructor, but it is probably my wish to vicariously relive my happy experience as a keenly aspiring instrumentalist in my high school band that keeps me from disengaging and giving Sybil the "space" she needs to declare her own mind.

* * *

Lois Chaber

In spring 1990, Neil again has to face a work-related crisis. Once resolved to remain in England, we decide to sell our small semi and buy a larger house, particularly so that the girls can each have their own bedroom—a must for their teenage years. After many months of negotiating the usual hurdles of the English property market, in April we finally move into a detached four-bedroom home not far from our previous one, to avoid having to change the girls' schools. The mortgage is a very stiff one, but Neil feels confident we can manage with his new Regalian position.

However, the global economic recession that had New Zealand in its grip has hit England in 1989, made worse by the punishingly high interest rates under the Tory government, a consequence of Britain being tied to the European monetary exchange mechanism. This recession becomes increasingly severe in early 1990, particularly in the construction industry, and rather suddenly hits the commercial property market, the sector around which Neil's new job revolves. Just a month after we've moved into the new house, Neil (one of the most recently hired Regalian employees) is abruptly informed, along with five colleagues, that he's been made redundant—to leave that day—with three months' salary.

Neil is in shock at the sudden loss of his golden opportunity, which includes the substantial salary that was to pay the new mortgage. He immediately begins an epic search for a new position, sending out more than fifteen hundred letters all told, exhausting every possibility. However, with the country in the vice of this recession and Neil with a minimum of UK work experience, he is getting nowhere, and gradually becoming discouraged and depressed. I, too, investigate job possibilities, but the market for American PhDs in English Literature—with no major books published—is very narrow, and I receive only one offer, to teach a small class in an American Student Abroad Programme. The pay is so negligible that, with the very real possibility that the family may have to relocate for

"THE THING INSIDE MY HEAD"

Neil to work, I decline the offer. We eventually have to go on the dole—the first time ever for both of us. Accordingly, we have to tighten our belts considerably, resulting in many privations in food, entertainment and clothing for the children, a situation unlikely to help Sybil's ongoing depression and compulsive behaviour.

A month after Neil's redundancy, the family suffers another loss, an apparently trivial one, but it has acute emotional implications for Sybil. Our little cat, Una, whom we brought all the way from Qatar and quarantined here for six months, has not adjusted well to urban life in England, and now, with our new house situated on a major road, she is run over in early June. The girls are inconsolable, especially Sybil. Every night brings prolonged crying jags and emotional upheaval when we try to settle her into bed. Cats are special for Sybil, and Una in particular has been more than a pet: she was a last link to Sybil's childhood of beaches, parties, nannies and sunshine in Qatar, the world we had to leave behind. The authors of *Third Culture Kids,* in fact, claim that "unresolved grief over the loss of things they had loved in their childhood" can be a major emotional problem for children who've had to make the transition from a foreign to a "home" culture.

Unfortunately, Sybil's therapist, Dr. Greenoaks, does not seem to realise this and, as an Asian, appears to lack empathy for Western attitudes to pets. When Sybil sobs out the loss of Una to her in their next session, she just chuckles uncomfortably; Sybil is shocked and upset. (This is the *only* detail that Sybil ever confides to me about her psycho-therapy sessions.) To assuage the girls' misery, especially Sybil's terrific grieving (most likely compounded by distress over her dad's recent setback), we very quickly obtain a new kitten, which Sybil is keen to name 'Ali Biba'—the Middle East still so much on her mind.

With the family situation going downhill, both girls' behaviour deteriorates.

Lois Chaber

Sybil's prolonged cleaning and repeating rituals are slowing her down tremendously, making it awkward to get her off to school and to put her to bed at night. Shortly after she finally gets to bed, we hear only partly stifled sobs and moans issuing from her room, and the crying gets insistently louder if we ignore it. I am for not reinforcing these bids for attention; Neil is the one who rises from our bed at an awkward hour and goes to sit by her side, coaxing her to divulge her woes. But Sybil refuses to confide in her dad, bottling it all up inside, or just revealing the absolute minimum to keep him engaged by her bedside late into the night. The most he can elicit from her is that she "has horrible thoughts"—with no indication of what these are.

I find myself getting angry at these blatant nightly appeals, rather than sympathetic, and allow Neil to wholly fill the role of comforter, so that, as the months go by, Sybil and I become increasingly alienated. It is a replay of Tehran! Of course, I am quite depressed myself, despite my medication, about our finances, about the prospect of losing the house, about Sybil's difficult behaviour, and about Neil's future—the future of the whole family. Perhaps I unconsciously feel it is I who should be receiving this nightly comfort from Neil. Once again, Sybil mirrors my own weakness, and I am repelled.

Molly, meanwhile, though only about ten, has not only by now grown larger and stronger than Sybil, but is manifesting all the classic behaviour of adolescent rebellion—balking at her family chores, defying her parents' instructions, and initiating dramatic standoffs between herself and us. Neil and I still believe in the usefulness of corporal punishment (before the thought-provoking debates over "smacking" children emerge in the UK); when Molly ignores our appeals and arguments, we resort to hard smacks or spankings, the latter mostly from Neil—or other severe punishments such as cancelling a birthday party. None of these tactics move her one bit; they only stoke her stubbornness, and she bitterly nurses her resentments, building up huge grudges she is to hold onto in later years. Nor do we try to understand the feelings that are underlying Molly's anger and recalcitrance. Discordant and dysfunctional family 'scenes' centring on Molly become increasingly prevalent, greatly distressing Sybil and increasing her depression. Pipher says of adolescent girls experiencing troubles, "Those who blame themselves feel depressed, while those who blame others feel angry"—a formulation which precisely describes Sybil and Molly. As Neil puts it, "Sybil implodes; Molly explodes." We badly need help with our parenting strategies.

With Neil unemployed and thus available, the Child Guidance Clinic offers us family counselling with a psychiatrist, Dr. Evron Pamuk, beginning in January 1991. Neil and I initially have high hopes. At our very first meeting, Dr. Pamuk insightfully asks Sybil, "Do you feel you are treated like a big sister?" The answer is "No." In subsequent sessions he gives Sybil "homework"—"Try to be naughty this week." He makes it clear that he is concerned with the dynamics of the whole family, however, not just Sybil's problems, and when he puts the spotlight on Molly's behaviour and attitudes in the third session—albeit in a genial and gentle manner—she reacts churlishly. From then on, she adamantly refuses to attend the sessions, expressing aversion to Dr. Pamuk and cynical contempt for the whole process. Dr. Pamuk advises us to stop punishing Molly lest she run away from home all together; to a large extent we now follow his advice, but, without her participation, he is not able to effect changes in *her* behaviour. The three of us continue to meet weekly throughout 1991, but, with the 'family' incomplete, the sessions are broken-backed.

* * *

One apparently good thing happens. Having learnt from our mistakes with Sybil's schooling, we register Molly in 1990 for the highly-subscribed entrance exam to the

Lois Chaber

Latymer School, a state grammar school, where the behavioural and academic standards are much higher than Ashmole; much to our delight, she makes the cut. We put Sybil on the waiting list, and, with a high score on a special exam and a sibling now in that school, in the spring of her second year at Ashmole (1991), she is invited to take up a newly vacant place at Latymer after the Easter holidays. Without insisting, we strongly encourage Sybil to take this opportunity, and, eventually, she agrees. But a few weeks after making the changeover, she expresses her ambivalence in a diary-like page pasted into her 'events' scrapbook:

> *In the spring term on a Friday 2 weeks before the Easter holidays 1991 Mummy said there was a surprise for me. I WAS EXCEPTED [sic] INTO LATYMER. I took two weeks to decide. On Thursday before Easter holidays I told Purnimi. We were crying. I felt so bad. Our friendship had just been at its best…*

> *I miss [Purnimi] so much I feel like I don't fit in with the people at Latymer. There are already two people who don't like me. I feel so lonely. I think back to the time when Purni and Eve were against me and I came home and cried every day. I hope I don't lose my friendship with Purni… Sometimes I think she and Eve are trying to sort of dump me when they say "Oh you'll make friends at Latymer [and] what about Opheera [a girl in her new class]" I feel like I want a friend at Latymer but yet, I don't because I don't want anyone to take Purni's place.*

154

"THE THING INSIDE MY HEAD"

The work is definitely better though and I'm hardly ever bored in classes. Science is so much better. I feel a bit snobbish saying this but I don't want to go back to Ashmole…

Starting mid-stream at Latymer, Sybil has to make up the work she has missed in this spring term, which is, moreover, the second term of the second year—a daunting task. Surprisingly, at this point she has the will and the stamina to do this, working hard and efficiently and greatly stimulated. She is particularly engrossed in a history project on the gunpowder plot, becoming quite indignant over the English government's anti-Catholic tactics. She astounds everyone—us, the school and herself—by receiving all A's in the end of year exams. For once, she feels really good about herself, and we all feel a surge of optimism.

In the summer of 1991, we anxiously request Dr. Pamuk to ask the uncommunicative Mrs. Greenoaks, still seeing Sybil, about Sybil's prospects for the future. He brings back the report, with which he blithely concurs, that she will probably grow up into a normal adult, but one that experiences more anxiety than the average person. Throughout these last couple of years, no one involved with the Child Guidance Clinic—presumably on principle—has explicitly addressed the issues surrounding Sybil's obsessive-compulsive disorder—increasingly manifested through her washing and praying rituals and 'repeating things'—or has given her any specific treatment for it.

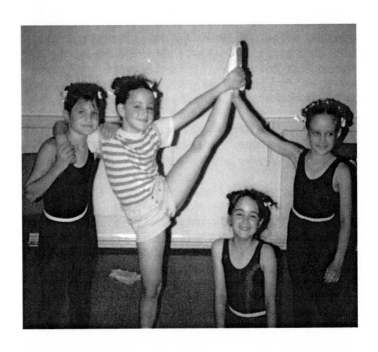

Sybil at 8 years with leg up at ballet class

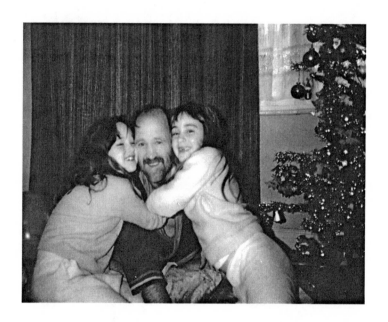

First Christmas in England: Sybil (left) with Dad and Molly

Lois Chaber

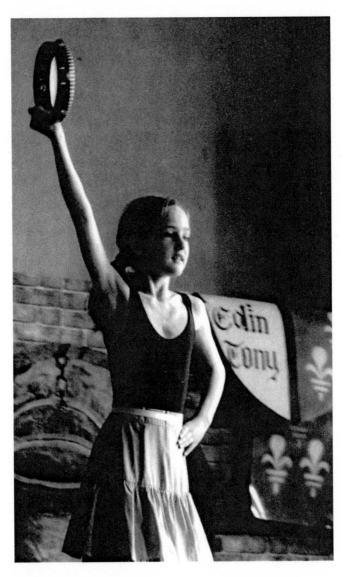

Sybil, age 10, performing a dance at school show

"THE THING INSIDE MY HEAD"

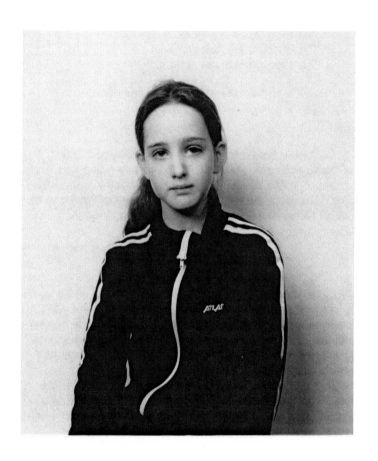

Sybil, age 10, feeling a bit 'down'.

Lois Chaber

Chapter 7: Molly Speaks

> For there is no friend like a sister
> In calm or stormy weather;
> To cheer one on the tedious way,
> To fetch one if one goes astray,
> To lift one if one totters down,
> To strengthen if one stands.

(From Christina Rosetti, "Goblin Market".)

Some time after Sybil's death, Molly recounted to me these episodes of Sybil's OCD behaviour she had witnessed in the 1990s. Neil and I knew nothing about the early ones at all. Molly's passionate loyalty to Sybil and their mutual sense of a secret sisterly alliance against their parents kept her silent.

* * *

[1989/90] Because we had bunk beds, I had to sit through Sybil's nightly prayer that she did, kneeling by the bed, before she went to sleep, that is, until Daddy made her get into bed. Her prayer would consist of endless apologising for every single thought, movement, or word that she had performed that day that was blasphemous or evil or bad towards someone she knew. She went into such minute detail, e.g. saying she was sorry for having possibly said a certain word with a slightly angry tone of voice which maybe could seem like it meant such and such, which could possibly amount to blasphemy, etc. Daddy used to come into the room and see her still up and get furious with her and force her into bed. I think she may have got out again and he'd get angrier and order her back into bed or even physically put her into bed, making her cry. She would get so frustrated if she couldn't get out again; then she'd lie in bed and tell me to make sure to wake her up if. . . . and then

"THE THING INSIDE MY HEAD"

*she'd reel off a huge long list of stuff: if I had a headache, if I
had a tummy ache, if I had a backache, if I was feeling
nauseous, if I couldn't sleep, if I had a bad dream, if I had
bad thoughts, if I wanted anything. I'd kind of know when
she'd come to the end, but sometimes she would start again.
It was like she knew it by heart, in the exact order as well.
I'd have to say "yes" at the right point, and I had to make
sure I stayed awake until the end to be able to say yes.
Even if I did, sometimes she'd start again anyway, etc.,
etc.—the whole list again.*

*I also remember a period in 1990 when every night, before
we went to sleep, she would come into my bed with her
Bible and signal for me to read out loud a particular passage
from Revelations. It was one about Judgment Day. I can't
remember exactly which one but it was hellfire and
brimstone about punishment and repenting. I would have to
read the passage over and over again because Sybil would
keep stopping me by making an upset sound; every time she
did, I would have to start again, even if I was just a couple of
words from the end. I had no idea why she would stop me
at those random points. I thought it was because of my way
of reading, my tone of voice, my annunciation, if I stumbled
on a word, etc. No matter how frustrated or angry I got, I
knew I had to keep calm and keep trying to read 'flawlessly'
until Sybil let me reach the end of the passage without
stopping. It was only then that she and I would be able to go
to bed. I don't know how or when this nightly occurrence
started or ended, just that it went on a long time, and is one
of my most vivid memories. Some nights it was over quickly,
and others it went on until we were both exhausted and at
breaking points.*

*It wasn't until years later, when I was eighteen and Sybil was
much better, that we talked about it again when I was doing
my Art A-level project on OCD, and Sybil was helping me
with my research. We discussed a lot of things about the
past—things we had felt guilty or confused about for years. I
brought up the reading of the Revelations passage, and she*

Lois Chaber

told me that the stopping and starting had nothing to do with the way I read it; it was her way—OCD's way—of punishing herself by trying to provoke me into getting angry with her.

* * *

[1991] When she got really bad, she had a habit of adopting a religious-type prostrated position on the floor—curled up in a ball but kneeling—at school and at home, no doubt connected to her obsessions with praying. Once, right in the middle of a crowded corridor at school, she just curled up into this position on the floor (a sign that her OCD had gotten so bad that it didn't matter who was around). I got really angry and said, "Get up!" A dinner lady tried to get her up. A lot of the cleaners, etc., spoke to Sybil and really liked her. They probably took pity on her because she was lonely. I remember a few times seeing her stuck, just standing. I felt angry and embarrassed. At that point, I didn't understand what she had. My parents never explained it to me properly, and I didn't know what OCD was until a few years later. At first, I was trying to be helpful and stick with her, but I guess I changed from being kind and helpful to ultimately being angry with her. She was acting weird all the time. People at school would come up and say, "Is she all right?" and I would just kind of shrug it off. I didn't know what to tell them because I didn't know myself what was wrong with her.

[1991] Once I had my friend Heulwen round and we were watching James Bond, and after dinner Sybil just curled up in her kneeling position, on the floor in the far corner of the room. And I was so embarrassed that I completely ignored her and when Heulwen asked, 'What's wrong with her?', I shrugged it off, mortified and furious with Sybil. My dad eventually came in and grabbed her and physically forced her out of the room. I guess this is around the time when she was standing on one leg, and doing all these weird postures for hours and hours and hours on end.

"THE THING INSIDE MY HEAD"

*I distinctly remember the moment I thought "my sister is
<u>actually, literally, full-blown crazy</u>". I guess I was about 11 or
12. I was watching from my bedroom window as Sybil ran
into the street in front of our house, and throwing her arms
into the air and shouting, 'Save me Lord, save me', and we
would run outside after her, shouting and trying and get her
to come back in. There was an awful look on her face, like
desperate fear, eyes rolled upwards to the sky: 'Save me
Lord, save me Lord'. I honestly thought she was completely
crazy. I had no idea what was wrong. I think I started hating
religion/Christianity then; I thought that it was largely to
blame for Sybil's condition. Years later Sybil told me that
when it came to her religion-based fears, she literally
thought the angels of justice were coming for her in chariots
of fire to cast their terrible punishment upon her—or
something along those lines.*

*[1992] I remember an incident when we called the police.
Sybil was doing something that made us all get so angry and
there was a huge terrible argument and I can't remember
who called the police. They came and spoke to her and the
situation calmed down. I wasn't very happy that the police
were called. There used to be these regular occasions of
clashes between the whole family. We'd all lose our
tempers at points with Sybil's compulsions and rituals.*

* * *

*[1992] Once, when we'd all gone to bed, Sybil was still stuck
in the hall on one leg. I was in bed and I suddenly got really
scared by a tapping noise in the wall by my head. I ran out
into the corridor and said, "Sybil, I'm scared," and then for one
moment she snapped out of it, after not having communicated
all day long, to come and help me and be worried with me.
We called Daddy out, who said it was nothing, and as soon as
she realised that it was out of her hands and she didn't have
to worry, she just went back into her posture again.*

Lois Chaber

I thought Sybil was crazy; didn't know what was wrong, didn't know what to say to people who thought she was completely mad. I felt everything: sadness, anger, embarrassment, pity, frustration at not knowing what was going to happen. Why couldn't I have a normal family, go to school every day and be normal? I'd just think of all these people with normal families who had no idea of the terrible scenes that went on almost every night or every week—just terrible scenes, everyone upset, screaming and angry. I suppose my parents were feeling all the same things; mum and dad would get frustrated and run out of patience and somebody would grab her and that's why the situation with the police happened. We decided that if we were firm with her, "Don't do this or that," or "Stop it," then it would stop.

My parents would argue a lot about what they had decided. I remember them discussing how they could make her eat properly. I got very confused after the incident where she suddenly stopped standing on one leg because she was worried about me. Why could she turn it on and off just like that when she wanted? I didn't realise it wasn't a case of what she wanted; it just happened. I guess my mum and dad were both fairly desperate and didn't know what to do.

* * *

In 1997, Molly, inspired and enlightened by Dr. Judith Rapoport's pioneering book for the general public, *The Boy Who Couldn't Stop Washing: The Experience and Treatment of Obsessive-Compulsive Disorder* (1989), embarked on a series of projects to provoke interest in and sympathy for this disorder from which her sister suffered. First, despite her public-speaking phobia, she volunteered to create an assembly on OCD before all of the Latymer School, preceded by an intriguing advertising campaign throughout the school with posters saying, "Can you make it through this door?" and "Have you washed your hands?" With an explanation of OCD and its symptoms plus excerpts from the

164

"THE THING INSIDE MY HEAD"

Rapoport book, the assembly, highly successful, stimulated the whole school into talking about OCD.

For her A-level Art Project the following year, Molly created an installation entitled "Reverence and Ritual", meant as a comment on the uncanny parallels between ritual 'cleansing' in established religions and OCD 'washing'. It consisted of a metal sink (found in a junk heap) with a towel and bar of soap with a definition of OCD hanging below; floating inside the water-filled sink was a laminated photo (by Molly) of a statue of Christ, overlaid with repetitions of a phrase from Psalms: "My sin is ever before me."

Some years later, for her photographic course at Westminster University, Molly, exploring this same theme further, replicated this installation with even more 'rescued' sinks in a darkened room. This was accompanied by a highly original short film featuring constantly changing images of hands, water, scenes and quotations from the Bible, quotations from Freud and others, along with a sound track collage of interviews with a priest, a mullah, a rabbi and OCD sufferers, sounds of trickling water and other haunting and appropriate aural effects.

Molly's interest in and concern for OCD is ongoing.

Lois Chaber

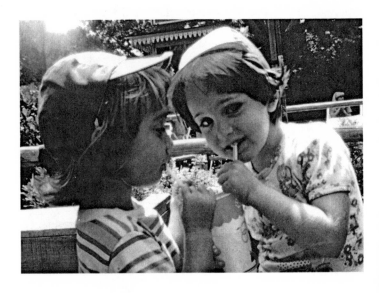

Sisters! (Sybil on right)

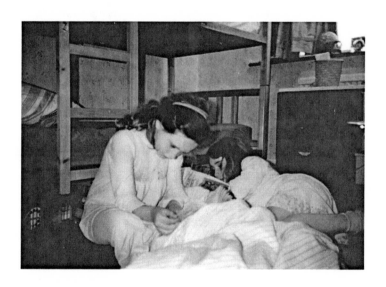

Sybil (left) and Molly near bunk beds at bedtime

Lois Chaber

Chapter 8: Crisis

Obsessive-Compulsive Disorder is a family illness.

* * *

Everyone in a family under the influence of OCD is exposed to ongoing, albeit intermittent, traumatizing circumstances.

(Herbert L. Gravitz, *Obsessive-Compulsive Disorder: New Help for the Family*, California: Healing Visions Press, 1998, pp. 17, 70.)

In later years, I discovered in the above book a remarkably accurate description of our family's plight in the girls' school year of 1991-1992. When the OCD of one member is allowed to dominate, Gravitz explains, a "family culture" of OCD—or "Para-OCD-ism"—develops, in which the other members subvert their own and the family's needs in order to adjust to the sufferer's behaviour. This Para-OCD-ism pulls the entire family into the turbulent orbit of the sufferer's OCD, so that all its members are overwhelmed by "chronic shock, chronic loss, chronic grief, and chronic exhaustion". We experienced this descent into chaos.

* * *

In the summer of 1991, following Sybil's brilliant performance at the Latymer School, we enrol Sybil and Molly in a 9-day summer holiday camp sponsored by the Scripture Union, an Evangelical Protestant organisation, partly because of our general ignorance about other camping options, partly in deference to Sybil's ongoing religious enthusiasm, and mostly because their Methodist Church, aware of Neil's unemployment and the family's straitened economic situation, agrees to fund them.

"THE THING INSIDE MY HEAD"

It will substitute for our traditional family holiday and give us and the girls a break from each other in this bleak time, Neil and I agree. But Sybil comes home from camp depressed and withdrawn; as usual, she will confide nothing, and Molly can only tell us that Sybil has been very shy in this coeducational camp (unlike her week at an all-girls' version the previous year), and has had an unrequited crush on a young lad.

It could well be that Sybil's experience at this Scripture Union camp has little or nothing to do with her current downturn; after all, the summer holidays are often a low point for her, and her disabling bouts of illness have been cyclical since childhood. At any rate, a pall of loneliness hangs over her for the rest of the summer, clinching this negative mood. Ties with her old Ashmole friends are weakening—she sees Purnimi infrequently—and she has no new Latymer friends. Her academic success at the new school had not been matched by a social one. There is no bullying at Latymer, and Michelle and Ivana, the girls appointed to orient her, have been kind and helpful, but Sybil has not been able to edge her way into the main friendship cliques of her class. Nor have Neil and I, with our lack of money and our stressed-out mood, been able to provide much stimulating family entertainment this summer.

In September, Sybil carries into the new school term her summer depression and malaise, and we soon become aware that sibling rivalry at Latymer is aggravating her condition. Our two girls, though very close and companionable, have nevertheless always competed fiercely for success and attention. Previously, the family had focused entirely on the fate of Sybil's transfer to Latymer—a new school with new challenges. Molly, having finished primary school and entered Latymer this autumn, is now in a similar position, and Sybil is no longer centre stage. None of this is openly discussed in the family, perhaps another mistake. Sybil, moreover, is still unable to find a close buddy in her class.

Lois Chaber

In alarming contrast to the previous term, Sybil, now listless, procrastinates in doing her homework and starts to fall behind in class. At home, we witnesses a recurrence of the disturbing behaviour from the Scottish holiday—prolonged hesitations, multiple repetitions, and grotesque posturing, such as standing on one leg with head tilted upward. Worse, as autumn continues, she begins to display these eccentricities at school as well, something she has not done before—perhaps a perverse way of claiming attention. We receive worried calls from Asha's father (who does the morning school run), and from sympathetic but troubled personnel at the school, inquiring about what is wrong: Why does Sybil stand all alone at lunch recess, holding her lunchbox on top of her head; why does she stop and stand in the middle of the road outside the school building, even in the face of oncoming traffic?

We are dimly aware that these disturbing actions and inactions are related to OCD, but totally in the dark as to the obsessional, anxiety-generating thoughts of Sybil's that drive such behaviours. We have conferences with the school, but no one is able to come up with a satisfactory way to help Sybil. They cannot force her classmates to befriend her; they cannot place her in the school band or the orchestra because there are no vacancies, and, furthermore, by now, her flute playing is too weak for the highly proficient musical ensembles of Latymer.

Molly becomes a distressed (and angry) witness to her sister's spiralling self-humiliation at school, feeling it will rebound against *her*. We do not explain Sybil's behaviour clearly to Molly because we ourselves are confused, mostly ignorant and in shock. Consequently, Molly is disturbed and resentful, in need of help herself, though still refusing to attend family therapy.

* * *

"THE THING INSIDE MY HEAD"

By late autumn, family routine is severely disrupted. Dinnertimes are an ordeal. Sybil spends long periods of time crouching by the toilet in the downstairs bathroom or standing on one leg, and we 'engage' by pleading with her to come out when the family is ready to eat, sometimes using force. Even at other times, she dawdles and refuses to come promptly to the table, washing her hands repeatedly, checking the cutlery we've laid out in order to make sure it's clean enough, again and again. The rest of us wait tensely at the dinner table, ignoring our food, disagreeing about what to do, till we are all frustrated and angry. When she finally comes to the table, she hesitates endlessly before starting to eat and eventually just picks at her food—very unusual for Sybil who has always had a keen appetite. We all hang on her every movement, tormenting ourselves and, probably, fuelling her craving for attention.

As for me, I am unable to cope with this dysfunctional family situation and resort to my old escape routes: threatening suicide, taking sleeping pills in the middle of the day, becoming hysterical—no matter that this behaviour shocks and threatens the children and provides an all-too-potent example for Sybil. I seem to be emphatically telling Sybil I can't bear her problems—not a great incentive for her to confide in me! I count on Neil to take control of the situation at critical moments. Once, when Sybil, Molly and I have become hysterical, bawling in unison on Molly's bed, Neil charges in resolutely and sharply slaps all three of us in turn, shocking us into silence. But Neil is often depressed himself and absorbed by his continuing inability to find a job, so shattering to his ego.

Sybil herself is opaque to us. As in so many times past, she refuses to talk about her feelings, her motives, her suffering. She must perceive that some people (including her family at times) believe her to be 'crazy', but, for whatever reason, is willing to bear this humiliation. Nor will she open up during our three-person sessions with Dr. Pamuk. The latter makes little headway with us, given

Lois Chaber

Sybil's reticence and Molly's absence, and he soon suggests to Neil and me, in private sessions, that she may need to be institutionalised at some point. His words shoot through me like an electric current: *"My* daughter institutionalised! Can this really be happening?" Dr. Pamuk speculates that Sybil, lacking a developed inner self, has created a hard carapace around herself, an outer skeleton, as a barrier between herself and the world. Sybil seems to be using her illness to form an identity.

Mornings are particularly tense all through autumn and winter. What with Molly's exaggerated lay-abed tendencies and Sybil's 'repeating things', they often hold up Asha's father in the school run, and everybody, including his own daughter, gets to school late. Hence, these daily episodes bear witness to a great deal of chivvying, scolding and even screaming on our part. We lose patience with Sybil's putting her jumper off and on, off and on again and occasionally try to dress her forcibly, or push and pull her down the stairs and out of the house into the waiting car. On February 14th, Valentine's Day, 1992, Sybil as usual is ritualistically prolonging her dressing routine; Molly is quarrelling with me over what she is or isn't doing to get ready. Finally, Molly sits down on the stairs and refuses to budge. Neil (at home of course) and I manage to hustle Sybil out the door, but Molly doggedly remains sitting, angry and stubborn, knowing this will infuriate me especially. Asha's father finally has to leave without her.

To me, Molly's behaviour is the ultimate violation of middle-class respectability: playing truant from school, something totally outside my own experience. It is the proverbial backbreaking straw in my dealings with these two increasingly difficult girls. Something snaps inside me.

I lie down on the floor, screaming repeatedly "I can't bear it any more from the two of them! I want to die!" Dr. Pamuk, whom Neil calls for emergency advice, suggests taking me to the mental health ward of nearby Chase Farm

"THE THING INSIDE MY HEAD"

Hospital. I end up staying there for a week, with no real treatment—but it is a peaceful retreat from the family turbulence. Eventually, I pull myself together, convince the staff that I no longer feel suicidal, and am discharged. However, I am secretly seething with resentment at the children and feel they are responsible for my going off the deep end, despite the fact that Neil reassures them, "You are not to blame for Mummy's illness." I am unable to take in the fact that Molly's extreme behaviour is a symptom of her own neediness and desperation in this critical family situation. In a follow-up appointment at the hospital, the consultant dismisses me as "just another menopausal woman", but the beneficial consequence of this episode is that Dr. Pamuk refers me to a well-known psychiatric treatment centre, the Tavistock Clinic in Hampstead. Any treatment for me is bound to improve the dynamics of the family and benefit the children, but the waiting list for treatment at the clinic is forbiddingly long.

* * *

As spring comes on, Sybil's awkwardness over her schoolwork increases; in particular, she has a major project for a science class that she refuses (in her passive-aggressive way), to work on at all. We are horrified at yet another breach of our middle-class expectations. Even exhortations from her teacher, in whom we confide, fail to prompt her, and things are reaching a critical point with Latymer, whose staff members have been exceedingly patient.

At the same time, it is becoming progressively more difficult to get Sybil to eat her meals. Finally, the day I have long secretly dreaded arrives. I serve a light dinner of banana pancakes with maple syrup, one of our oldest family favourites, and Sybil refuses outright to eat anything at all. My heart races with panic; this is surely anorexia nervosa! Terribly worried but also highly indignant, Neil and I try insisting that she eat, not letting her leave the table, coaxing

173

and threatening alternately, to no avail. Angry now, we tell her we are going to bring her to our local hospital, Barnet General, if she doesn't eat. She screams "NO!" but still refuses food. We force Sybil into the car, taking along the plate of by-now-cold pancakes. Sybil is crying piteously, but is adamant until we pull into the hospital's car park, when she finally agrees to eat something. Sobbing, she forces down her throat bites of a cold, sodden pancake, eating just one, but the impasse is temporarily resolved and we return home. This incident is part of a recurrent pattern that Neil and I have only half-consciously noticed: Sybil tries out some self-impairing behaviour, and, when it is met with threats or reproaches, backs down at first, only to go back to it later, with greater strength of will.

I am horrified but not really surprised at this development. The little booklet that I request later on from the Eating Disorders Association describes the child who might become anorexic as "introverted, conscientious and well-behaved". Sybil, with her passivity, her repressed anger, her low self-esteem, her diminished sense of self, was almost 'destined' to become anorexic within our family context, her own medical history, and our current financial crisis.

Thanks to my own earlier obsession with anorexia, we are very aware that Sybil's newly-emergent eating problem is not the 'slimmer's disease' of popular renown, but rather, as Julia Buckroyd defines anorexia, "using not eating as a way of expressing emotional distress and having a feeling of compulsion about that way of behaving" (*Eating Your Heart Out: Understanding and Overcoming Eating Disorders*). In other words, it is an expression of the crisis point Sybil has reached, and being a compulsive behaviour, also probably an outgrowth of her OCD. All the various theories about this eating disorder agree that for the disturbed teenager, controlling her food intake, controlling her body, appears to be a means of gaining control over her life. It is also well known that becoming anorexic is a way of

"THE THING INSIDE MY HEAD"

halting sexual development for girls—periods stop, and they lose other secondary sexual characteristics such as rounded hips and breasts. This is 'perfect' for Sybil, who has shrunk from growing up anyway.

But at this time, Neil and I are more concerned about her physical survival than about psychological theories, aware as we are that anorexia can be fatal (it has, in fact, the highest fatality rate of all the psychiatric disorders). Our family life now centres around trying to get Sybil to eat, just as it has previously centred on coping with her OCD symptoms (still present). We manoeuvre to have a classmate of Sybil's or her old friend Asha over for some of our family dinners without Sybil's prior knowledge, just springing these 'visits' on her. This strategy works temporarily, for she is too embarrassed on these occasions to create a fuss by refusing to eat. At other times, we manage to keep her in check by reviving the 'hospital' threat and repeating the 'pancake scenario'. But finally, the threats and the drive to the hospital car park lose their power and we really have to drag her into the Accident and Emergency Department and explain her persistent food refusal. When staff there cannot talk her out of it, they admit our fourteen-year-old daughter to the "Sunshine Ward" for children.

In the children's ward, the nurses coax and coddle her, and, safely removed from the threatening, ever-looming pressures of home, she gradually begins eating normally again. They then discharge her, but when she returns, the eating trails off till we are back to square one, and we feel we have no recourse but to re-admit her. In between hospital admissions, Dr. Pamuk speaks sternly to Sybil in his office, and Mrs. Greenoaks even goes once to the "Sunshine Ward" to have a therapeutic session with her, but the same cycle is re-enacted all throughout April and May of 1992. Of course, with her frequent hospital stays on top of her disinclination to do homework, her school term is rapidly becoming a disaster. We make Latymer staff privy to what has been going on, and they are very sympathetic but feel

Lois Chaber

that Sybil is unlikely to complete the term satisfactorily. She is due to go on to GCSE work next year—yet another rite of passage that she may be consciously, or unconsciously, striving to avoid.

* * *

Our family crisis is further complicated by Neil's changing situation. By 1991, the recession had become deeply entrenched in England; employees in the construction and property industries were being laid off by the thousands, and other companies were either not hiring or deeply suspicious of anyone trying to change professions. After several months of relentless but ultimately futile job hunting, Neil, not the sort of person who could just live on the dole indefinitely, undertook selling on commission only for Sun Alliance Pensions and Life Insurance—yes, that terrible cliché and last resort of the unemployed, flogging insurance—a desperate attempt to maintain his self-respect. As a part-timer, Neil still receives some dole money, and, luckily for us, at this time the unemployment benefits include payment of mortgage interest, for a limited time—a policy soon to be ended during the Conservative period in government. But before mortgage relief kicks in, things are so shaky that one day I find a bank representative on my doorstep, wagging his finger at me for our non-payment of the mortgage! Neil is sliding into worse misery, however, for the insurance peddling is uninteresting and unremunerative, and his 'clients' treat him like crap.

Hence, in 1992 we make the painful decision—without consulting the children—that Neil will make himself available for work overseas in his own profession, project management, rather than see the family sink under financially and his own soul wither and die, even if it means splitting up the family, with the girls and I staying behind in England. In late April, right during this tense period of confrontation with Sybil over food refusal, Neil receives an offer from a 'body shop' to be seconded to Shell Petroleum on a building project in Port Harcourt, Nigeria. Neil and I agonise over the decision: On the one hand, it will save our home, lift the family out of a strained subsistence existence, rescue Neil from desperation. On the other, there is a great unknown: Will this crime-and-corruption-ridden country, under a military dictatorship, prove too dangerous for Neil? What effect will his working abroad have on Sybil and Molly? Will I be able to manage competently for both of them alone at home? In the end, we follow Dr. Pamuk's strong recommendation that Neil take up the Nigerian offer as the best of a bad situation for the family.

Dr. Pamuk also advises me, under the present circumstances, to write to the Tavistock Centre and ask for emergency psychiatric help. I explain everything—the extreme anorexia, the aggravated OCD, Neil's imminent departure for Nigeria, my own lack of confidence—and, sure enough, I am moved up the waiting list and granted an assessment within a week. Once again, Sybil's plight has affected my own medical care, this time positively. Dr. Pamuk, moreover, now urges us to consider admitting Sybil to Hill End, the NHS adolescent psychiatric unit for our region, thirteen miles north of us in the town of St. Albans. About the same time as we break the news to the girls that "Daddy is going to work in Nigeria" (they are both extremely upset, despite the advantages we spell out), we also begin having exploratory family meetings, both in St. Albans and in the Sunshine Ward, with a team from Hill End. The staff members seem reasonable and pleasant to us, and we are vague and evasive with the girls about whether Sybil will actually have to take up residence there.

At one of these family meetings in May, we negotiate an agreement with Sybil: we will not finalise anything with Hill End provided she starts to eat normally. This motivates her for several days, and we are hopeful, but gradually she resumes inflexible anorexic behaviour. Again, after an initial retreat, she has then wilfully gone over the edge. We now feel incapable of solving the problem at home, and, in view of the fact that the *two* of us cannot budge Sybil now, *I alone* will certainly not be able to cope when Neil goes off, soon, to Africa. His looming departure makes us desperate, and we do something we probably would not do under other, less acute circumstances: We are informed that children under sixteen have no say in mental health admissions decisions their parents make for them. Thus, we secretly arrange for Sybil's admission to Hill End, secretly pack a suitcase for her and tell the girls only that we are going up to St. Albans for one of the usual meetings.

There in Hill End Hospital, a shabby brick building that has seen better days, after a family discussion about Sybil's eating that does not come up with any new solutions, we suddenly tell Sybil we are leaving her there. A terrible scene ensues, and we leave amidst screaming and sobbing from both girls. Sybil's subsequent resentment is never *directly* articulated by her but can possibly be gauged from Molly's intense reaction:

> *Regularly, before Sybil went to Hill End, we went to see a psychiatrist there. I hated going to these sessions. One day we went and the session finished and suddenly I saw a funny look on the face of the adults, and mum and dad said, "We've brought your bag, Sybil; you're going to stay here." They [staff members] almost dragged her off while she was screaming and crying. This was one of the worst days of my life, seeing the look on her face when she was dragged off—betrayed, scared, terrified. There was nothing I could do and I was just shouting at my parents when we got back in the car. Just because I was young, nobody would listen to me at all. I was so confused and didn't understand why my parents would do something so terrible; I hated them for*

"THE THING INSIDE MY HEAD"

it. I didn't know how they could do it, when they saw her face. I hated these people there; they were horrible; they were nasty people who didn't care at all.

Feeling utterly miserable, Neil and I nevertheless steel ourselves against second thoughts as we drive home. We genuinely feel we have placed Sybil where she will receive helpful therapy, albeit against her will. I am so panic-stricken about Neil's impending departure that I can only focus on my own neediness in the days between our 'betrayal' of Sybil and his take-off. He has been spending the whole month coaching me in how to survive without him: how to care for the machines in the house, how to get to the places *he* usually drives to, how to handle financial matters, and so on. I, like Sybil, have been extremely dependent for so many years. When I finally part from Neil, my stomach is turning somersaults, and I feel the ground giving way under me. I am really on my own now, for the first time since our marriage in 1976.

* * *

Sybil's coerced admission into Hill End Adolescent Unit does not mean I am entirely free of responsibility for her, since their policy is that the young patients must go home at weekends. Depending on the reports of their behaviour at home, they either continue there as patients, or are discharged. Neil and I have optimistically hoped that Sybil can carry on her home activities during these weekends as if nothing has happened, the better for her to re-enter the 'normal world' when she recovers—which we assume will be fairly soon. We have arranged for her to participate in the Borough of Barnet music programme on Saturdays, which Molly attends, and with great difficulty I manage to get both girls out the door and to the music centre on the first weekend, where various band ensembles practice. But Sybil cannot be happy about the fact that she is placed in a band two levels lower than Molly's. Sybil eats virtually nothing during the weekend and communicates little as well, divulging nothing of the feelings that must be churning within, except for her endless sobbing at bedtime. I don't know how to get through to her and am relieved to bring her back Sunday evening.

The following weekend, still bent on 'normalising' Sybil's time at home as much as possible, I arrange for Asha, her old friend, so mature and understanding, to come over for dinner, but, as Asha describes, it becomes an awkward occasion:

Sybil sat down for the first bit of the meal; then she left the table and we carried on eating. The time that she was in the bathroom got too long, and Lois went to check on her. She wouldn't come out. Lois came back, and then we ate for a while. Then Lois went to the bathroom again and tried harder to get her to come back, but Sybil was more adamant; I think she was screaming 'No!' There was a bit of a struggle and she came back to the meal, and it was almost completely silent. Then I turned to Sybil and asked her to tell us a Bible story (Sybil was always what I would describe as religious). She began telling a religious story, and after talking for about five minutes, she got to a certain line—something about a man looking out to the sea and the sky—and just kept repeating this line over and over again without seeming to realise that she was; then Molly interrupted her and said, "Oh, Sybil, you said that before." Sybil paused and then she said the line over and over again.

"THE THING INSIDE MY HEAD"

On Sunday Sybil won't leave her room, won't eat at all. When it is time to bring her back to Hill End, she refuses to go down to the car; just stands there, silent, hyperventilating and with unfocused eyes. I try to reason with her, but don't really know how to deal with this daughter who has become a zombie-like stranger. I panic, unable to face the thought that she may remain here on my hands in her present state, unable to offer her unconditional love and reassurance. I am obsessed with my own survival without Neil at this point, my heart beating with fear—fear of my own daughter!! Like any animal, she must be sensing this fear— and what must it be doing to her psyche?

I phone both Hill End and our local Social Services, pleading for help in getting Sybil back to the adolescent unit, but neither have any available staff on the weekend. In desperation, I call a nearby friend of ours, Jane, whom Sybil has known since primary school days. When she arrives, Jane speaks a few words of gentle persuasion, and Sybil, reluctant to create a scene in front of this family friend, complies and walks down into the car. I have no option but to give a 'bad' report about Sybil's weekend behaviour to the person in charge back at Hill End.

Unfortunately, during these two weeks or so that Sybil has been an in-patient at Hill End, I have come round to Molly's view of this unit, not at all the nurturing, therapeutic temporary home we had imagined it was going to be. "The place is run in a military sort of style," in Molly's words, with a minimum of comfort or cheer and, as we discover, a punitive philosophy. The first time I brought her back on a Sunday, dismayed by the bleak, bare walls of the reception hall, I asked the waiting staff member, "Are patients encouraged to put up posters and pictures to make the place more homey and cheerful?" He grinned and answered: "It's not meant to be homey. We don't want the young people to be comfortable here, otherwise they won't be motivated to behave better and return to their homes."

181

Lois Chaber

Hence, even over this short period, a revised picture of Hill End emerges: a stringent institution mainly for delinquents and substance abusers, an institution not physically, but mentally harsh. We have made a big mistake. However, we had been told this was the only NHS psychiatric centre for adolescents where Sybil was eligible for treatment, given our North London residence, and the family meetings we'd had provided no clue to its dismal atmosphere.

In the middle of the week following Sybil's resistance to going back, I receive an emergency call from Hill End staff; Sybil hasn't eaten or drunk anything since the weekend, and they are at their wit's end. Would I please come to the unit right away and try to feed her? When I arrive, they take me to a room and bring in Sybil, pale, thin, silent, sullen. I am asked to hold her in my lap and feed her, like a baby. They seem to believe that re-enacting a primal mother-daughter scene will trigger some emotional response in Sybil and break through the barrier she has erected. But it is an abysmal, embarrassing failure. When I try self-consciously to cradle her in my arms (with two staff members watching, almost voyeuristically), she strikes out violently at me with her arms and legs, yelling "Get Off!", and the staff members rush to restrain and reprimand her. The consultant psychiatrist asks my permission to transfer Sybil to a nearby hospital, where they can force-feed her. I manage with difficulty to get through by phone to Nigeria and tell Neil the bad news.

Sybil has been placed in the children's ward of Queen Elizabeth II Hospital, in Wellwyn Garden City, and fitted with a nasogastric feeding tube that goes through her nose down into her stomach. Earlier, Dr. Pamuk had predicted that Sybil was sure to reconsider her anorexic behaviour if this very uncomfortable device were installed, but now Sybil seems prepared to tolerate this and any other 'torture' to sustain her 'hunger strike'. Stricken with guilt, and shocked into intense concern for *her* survival now, I

"THE THING INSIDE MY HEAD"

make the forty-five minute drive up to this hospital every day,
like clockwork, to visit her and to try by my presence to
assure her of my love and concern. But it is too late. She
stands dumb and unresponsive in the ward, pointedly
turning her back to me day after day. I begin each hospital
visit by having a one-way 'chat' to her, regaling her with
family news. This gets no reaction, so most of the time I
remain sitting as close to her as she will let me for a few
hours, writing long letters to Neil. I also try reading aloud
Neil's letters to the family, but she covers her ears; so, at my
suggestion, he starts sending postcards and short letters
exclusively to her, which I leave at the hospital. These brief
but regular communications from afar, filled with tenderness
and anguish, represent Neil's utmost efforts to break through
Sybil's shell of resentful indifference, massage her abject
self-esteem and exhort her to more reasonable behaviour:

*27/09/92: Never fear Daddy is here and
thinking of you always. You are worth so much
to me.*

*05/08/92: I think about you my dear Sybil
all the time. Do let the hospital staff take care
of you. I am certain there is nothing to be
frightened of. They only want to help you and
they will help you all the more if you help them.
Please do that honey. I am sorry I am not there
to bring you roses from our garden or to have a
nice chat with you. My job, which is so
important to our family, is going very well. I can
see that I will continue to work very long hours,
which helps me not to think about missing you
all too much. You do have the strength, you
are not powerless to help yourself and to let
others help you to get better. I know my Sybil
has the strength.*

Lois Chaber

8/08/92: Do get better soon. I think you are such a terrific person and so many other people do too. I want my Sybil back. And so do Mummy and Molly. I want to know that you are letting other people enjoy being with you. I know I am not with you, but you are with me in my thoughts, and I trust and believe in you being such a good person.

Sybil remains at Queen Elizabeth II several weeks, obdurately refusing all food and drink, hardly ever uttering a word, unswervingly hostile to me despite my daily visits. Even with tube feeding, her weight sinks very low—down to the third percentile of children her age—and she is in critical danger at points. Hill End staff, still in charge, finally decide that it's best to move her back to the Sunshine Ward at our local hospital, where the nurses have previously established a rapport with her, and where it is more convenient for me and Molly to visit her. Molly has just returned from a visit to my sister Madelyn in California where I sent her to provide a much-needed break from her now-claustrophobic relationship with me in our 'deserted' home. Even in the Sunshine Ward, Sybil continues to show an implacable aversion to both of us, even ignoring my sister and her baby son when they come to London to lend me emotional support. She appears to be 'acting out' the adolescent defiance that she was never able to muster in conventional ways in our home, the 'naughtiness' to which Dr. Pamuk had tried to prompt her in the past. But it is also more sinister. When she finally begins to talk just a little to some of the nurses, she tells them she believes I'm actually a "devil in the shape of her mother"—the first glimpse of shocking, *seemingly* psychotic thoughts that are to surface again.

Some of the more kindly staff at Hill End visit Sybil in Barnet for therapeutic talks with her; this, plus the anti-psychotic medication she is now receiving and the patient

"THE THING INSIDE MY HEAD"

care of the paediatric nurses, results in improved self-care
and more willingness to talk as August draws to a close.
However, she still refuses food and drink, confiding to the
nurses that this is now mainly to forestall her return to Hill
End, which she declares she loathes. The doctors strike a
bargain with Sybil: if she starts eating immediately, she can
remain in the Sunshine Ward for an indefinite time, but if she
doesn't, they will send her back to Hill End and teach staff
there to operate the nasogastric tube. She commences
eating—hooray! But there is no letup in hostility to Molly and
me. Her feelings towards Neil are unclear; she evades
talking about him explicitly but evinces feelings of pain at his
absence. Meanwhile, not yet eligible for leave, he continues
relaying epistolary pep talks:

> *16/08/92: Mummy tells me how you are
> and that she sees you often. Do talk to her. It
> will be talking to us both, both Mummy and I
> love to hear what you have to say. I have now
> been here 7 weeks and so in less than 6 weeks
> I will be seeing you. You can't believe how
> much I'm looking forward to it. I have not
> deserted you, but I have to do my work
> separate from all of you for the time being. But
> you and I and all of us have a right and need to
> be separate at times, for ourselves or for the
> benefit of others. It doesn't mean we love and
> care any less.*

Painfully aware of Sybil's present aversion, I cannot
envision our family functioning in a wholesome way if she
returns home, even eating and talking; she herself,
moreover, tells the nursing staff she doesn't want to go
home, especially without her dad. One day late in August,
by sheer accident, in our local newspaper, I notice a social

service advertisement inviting the public to offer a foster home for a young boy, pictured on the page. Maybe this is a solution for the time being: put Sybil into a foster family so that she can heal psychologically and have a 'life' again. It would be painful for all of us, but certainly better than the chaos of our home that preceded her admission into Hill End, damaging to everyone concerned. Neil sadly agrees.

Sybil responds eagerly to my idea, conveyed through Hill End staff, and soon Barnet Social Services is arranging the legal and administrative side of things. We all decide it would be better to arrange the fostering privately with some family that Sybil already knows, given her sensitivity and precarious psychological state, even though it means we have to finance it instead of the borough. After one family politely turns me down, I can't think of anyone else we know likely to take up such a burden except Mr. and Mrs. Wells of the Methodist Church parish, they of the Sunday School and the Bible Study. They consent to the fostering, thanks to their strong Christian principles and their fondness for Sybil, and presumably the four hundred pounds or so a month we will be giving them for her room, board and care is an additional incentive to this not-very-wealthy family still paying private academic fees for two children. I am aware they are quite evangelical teetotallers, but I assume this will suit our pious daughter to a tee.

With a profound feeling of failure and desolation, I make one last hospital visit the night before she is due to move to the Wellses's home. With Sybil's slumped back turned to me, yet again, I try, sobbing, to convey some of my mixed feelings: "Sybil, I can't tell you how much pain we feel at losing you, but we so much hope this will help you to have a good future. Goodbye. I love you." This is the last time I am to see her for several months.

* * *

"THE THING INSIDE MY HEAD"

At the Wellses', Sybil is to reside in a tiny spare room up in the loft, sharing the home with Richard and Phyllis and their three children, Sybil's age and upward, all of whom she knows through church activities. The plan is for Sybil to resume her classes this autumn at the Latymer School, which will undoubtedly be very uncomfortable for her because of her 'weird' behaviour during the previous term and her abrupt departure before it ended. All of our expectations—and that includes the professionals who approved this arrangement—are possibly too high. She has been through a year of trauma and now she has to adjust to a new home, a new family, and a new term at school.

Mrs. Wells is a greying, middle-aged woman, with a plain, strong face and a no-nonsense, forthright manner that carries over into the conservative skirts and blouses she unfailingly wears. Though not openly emotional, she frequently allows the fourteen-and-a-half-year old Sybil to sit on her lap. Sybil, I believe, sees in her the sensible and stable 'mother' that I have failed to be. Mrs. Wells' description of the early fostering days indicates that Sybil is not 'back to normal':

Sybil always got on well with our family. Catherine, the middle one, was the one who did most to help Sybil. She would help her with her homework and would encourage her to do things where Sybil would have sat and done nothing. She remembers Sybil as being very forward to come and help with the washing up. Yes, Sybil was always very helpful and obliging.

But Sybil was always a bit reluctant to get down to doing homework. The very first day Sybil was with us and was going to school, she came in and said she had homework to do. I settled her down at the table to get on with it. I said to Sybil that I was only going to be in the next room because I was teaching [private lessons]. I went in to see how she was getting on a little bit later, but she was in tears and not doing anything. So I brought her in to sit in the same room as me. But it wasn't till somebody actually sat down with her that she would actually get down and do it.

For a while I took her to Latymer by car, but that wasn't very satisfactory because of traffic conditions going over that way. And then she started going on the bus. There were three buses, but that wasn't very satisfactory because there were so many changes and so much waiting around time. One day she didn't come back from school and we had a great panic as to where she'd got to. It was at that point that the borough of Enfield decided to provide some sort of transport for her.

The Child Guidance Centre is still supposed to be looking after Sybil, seeing her with the Wellses as a 'family', but Sybil is as unforthcoming as ever, from what Mrs. Wells says: "I know we saw Dr. Pamuk two or three times, with and without Sybil;. She wasn't responding at all to anything on that occasion when we brought her, just sat and didn't say anything or answer any questions."

I phone Mrs. Wells every week to find out how Sybil is doing. I am not very happy that she is unwilling to battle the morning traffic to bring Sybil to school; Asha's father had always done it. However, I am careful not to criticise the Wellses in any way; I don't want to jar this delicate fostering setup or create any bad feeling. A few weeks into Sybil's stay there, I go to the Wellses home, hoping to have a brief visit with Sybil and sustain the threads of our family's relationship with her. However, as soon as she sees me in the doorway, she turns her back and walks slowly, silently, but decisively up the stairs away from me.

Neil, who has been looking forward eagerly *and* anxiously to seeing Sybil on his first leave home from Nigeria at the end of September, does not fare much better. She vetoes his visit when he tries to arrange it with the Wellses. As determined as ever, Neil, one Sunday morning, quietly joins the Wells family at the Methodist Church in hopes that Sybil will relent, but she gives him the cold shoulder. We are hurt and frustrated, but we certainly understand her anger at the family after the Hill End episode as well as her inevitable feelings of abandonment by her beloved dad.

As the autumn advances, Mrs. Wells has to deal with a marked deterioration in Sybil's already precarious behaviour:

> *At first she did her homework if she was sat with. But it got more difficult to get her to actually do anything at all. At school, they told me, first of all, she got on with the work if encouraged very positively. But it got more and more difficult to get her to do work unless someone stood over her. She sat and didn't do things and she would go and sit down in one place and then another and stall. Some of the children there were very good to her; they tried to look after her and encourage her and help her along, but I don't think that she was really responding very much to their advances. Latymer were prepared to have her go on going there even though she wasn't really doing what she ought to. But I think they were getting worried that she was becoming a bit of a liability*

to herself, like stopping in the middle of a corridor when people were streaming past. I think the school as a whole was very understanding of the problem and I give them credit for that.

I started getting particularly bothered when she would stop in the middle of the staircase; I was afraid she might just fall down it. Then it got to the point where she would lock herself into the bathroom, supposedly washing, but in fact she wasn't doing anything and we had to take the lock off the toilet door because she locked it and just sat, and in fact we were not able to get her out. It sounds terrible, but at that time I had to wash her after a while because she didn't do it herself.

Getting dressed was another thing that she did to start with, but again, like everything, she just needed to have some help, to get things going. She ate reasonably well to begin with, I remember, but that went off, like many things. I don't know whether it was really an eating problem because it was like getting dressed and washed and everything else; it was getting to the point where she needed to have everything done for her and she was being a danger to herself in these trance-like attitudes in different places.

It was as much the fact that she was becoming a full-time job to look after really, because we didn't feel we could leave her at all. We did talk to her about it and tried to get her to say what was in her mind and what might be worrying her. If she could have expressed what her feelings and her problems were it would've

"THE THING INSIDE MY HEAD"

*been easier for everybody perhaps and easier
for herself as well, but she couldn't.*

Mrs. Wells tells Sybil and the Child Guidance Centre
that she can no longer cope, especially as she has high
blood pressure, and she is advised to admit Sybil to the
Sunshine Ward—yet again. I am terribly upset and wonder
to myself if Sybil feels betrayed by Mrs. Wells, to whom she
obviously had grown very close—but *I* am certainly not in a
position to accuse! The Wellses are still being treated as
her legal guardians, and, moreover, given Sybil's hostility to
us, we feel helpless. We learn from Mrs. Wells that Sybil is
just as unresponsive and inactive in the hospital, and,
besides, she is really too old now for the children's ward.
When she, inevitably, goes on 'hunger strike' again, she is
soon sent, unwillingly, back to Hill End, where staff learn
how to feed Sybil through the nasogastric tube.

* * *

Neil and I are now grimly determined to 'rescue'
Sybil from the Hill End Adolescent Unit. In addition to her
extreme anorexia, we understand she has reverted once
again to 'mutism' and rigid posturing. We start investigating
alternative treatment centres and learn of a highly regarded
unit for adolescents at the Bethlem Royal Hospital in Kent,
run in a totally different manner by the Maudsley Trust, one
of whose specialties is adolescent OCD.

For the next two months both of us do our utmost to
have Sybil transferred there. I have finally been assigned a
therapist at the Tavistock Centre in November, a thirty-ish
Brazilian woman, and I am receiving *real* psychotherapy for
the first time in my life. My therapist is very supportive when
I have to deal on the front line with great bureaucratic
resistance in the NHS to a transfer (Neil has returned to
Nigeria by now). The various health authority jurisdictions

Lois Chaber

and the medical profession's institutionalised sense of territoriality are the main stumbling blocks; the health care community, it seems to us, is led more by these considerations than by the patient's needs. Phone calls and letters fly back and forth between Neil (in Nigeria) and me (in London), Hill End, and the Bethlem Royal Unit throughout November and December. In excerpts from a letter written by the Hill End Consultant to the Consultant at the Bethlem Royal in November, something of Sybil's life at Hill End can be glimpsed, as well as this latter unit's somewhat sceptical attitude towards her symptoms:

> The being 'completely rigid' described early in the second paragraph of Dr. Pamuk's letter [to the Bethlem Royal Consultant] is not constant here. She has been noticed to respond quite appropriately when a male member of staff entered to assist in dealing with her tube while she was not fully dressed and she has been noticed agilely to whisk her body through a door before it closed. However, as we increased the dose of Chlorpromazine [an anti-psychotic drug] to 400 mg, her posture has become twisted and we have added Procyclidine [reduces side effects of former].

> Sybil changes very slowly. She still does not talk but has accepted the occasional holding by her peers, has gone to the W.C. by herself and has been more co-operative with her dressing and school attendance. She sometimes sits quietly during meetings, sometimes she gets up repeatedly.

"THE THING INSIDE MY HEAD"

At a certain point, Hill End becomes receptive to the idea of transferring Sybil—presumably they are by now exasperated and exhausted by her extreme passive-aggressive behaviour—but the Bethlem Royal Adolescent Unit remains reluctant to break medical protocol. On top of pleading phone calls from me to the Maudsley, Neil writes to the Bethlem Royal Consultant tactfully voicing some of the issues behind our wish for a transfer:

> *My concern and love for Sybil are very deep, and it disturbs me that economic circumstances of a long redundancy and now having to live a long way from my family have contributed to Sybil's difficulties. In my view, there is an accumulation of many circumstances, which together have brought Sybil to her current state. The two things I want to mention concern solutions.*
>
> *Firstly, there is Sybil's anorexia, her defence against situations that for whatever reasons, threaten her; to fend off these, and to avoid being swept away by the resulting overwhelming uncertainties and fears, she brings forth anorexic defences to create for herself a shell and a 'secure hideaway'. Sybil is slow to trust. Perhaps experiences have made her that way. With Mrs. Greenoaks, her counsellor at Vale Drive Clinic, it took almost a year for Sybil to become open. Hill End, because of its short-term approach, cannot move in such a way that Sybil can develop trust and be receptive to what they have to offer.*
>
> *It has been said to us that Sybil is using devices, including anorexic ones, to control situations and people, and I think that can be*

193

Lois Chaber

the case. I am not too sure about Sybil's awareness, but I think from the other side people are seeing Sybil's 'control behaviour' through their own emphases, and I am just not so sure that this concern shouldn't have a lower profile.

When Neil returns home for his Christmas leave, we immediately arrange to attend a review session with Sybil at Hill End, having now determinedly offered to take back her guardianship from the Wellses, who are happy to relinquish it. Not having interacted with our daughter for so long and conscious of her six months of hostility towards us, we await her presence in the sombre, unadorned meeting room with almost suspended breath. She enters, helped by attendants, staring up at the ceiling, body twisted, pale-faced and ghastly-thin. Wordlessly, Neil and I each instinctively reach for one of her almost skeletal, bluish hands; she grasps ours, and we are flooded with immense relief and pleasure. We are *almost* a family again.

The Bethlem Royal Unit finally consents to hold an assessment of Sybil for possible admission on the 27th of December. Neil, Molly and I collect Sybil, with her feeding tube, from the Sunshine Ward, as well as a nurse from Hill End to help us manage Sybil, and travel down to Kent. Neil and I are extremely tense since the decision about her admission depends on this interview. The professionals from the unit, including a psychologist specialising in OCD, ask *all* of us various questions about the family and about Sybil (though Sybil remains mute). The nurse from Hill End unexpectedly plays a crucial role in the outcome. When the Bethlem Royal staff query us, "Why do you think Sybil would be better off at this adolescent unit than at Hill End," she points out that the peer groups of the two are markedly different, the ones at Hill End being primarily substance abusers with Sybil quite distinct from them.

"THE THING INSIDE MY HEAD"

Excerpts from the Official Report:

III. Patient Profile:

Physical: Small, thin (said to be 36 kg.) girl obviously malnutritioned. Peripherally blue, postural oedema [swelling, inflammation], noisy breathing, standing with arms rigid and head extended backwards. No solids since 09/11/92. n/g [nasogastric] feed tube in situ, incontinent of urine. Immobile.

Emotional: Appeared sad, did cry when being told how we assumed she must be very sad.

Social: No social contact at all—isolates herself, total gaze avoidance.

Language: Mute since admission [to Hill End].

Family: Mother has history of depression.

Peer Group: No interaction with peer group.

Personal System: Ritualistic behaviour: 360 degree turns, door passage difficult. Sad. No verbal communication. Thoughts obsessive/ruminations possible.

Summary: Sybil is a 14-year-old girl with an extremely disabling and risky mental health problem. She has withdrawn and regressed to a point where she now receives care appropriate for an infant. This it would appear protects Sybil from other psychic constructs and brings her parents together where otherwise the family would fragment.

Admission offered.

One major victory for us!

Lois Chaber

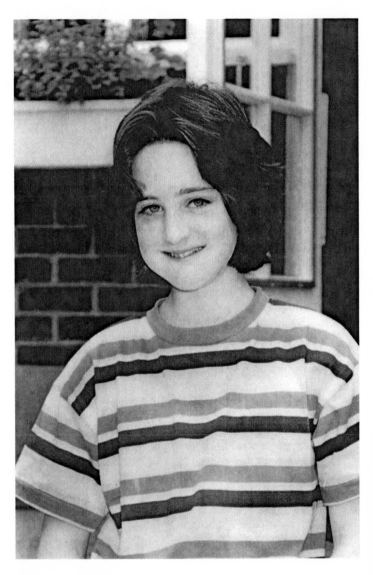

Sybil, circa 1990

"THE THING INSIDE MY HEAD"

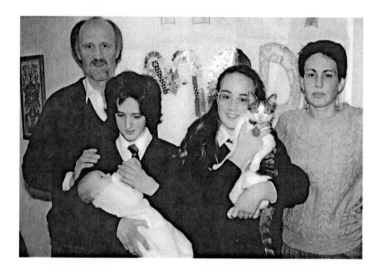

The family, with Ali-Biba and our infant nephew Charlie, during Neil's unemployment, 1991. Sybil and Molly wearing Latymer School uniforms.

Lois Chaber

"THE THING INSIDE MY HEAD"

PART II

Lois Chaber

"THE THING INSIDE MY HEAD"

Chapter 1: Ups and Downs

Sybil at the Bethlem Royal Hospital

> Lautice held the leaf out so that Saunat could see it and said, "This is the leaf of the Copa tree which grows in the Jungle of Wonders. It is a magic leaf and if you hold it and wish, it will keep you and anything or anyone safe. You have a long journey ahead of you, the quest for peace; get ready for this journey and use your power and the leaf well.
>
> > (From "Peace from the Past," a school project by Sybil, 1989.)

> We . . . have been led to distinguish two kinds of instincts: those which seek to lead what is living to death, and others, the sexual instincts, which are perpetually attempting and achieving a renewal of life. . .
>
> > (Sigmund Freud, *Beyond the Pleasure Principle* . . ., trans. James Strachey with Anna Freud, *The Standard Edition of the Complete Psychological Works*, vol. xviii (1920-22); the Hogarth Press and the Institute of Psycho-Analysis, 1955.)

Sybil, now going on fifteen, is to spend almost two years, the better part of 1993 and 1994, in the Adolescent Unit at the Bethlem Royal Hospital, a direct descendant of the notorious 'Bedlam' originally (1247) at Bishop's Gate in London, and twice relocated. 'Bedlam', which has become a byword for chaos and madness, is a corruption of 'Bethlem', itself shorthand for 'Bethlehem'.

The Adolescent Unit, along with a separate unit upstairs for children, is located in the East Wing of Tyson House, a two-storey nondescript but not unpleasant brick building, in a corner of the hospital grounds. The Unit, with facilities for fourteen in-patients and three day-patients, is staffed by a multi-disciplinary team of professionals: psychiatrists, nurses, occupational therapists, clinical psychologists and social workers. It accepts teenagers suffering from severe mental health disorders such as schizophrenia, obsessive-compulsive disorder, and severe mood disorders, but, in contrast to the Hill End Adolescent Unit, it excludes teenagers involved with drug abuse or violence. The nurses perform most of the daily therapeutic work of the Unit, mainly through individual counselling and group discussions.

Throughout these two years, the medical professionals at the Unit have their own perspectives on Sybil and our family, as excerpts from Sybil's medical records, which were not accessible to us at the time, will illustrate.

* * *

Although Sybil has been accepted into the Unit in late December, a bed will not be available till late January, and with her refusing to spend any more time at Hill End, a special arrangement has to be made with the staff of the Barnet General Sunshine Ward. Weary of caring for such a demanding patient, they agree to feed her through her nasogastric tube in the morning and night, and to bathe and dress her, but I must collect her in the morning and bring her back each evening, caring for her on my own, as Neil has returned to Nigeria after the holidays.

Sybil, with the other end of the intrusive feeding tube that goes down into her stomach protruding from one nostril—a sight I am not yet inured to—continues to reject all food and drink, remaining totally mute, dysfunctional and locked all day into a position with her head bent backwards to stare at the ceiling, even when resorting to other postures such as standing on one leg or crouching on the floor. She also refuses to swallow her saliva, believing it is poison, a throwback to early childhood. She lets it collect in her mouth, cheeks puffed out, till it overflows, dribbling all over her face and down onto her clothes. I have to jump up roughly every ten minutes and try to collect the saliva in a bowl, wiping her face and clothes.

Unable to read or watch television with her head thrust back, Sybil needs to be amused if she is not to become distressed. Although I can read to her for short periods, I am very busy during the day doing housework, collecting Molly from the Latymer School several miles away, and attending to the family paperwork that Neil's return to Nigeria has left on my hands. Wracking my brains to think of ways to keep Sybil occupied, I eventually hit on the idea of supplying her with some paper and coloured pens. She takes to the idea of drawing pictures, particularly Biblical scenes, just using her sense of touch. It is very difficult for me to leave the house at all as Sybil cannot use the toilet by herself, so when I do, for such absolute necessities as my trips to the Tavistock Centre for therapy or to the supermarket, I have to find a 'baby sitter'—my very kind and gentle cleaning woman, Lily, or Phyllis and Richard Wells, her former foster parents. My daily ministrations are forging a new bond between Sybil and me, and sometimes I think her regression is aimed at reclaiming the devoted attention from me that she didn't get enough of as a baby.

Molly, chubby and bespectacled, disaffected from secondary school and generally immersed in adolescent sullenness, at first virtually ignores Sybil when at home, just saying hello and goodbye and remaining glued to the TV set. But Sybil, frustrated by my inability to recognise New Testament scenes, takes her drawings into the living room for Molly, with her shared Sunday school background, to identify. Her face lights up with a big smile when Molly correctly guesses the Biblical incidents from the crude pictures, and from then on Molly starts taking more of an interest in Sybil's daily drawings, even volunteering to read aloud from the Bible.

One day not too long before Sybil has to leave for Kent, I secretly arrange for her former Ashmole friend Purnimi to pay a short visit. I warn Purnimi what to expect since she last saw Sybil, about six months ago, before her shocking deterioration. I wait in another room, listening, while she speaks tenderly to Sybil, telling her that she had always wanted a best friend and Sybil has been that best friend. She promises to write to Sybil and has brought her a cuddly teddy bear with valentine hearts on it. Sybil, very nervous throughout this short visit, of course doesn't respond, but after Purnimi leaves, when I hold up the teddy bear to her tilted-back head and read the lovely message in the get-well card, she breaks out into a big, happy grin.

Sybil becomes more tearful and tense as the time to go to the Bethlem Royal approaches. She has become used to coming home each day, has bonded with me, and seems to think she can remain here indefinitely as she is. On her last day but one at home she cries and prays all day, and it proves extremely difficult to get her back to the Sunshine Ward where she must be fed through her tube. In the hospital car park, she refuses to budge from the car, and I am in the process of virtually dragging her into the building when a visitor offers to help. Once again I am perhaps overanxious to get Sybil off my hands.

I strongly consider not bringing her home the last day, but decide it could destroy our renewed relationship, so I collect her. The trust I have shown touches her; she doesn't make a struggle going back, although I can see it is costing her a great effort. These past few weeks turn out to be the last period of extended time that Sybil spends at home for a very long while. The next day, January 26th, 1993, Phyllis Wells drives us to the Bethlem Royal in Kent, where, sorrowfully but hopefully, I leave Sybil to begin her new course of treatment.

"THE THING INSIDE MY HEAD"

* * *

Excerpts from Sybil's Medical Notes—the early days at the Bethlem Unit:

February 9, 1993—[*Sybil's first doctor comments on an interview with me two weeks after her admission*]: "Both girls have intimated severe anger at parents but not specific abuse allegations. One wonders whether there have always been difficulties with emotional separation from Lois who herself had an abusive background [reference to my stepfather]... Lois encouraged Neil to seek anti-depressants when he began to appear 'angry and grumpy around the house' (Is any expression of anger unacceptable in the household?) ... Lois's main concern is whether Sybil will be able to 'function again as a normal teenager'."

February 11: "Settling well into ward, enjoys company of other young people. Communicating via written messages with staff. Still requires much care in dressing, toileting, etc... Communication skills gradually improving as is her trusting in other young people here."

February 11—[*From Sybil's first Clinical Review*]: "... Sybil has indicated that she finds the regime here more friendly and relaxed in comparison to that at Hill End...

"Her medical team is considering a possible diagnosis of 'pervasive refusal disorder'—as described by Dr. Brian Lask in the 1991 Archives of Disease in Childhood: 'Such a disorder has usually been described in the context of sexual abuse, not necessarily interfamilial, accompanied by threats of major violence...'"

February 23—[*From Sybil's doctor's first extended interview with her; still mute, she writes her answers on a pad here and in subsequent interviews*]: "She is occasionally upset by her own voice saying 'nasty things' in her head. This seems to happen when she is angry. Admits she feels

205

angry at herself and also at her mother. Worries that she is going 'mad' because of the voice... No suggestion of psychotic overlay... Sybil found it 'too difficult' to explain why she began to refuse food and became mute. Described how she didn't want to undergo adolescence as she felt unready for it... Felt her mum had always placed too much emphasis on academic achievement and 'too many rules and punishments' at home."

[*After the interview the doctor comments:*]

"—? Any traumatic sexual assault in past. ? Had mother abdicated parent role? Ever been good communication between Sybil and mother? ? Had Sybil been empowered previously by seeing her mother giving way to defiant/manipulative behaviour from Sybil or Molly ..."

March 4—[A*nother interview with Sybil*]: "[Sybil] denies any sexual abuse, parental split had become more accentuated, since arrival in UK, over how to respond to and discipline difficult behaviour from Sybil and Molly... Sybil agrees that the illness role has both allowed her to avoid issues of sexuality (as seen in anorexia nervosa) and also to receive more consistent handling from her mother..."

* * *

All this time I have been visiting Sybil in Kent every Saturday or Sunday. These journeys—a combination of tube, rail and bus—are fraught with anxiety-inducing contingencies. At about the same time, I have started seeing my psychotherapist at the Tavistock Centre three times a week. I am also visiting the Royal College of Obstetricians and Gynaecologists near Regents Park several times a week to research childbearing in the eighteenth century. Reading midwifery manuals, I am hoping to write the definitive article on the strikingly unusual portrayal of women's anxiety over pregnancy and birth in Samuel Richardson's novels, my interest being partly

"THE THING INSIDE MY HEAD"

academic opportunism, partly personal obsession. All of this creates a frantic schedule, but I come to feel that undergoing these difficulties is in some way penance and compensation, however inadequate, for my neglect of Sybil during the earlier stages of her illness. During these early visits, Sybil seems to be making slow but steady progress, despite not eating, drinking or speaking, and the love and trust rekindled during those three weeks she spent at home show signs of continuing.

Saturday, February 6th, is a typical visit to Sybil in her small, sparsely furnished room with its pale institutional colours. Sybil is communicating fairly readily by written word and disgorging saliva less frequently. I read aloud from Neil's last two family letters, escort her to the communal toilet facilities, take a walk with her on the attractive tree-lined grounds, and read from the library book I have brought for her. Together, we go through the drawings she has done on large, coarse paper—which have become an outlet for her—and I give her lots of cuddles and kisses. She writes, "Can you send some of my pictures to Daddy?" She marks ticks and crosses (yes and no) in response to my various questions. She ticks 'yes' she likes her doctor, 'yes' she likes her primary nurse, 'yes' she is going to the school, and 'yes' she likes it. I am elated. Towards the end, she writes, "Tell Molly I miss her," and, "If you talk to Purnimi, tell her I am thinking of her." My heart almost breaks and I am close to tears because I have to leave her. When I am kissing her goodbye, she draws a big picture of a heart and gives it to me.

During this period, I encourage Phyllis Wells to visit Sybil and offer to pay for her transport (sometimes including a little extra in my reimbursement). She, too, has a very positive visit in February and continues these subsidised visits at intervals throughout the two years, Sybil often drawn to sitting on her lap. Eddie and Edna, Neil's cousins from Essex, also visit Sybil from time to time during her 'up' periods. We all agree that the Adolescent Unit here is a huge improvement over the one at Hill End. The other teenage patients have problems more akin to Sybil's, though none so extreme; the nursing staff is kind and compassionate, and the whole atmosphere is relaxed, friendly and caring.

Typically, I am from the very beginning concerned about Sybil's interrupted education and am gratified to learn she is getting some basic instruction at the Unit's little schoolhouse. Gwendolyn, one of the teachers, explains what a challenge it is teaching this disturbed teenager who won't speak and won't look directly at anybody or anything:

Generally you taught kids here to the level of their individual achievement. So, if you were teaching them, and maybe at the time, they weren't able easily to learn, weren't able to do the work they were used to, you taught them what you thought they were able to achieve, and then, if they were successful, you worked up to what would be their kind of GCSE work.

I remember when Sybil first came she was looking up in the air and she couldn't say anything because she had her tube. And I remember thinking to myself, "How was Sybil able to get from A to B?," because she wasn't looking ahead to see how she was going to get there, but she always managed to get into school. I thought, "How am I going to get Sybil to do some Maths if she isn't talking?" And I don't think she was writing either at first. It was very difficult to actually do any work at times; sometimes she'd just sit there. She had to get up and 'posture' as well.

"THE THING INSIDE MY HEAD"

*The first bit of Maths involved using a
Walkman. The other method was explaining it
to her and getting her to nod if she understood
it. People would ask questions and then get
Sybil to signal if that's what she wanted.
Sometimes she couldn't make a signal—she
just found it very difficult. Most of the time, if I
wanted a direct answer, I'd say to Sybil, "Oh, do
you want this?" But sometimes I'd say, "Oh, I
think this might be what she wants," and if she
agreed, then I'd look at her and say it directly as
well.*

All this time, Neil has been writing regularly to Sybil,
both colourful postcards and brief letters, which pile up,
unread, on her night table. She sometimes 'allows' me to
read them to her when I visit. He telephones her once a
week from Nigeria, and when they call her to the nurses'
phone, she comes eagerly. Although she doesn't speak to
him, her face lights up as she hears his voice talking to her
soothingly. However, as the time approaches in March
when Neil is due to return home on leave—his first one since
Sybil has gone to the Bethlem Royal—Sybil begins to take a
downward turn that appears to correlate with his upcoming
visit.

* * *

*Excerpts from Sybil's Medical Notes, March 1994—Neil's
first leave since her admission:*

March 18—[*From team meeting before Neil's visit*]:
"[S]ince she found out that her dad is returning from Africa
… [i]ncreased obsessional slowing of movements and
hesitation. [Sybil] agrees that she feels anxious much of the
day."

Lois Chaber

March 21—[*After his visit*]: "Sybil initially tried to avoid [Neil] but then stayed with him."

They note that she spent the next day kneeling on the floor and wailing.

March 24—[*From notes on the Family Review, where Sybil's team, Neil and I are present*]: "Fed back [to parents] how Sybil had been making progress up till she knew of her father's imminent return."

March 29—"[Sybil] continues prolonged kneeling on mattress in room. Intermittent incontinence of urine/faeces, needs to be physically carried to toilet, etc... Had brief home visit 27/3/93 & on Sunday 28/3. Plan: Recommend that Sybil should stay in A.U. [Adolescent Unit] over weekends, etc."

* * *

Neil and I are bitterly disappointed at the apparent connection between Sybil's dramatic downturn and his home leave; we infer that Sybil's great love for Neil has turned to anger at what she perceives as his abandonment of her. As I resume my solo visits in the weeks following Neil's return to Nigeria, I am dismayed and saddened by her ongoing regression and by her renewed hostility towards me.

Sunday, April 18th—another dismal visit to Sybil: Her room smells of urine and stale spittle. She is sitting on the thinly-carpeted floor, with head tilted way back and arms held out rigidly, her entire physical being radiating aversion to me. I try getting her to sit or lie on the bed with me, but she resists strongly and just slithers to the floor again, so I sit near her on the floor. She turns her back to me and shrinks from my kisses. She slobbers out saliva violently into a small plastic bowl every fifteen minutes or so. I spend some time talking and reading to her. She remains impassive, but towards the end of my visit, tears appear in

210

her eyes. Several times I put pen and paper on her lap, hoping to induce her to write something—anything—but there is no response, just as there is no response to my affection and reassurances when I leave. Visits continue in this mode throughout the next month.

*   *   *

Excerpts from Sybil's Medical Notes—the team's concerns in May:

May 13—[*From Sybil's Clinical Review*]: "She is no longer spitting at staff. She requires a toileting programme for incontinence. Her refusal to 'mobilize' on her own is causing strain to the nurses' backs...

"... She has intimated to Jane [her primary nurse] that she has a 'secret' that nobody else will understand. She appears to still have obsessional religious thoughts, based on which she is often to be seen extending her arms in the air."

The team reports that Hill End has said that they found "no evidence" *for c.s.a. [sexual abuse]; the note goes on to say,* "However, some of Sybil's ongoing behaviour and communications (the 'secret') seem to indicate that c.s.a. may be a possibility... Jane to explore issue of c.s.a. [sexual abuse] directly with Sybil."

*   *   *

A turning point, or 'up', for Sybil comes with the advent of her fifteenth birthday on May 18th, 1993. Yet again, for me, there is the difficult decision about whether to 'sacrifice my time' for Sybil's sake—the old, haunting crux of my life. Should I visit Sybil as usual on the weekend and bestow her birthday gifts then, or should I make a special trip as well on Tuesday, her birthday day? I go for the latter option, fortunately, as it turns out. I enter the Unit with great trepidation due to the many weeks of her discouraging behaviour and arrange with her primary nurse Jane (who has a light touch) to preside over the opening of Sybil's presents. When I walk into her room, by now filled up with the fluffy toy animals, small pot plants and miscellaneous bric-a-brac that well wishers have sent her, and say "Happy Birthday," Sybil actually gives a prolonged, embarrassed smile and looks directly at me for the first time in weeks! Jane opens Sybil's presents, affectionately teasing her as she does so, even coaxing her to participate ever so tentatively. Sybil alternates between smiling and looking at us and throwing her head and hands back with her mouth agape like a frozen scream. There are gifts from relatives and friends, but best of all is a *huge* card from her old class at the Latymer School, individually signed by each member, with their generous gift of a stylish denim shirt and toiletries. And the Unit has planned a little party for her later that day. Sybil appears quite touched that so many people have affectionately remembered her day.

This improvement continues, though erratically, in the ensuing weeks.

* * *

Excerpts from Sybil's Medical Notes—the team's comments on Sybil and family in June:

June 1—[*From inpatient medical notes*]: "N.B. Sybil has been saying she's embarrassed that everyone is asking her if she's been sexually abused because she has not."

June 15—[*From the doctor's interview with Sybil*]: "She wrote that her main fear is of being sent to Hell. She believes in this concretely as somewhere you go if you are bad, where you are tormented forever and separated forever from God. She then 'said' she did have 'angry thoughts' and she had to engage in rituals to 'undo' them... Has told

"THE THING INSIDE MY HEAD"

Primary Nurse she believes she will give people cancer and viral infections..."

June 17—[*From Sybil's Clinical Review*]: *In a* "Reformulation", *the team summarises their understanding of Sybil so far:*

"Sybil seems to have a full house of etiological vulnerabilities:

1) Genetic—mother has psychiatric disorder

2) Organic—early birth trauma

3) Psycho-dynamic factors—no early attachment to mother left her feeling that angry thoughts were not allowed as her early representation of mother was someone with no resilience or capacity to withstand angry feelings. Early on she defended herself by being a model child, but when her father became absent (preoccupied with work) her angry feelings were combated with obsessional rituals. When father left for Nigeria the obsessional rituals were unable to defend her against a further escalation of angry feelings. The angry feelings were then driven underground by a regression to a state of complete psychological, social and physical withdrawal; this state had the effect of making her parents feel as if she were angry with them by her refusal to have anything to do with them... "

"Treatment": *The team decides there will be no OCD therapy, as they feel Sybil does not at this time wish to stop her rituals.* "Psychodynamic type treatment has been tried, and currently would be over intrusive and likely to do more harm than good." *They decide that no family therapy is possible because of Neil's residence in Nigeria.* "The current milieu therapy of a resilient and robust network of staff who are able to tolerate her may make her more able to accept her angry feelings. In the future some cognitive programme of graded exposure to angry feelings, starting

213

with ones which would seem totally benign to most people could be attempted."

* * *

In June 1993, despite her birthday upswing in May, Sybil begins to deteriorate again. On Saturday the fifth I have a very mixed visit. The visit begins well, but true to her old pattern of self-affliction and self-degradation, much of the time she kneels on the floor, head held back, letting the mucous from her nose (she has a cold) drip into her mouth while saliva drips out of it. After a long period of non-communication, I make, near to my departure time, a final desperate effort to engage her emotionally. I start crooning to her, "I love you darling, I'm here for you honey, I'm thinking about you all the time..." When I climax by saying "You're a great girl," she bursts into tears, but lets me hold her and massage her back, continuing to cry for some time. At an earlier point, when she left her room briefly, I had glanced at some of her scattered scribblings about 'voices' in her head, which end on this disturbing note: "Sometimes I wish I had never been born... I hate myself."

By August, she is spending so much time kneeling that her knees are swollen and inflamed, and the doctor is worried about possible arthritis. During my visits she often is incontinent in front of me and the nurses have to wash and change her in her room. They tell me this is happening about four times a day.

On August sixth I receive a phone call from the current registrar conveying some of the conclusions of a staff meeting. With regard to the vexed issue of Neil's home leaves, they now want us to meet with staff before Neil sees Sybil to discuss some ground rules for his visits—their length, frequency, and so on. They suggest that Neil only visit Sybil when accompanied by me, so that we present a "united front", for Sybil may see me as a "rival" to herself. He tells me they'll soon begin a trial period of using the drug

"THE THING INSIDE MY HEAD"

Clomipramine on Sybil (the medication for OCD that I first read about in 1991).

Around this time Sybil revives the 'toilet syndrome' to which she had resorted at home: retreating into the toilet to isolate herself and to associate herself with what is repellent. On a typical visit, she'll flee from me into the Unit's girls' washroom, crouching on the floor by the inside door, and then lock herself into a toilet cubicle if I try to follow her.

Another phone call from the same registrar in early September leaves me very distressed. The doctors are now beginning to wonder if Sybil has become psychotic and want to give her an increased dosage of Chlorpromazine, the anti-psychotic drug. Up to now, he says, the 'voices' she refers to frequently have been assumed to be obsessive-compulsive urges, but now they wonder if they are actually delusions, for she has mentioned some apparently psychotic beliefs: she believes the stars in the sky are actually people from alien planets who are sending her special messages through the television set. The issue of whether Sybil is psychotic or not will continue to haunt her care.

Even more disturbingly, he tells me, cautiously, that they have decided to make inquiries in our local area about possible options for Sybil's residence, in the near future: either an institution of some kind or the possibility of living at home. I ask, "Does this mean that if she doesn't improve soon, you'll consider her a hopeless case?" The registrar assures me they are still working very hard with Sybil, but he doesn't actually deny my inference.

I at once become panic-stricken and depressed, first, to think that Sybil may actually never get better after all, and second, to think that I may have to become her full-time carer. How could I possibly cope, with Neil abroad, when now on the ward it usually takes two nurses plus a wheelchair to deal with Sybil? I think of her room at the Unit, usually reeking of stale urine and saliva... When I talk to my therapist about it, later, she tells me I *should* consider taking care of Sybil at home—maybe she needs to get away from the hospital. My fear of being able to cope is in fact a repetition of what happened in her infancy, she admonishes.

In fact, the most helpful and successful aspect of my intensive therapy so far has been my Brazilian doctor's pragmatic counselling about my interactions with Sybil at the hospital and with the persistently pugnacious Molly at home. She has helped me to foreswear violent and degrading physical entanglements with Molly consequent upon her most extreme behaviour, among other valuable counsel. Sadly, less progress has been made in digging out and tamping down the core of my anxieties or in convincing me to withdraw from my medication.

At the Bethlem, the staff is trying new tactics with Sybil in October. She has recently taken to wrenching out her nasogastric tube, a worrying and potentially very damaging new habit, which has led staff to believe that maybe she needs to, or wants to be, force-fed orally. Pat, Sybil's new primary nurse, Jane having left the Unit, is particularly enthusiastic about this experiment. They want Sybil to experience 'taste' again, so they will try getting some liquid food down her throat, even if it is only a dribble. Sybil is extremely uncooperative, mostly refusing to swallow, but they carry on regardless, and then proceed after a while to feed her through the tube.

During the latter part of this year, Neil has continued communicating with Sybil from distant Nigeria with a stream of upbeat and affectionate postcards, using the irregular and unreliable mail services of various companies or friends going on leave. He persists in telephoning as well:

"THE THING INSIDE MY HEAD"

Making an international call from Port Harcourt was very difficult, especially during the first year I was there. Few phones had international access, so queuing for a call of predetermined length at the national telephone company was the most common, and half the time I would come away disappointed as there were no lines available. The French contractor on the project I worked on had an international line, but getting through could take up to two hours of dialling. Sometimes I would get through to the hospital, but the operator could not connect me to the Adolescent Unit. If a nurse on the Unit was available to pick up the phone at night, Sybil might not want to come to the phone. If she came to the phone, I would chatter on, perhaps hearing her breathing heavily (for she was not talking), willing my words to bring cheer to her heart. At any point in all of this, the line might go dead.

And during the autumn, Neil begins in earnest to search for a job back in England, despite the ongoing recession, impelled by Sybil's need for him. He is immensely frustrated by her unpredictable, usually hostile and regressive behaviour during his leaves and feels helpless, not knowing what to do, how to react, other than to be patient and, however awkwardly, try to physically demonstrate his commitment and love.

* * *

Excerpts from Sybil's Medical Notes—parental issues in October

October 21—[*From Sybil's Clinical Review*]: "Just prior to this Clinical Review, Sybil's father had been in the country for two weeks and had visited her quite frequently. Previously this intense contact had been thought to be associated with a deterioration in her behaviour, but on this occasion her clinical condition appeared to improve somewhat in the middle of the stay, in that Sybil started to communicate with members of the nursing staff by signing [using improvised sign language], which was something she had not done for some time. It was felt, however, by the nursing staff, that some of her parents' behaviour during their visits might be difficult for Sybil to cope with, e.g. they tend to follow her around the Ward and sit on the floor when she does. Her father also 'pets' her, touching her face, which she does not appear to like very much and on one occasion during this visit she had become quite angry and had hit her father. Just prior to the Clinical Review, her father had said goodbye to her before returning to Nigeria and it was unclear whether this was connected with Sybil once more becoming quite uncommunicative.

"The differential diagnosis [for Sybil] appears to lie between a possible but unlikely organic or neuropsychiatric disorder, a form of pervasive refusal syndrome, a gradually worsening psychotic illness or possibly an affective problem with a depressive/hysterical component."

The team decides it will try to exclude these possibilities, one by one.

* * *

On Friday, October 22nd, I receive a call from a different registrar, who tells me that they are currently investigating the possibility of organic damage. Sybil has already had a brain scan, which was normal, and now they're going to give her an ECG and several blood tests for neurological possibilities. All this testing comes to naught.

Meanwhile, the oral feeding experiment continues, and the nurses have asked me to participate, hoping this will

"THE THING INSIDE MY HEAD"

have a beneficial effect on Sybil; however, this backfires—like the similar 'feeding scenario' at Hill End—for she is even more adamantly resistant, as well as resentful, when *I* hold the cup to her lips. Taking a cue from Sybil, I try to back out of this programme, but my therapist compares this to appeasing Molly when she is difficult, and Pat the nurse is cross, so I carry on, ruefully.

Around mid-November 1993, Sybil begins to improve again. I come bearing a letter from Purnimi and reading it to Sybil, which brings lots of smiles to her face, is the highlight of my visit. But there is a telling moment when Purnimi recounts how she bumped into Asha, Sybil's old primary school friend, one day. Asha, she says, "told me that the kids from Latymer really miss you!" Suddenly, Sybil takes up her pad and writes: "How could they miss me?" "Because you are a lovely person," I say to her, and I tell her how Miss Melzer, her former teacher, has told me "that Sybil had made a strong impression on the class". Sybil looks at me quizzically, obviously finding this hard to take in. But a week later she shows me what she's made during the interval: a huge birthday card for Purnimi with writings and drawings all over it, which she nervously gives me the go-ahead to deliver. Then, on an impulse, she writes brief notes to Purnimi's younger sister and to Molly, as well. These are her first attempts at communication with the outside world in the ten months since she has been in the Adolescent Unit.

Throughout the year, Sybil's participation in the Unit's school has followed the course of her cyclical ups and downs. At times they've literally had to carry her there or forcibly transport her in the wheelchair, just on principle, but now she is once again taking part, though still posturing frequently. During a visit at the end of November, the nurse Meg tells me that every Friday the schoolteachers, in conjunction with the students, formally assess each patient's efforts that week, and for this past week they have awarded Sybil an 'A' for the first time.

Lois Chaber

Molly has sometimes accompanied me in my visits to Sybil during the year but has found the long boring journey on public transport and the uncertain reception from Sybil at the other end very off-putting. Each time, I've had to struggle to get her up and out of bed on a Sunday and 'bribe' her with a couple of teenage magazines. Molly comments:

I felt a mixture of feelings about going to see her: going was like a duty; staying at home made me feel guilty. Mum and Dad would go on at me and say that I would have a stronger influence on her, was closer to her age and could bring her out of herself more. I just didn't go enough really. It was hard when she wasn't communicating. I guess I was just being selfish and not really thinking about her, just being bored there. We'd tell her about things and give her letters and she'd get a lot of gifts, especially soft toys. Sometimes she was worse and sometimes she was better. My mum tried to explain to me what she had, but I didn't really understand much. I knew she had mental problems.

One picture of the Bethlem I have in my mind is Sybil sitting in her room, not speaking. She was collecting saliva in her mouth and she had a bowl, which she would spit it out into. She was communicating at times with hand signals. The young people in the ward seemed to be really nice friends, and there was a boy there whom I think she was friends with, who would come in while we were talking to her and talk to us. He made her a friendship bracelet and made me one too. It seemed like a nice place, as opposed to the Hill End Adolescent

"THE THING INSIDE MY HEAD"

Unit, the staff helping her to go to the toilet,
washing her and generally trying to help her.

Molly's last visit to the Unit for this first year is in December, to celebrate the beginning of Chanukah, the Jewish festival, with Sybil (a cherished family tradition, despite the girls' Christianity). At one point, coming back to Sybil's room after getting some tea, I find the two of them engaged in an animated 'conversation' in sign language about a picture of one of the popular 'boy bands' in Molly's teen magazine. They are exchanging views about the good looks of the members of the band and, much to the pleased surprise of Molly and me, Sybil points out her favourite one. Welcome to adolescence, Sybil! Later, in the toilet with me, washing her hands from saliva, Sybil tells me in sign language that she "loves Molly so much".

Neil is home from Nigeria for Christmas, and Sybil is deemed well enough to come home on two separate days. Having been instructed by staff, Neil and I manage to feed her through her tube while returning her to the unit for her night-time meal. She is delighted to be home for the holiday at first, but engages in a lot of posturing rituals, and by the end of the second day she has deteriorated considerably, descending into misery. It was a big step, perhaps too big.

* * *

January, 1994: It has now been one year since Sybil joined the Adolescent Unit. The force-feeding experiment has not been a success, and Sybil's primary nurse is changed, with Pat transferring to a different ward; I wonder, sadly, whether that's due to frustration over Sybil's lack of progress. Although a young woman, Mary, is designated the new primary nurse, it is actually the more mature and experienced Nicola, appointed as associate nurse but in fact senior to Mary, who is supervising the team. A second

221

Lois Chaber

associate, Debbie, has also been added to Sybil's nursing team; it is rare in the ward for someone to have three key nurses, but Sybil's extreme, unique case warrants it, and the three make a point of showing Sybil that they are all standing together. Nicola, a heavy-set blonde who appears to be in her thirties, with a pleasant face and a good sense of humour despite her sometimes quite firm manner, has strong views about what Sybil needs at this point:

When Debbie and Mary and I took over, I think the feeling was that Sybil had been diagnosed with so many different things; she had been treated for an eating disorder, OCD, depression and early onset schizophrenia. We felt that everyone else had given up on her. All these treatments had helped to different degrees, but it felt as though we were hitting the wrong spot. I felt that we should deal with the core, not the symptoms that she threw off at times, so I was very keen that we look at it differently. We described to Sybil what we felt this core was, and that, via the [therapy] sessions she would have, she would find words for the feeling she was unable to presently give words and meaning to. I remember when we first all met, we agreed that what we took on with Sybil had to be a clear plan for her to take responsibility for herself now. We felt that the pulling out of the tube was just a cry for help really, and we felt that we needed to give her the control back. We'd say to her that she would be leaving in eight months regardless of what state she was in and would have the opportunity to move on with her life, although we acknowledged that would be very difficult.

"THE THING INSIDE MY HEAD"

*There were things we needed to be very
clear about, like, when we bathed her* [after
incontinence], *that we all wore gloves and didn't
speak to her and things like that; it needed to
be a matter-of-fact thing so that there shouldn't
be a positive reward for negative behaviour.
The same with the wheel chair: it was OK for
using to move from A to B, but it shouldn't be
left outside as something for her to move
around in all the time. She needed to be
motivated to be normal and get out of this sick,
bizarre role she had taken on. Also, I think
people needed to be honest with her. In the
past, she'd sometimes release everything that
was in her mouth down people's trousers or
shoes. It was this sort of behaviour which got
people into the anger thing, and I always used
to say, "Don't just not say anything, but come
across angry; just say to her, 'Why did you do
that to me? I'm just trying to help you'." We
should try to get across to her that it is
unacceptable and it does make us angry.*

Nicola also has her own opinion on the cause of Sybil's
present illness:

*There was some feeling before that there
had been a major trauma, and this was the
result of it. I suppose I just didn't really believe
that. I think it was a case of a combination of
things that had happened. She would often say
quite shocking things, like, "Do you think my
father sexually abused me?" And I'd say, "No, I
think what has actually happened and why you
find it so hard to talk about it, is that it all seems*

like nothing." And one of the things was the family being in Qatar and unable to leave because Neil's passport had been taken away. I think it was things like that, which when she told them, it felt like they weren't anything major. Why should that have upset her? But it obviously did. She was very worried about her mother and father in the case of Neil's passport. And it was by her bringing up things like that, that gradually she realised we weren't expecting a big disclosure.

And Nicola describes how difficult it has been to care for Sybil:

We had problems because she used to constantly kneel on the floor and then stand up and repeat this all day; the skin on her knees was breaking down and she would not stop. That was the worst time we had with her, really, when she was doing repetitive behaviour, when she was being doubly incontinent, etc. Nursing her was really hard; you were trying to work, but you had to bathe her and change her and everything. Then you'd put her on the loo to make sure it wasn't going to happen again— and you knew that she had control of it, yet, five minutes later she'd be wet again. I remember trying in supervision to get people to think round their anger and understand why Sybil would want us to feel this for her. I think she was projecting a small amount of how awful it was to feel the way she did; she wanted us to react.

"THE THING INSIDE MY HEAD"

When she got a bit better, she'd do roly-polys down the corridor; she had this habit of crouching down, and I think she'd roll to move on from that. She used to have this network, down the wall, which we could never quite understand. She'd say that it was because there was a certain sort of electric field that goes down the wall, so she'd move to certain points or she'd twirl around every now and again. I remember when she was getting better, I used to joke with her that I would electrify those pathways: "That will give you a zap, every time you walk on one."

Once when I was talking to some friends about her, I said, "I can't believe one person stirred up such extremes of emotion in me: one minute I absolutely adored her and loved her, and the next thing, I couldn't stand her because of what she did and what she physically put us through in having to take her backwards and forwards."

Unfortunately, this changeover in Sybil's team has adversely affected her, as does most change, and she is 'down' again, hiding in toilets, posturing, and showing hostility towards me, although this fluctuates. All I can do is keep visiting, reiterating my love and support.

* * *

Lois Chaber

Excerpts from Sybil's Medical Notes—the team's view of Lois in January 1994:

January 13—[*From the Clinical Review Management Decision Sheet*]: "There has been some concern about [Sybil's] physical state, in that she looks quite pale and unwell at times... The consultant reported his impressions of Sybil, in particular that when she was at her best she appeared very in touch, with a good sense of humour.

"There have been two family sessions in the past two weeks, since Mr. Macindoe has been on leave in this country. On the second occasion Molly came and the consultant was impressed by how thoughtful and sensitive she seemed and how aware of how Sybil might be feeling about things. In particular, Molly was very angry that Sybil had been put into Hill End Hospital against her will and she thinks that Sybil's current presentation is because of her anger and frustration rather than mental illness. Sybil's mother has appeared quite 'drugged' in the sessions, and it is clear that she has severe psychological/psychiatric problems of her own. She appears to have difficulty appreciating how things may be for either Sybil or Molly and Molly talked at some length about being persistently nagged by her mother, who admitted this.

"Mrs. Greenoaks who had seen Sybil for individual weekly therapy for some time prior to her admission to Hill End Hospital then [in the Clinical Review, not the Family Session] gave her impression of the problems. She felt that Sybil probably felt that she could not win with her family and that she finds her relationship with her mother impossible. She gave a couple of poignant examples:

"1) Sybil's mother appears quite obsessional in her own right, and would want Sybil to brush her teeth at a particular time. If this was questioned, she would say 'How do I know if she has brushed her teeth when I don't know

226

"THE THING INSIDE MY HEAD"

when she is doing it?' 2) She had also been as much as a half-an-hour late on several occasions picking Sybil up from psychotherapy, because she had become involved in a library. When Mrs. Greenoaks wrote to Dr. Chaber about this, her mother then confronted Sybil and blamed her, and Sybil was left feeling very angry. The psychiatrist felt that Sybil had great difficulty expressing her anger with her mother, whereas Molly is able to be more direct about this.

"... Dr. Pamuk [the former family therapist] had been worried about Dr. Chaber's mental state and had referred her to the Tavistock, where she is currently being given individual psychotherapy of her own, three times a week. While he had been seeing the family, Dr. Chaber had had a 'breakdown' requiring admission to Chase Farm Hospital. The reason for her extreme distress had been because Molly had refused to go to school that day, but Sybil then felt very guilty because her mother in some way blamed her for her illness. This had been in late 1991 and then in spring 1992 when her father was due to go abroad, Sybil's hunger strikes started. It would seem that being left to cope with her disturbed mother was more than she could bear. This was elaborated on by Mrs. Greenoaks, who said that she thought the fact that Sybil had started menstruating at this time was also significant. She had said that she did not wish to grow up as she was afraid of becoming like her mother.

"Dr. Pamuk reported that Sybil had appeared most 'normal' when she was a patient at Barnet General Hospital, having been transferred there from Hill End when she was not eating. She had apparently functioned well there and had looked after other children with problems. She had begun to talk to nurses about her problems in a way that was showing her difficulties, e.g. her anxiety about feeling so angry with her mother that she wanted to hit her. Both the family therapist and the child therapist gave further details about Sybil's time with foster parents, the Wellses. It had previously been thought that they were a very ordinary family, and Sybil's inability to live there was indicative of her own mental illness. Apparently, however, they also had their own difficulties, and in particular were religious in quite an evangelical and controlling way, which may have given Sybil further dilemmas.

"Discussion focused on the fact that more information had been presented by both Dr. Pamuk and Mrs. Greenoaks which gave more emphasis to the family pathology, and in particular the problems Dr. Chaber has which may make it difficult for Sybil to interact with her in any normal sort of way. There was concern expressed about how unwell Sybil is at the moment and how, if something does not change, her life is literally at risk, as the times when she is not communicating appear to be very stressful and tiring for her...

"It was thought unlikely that more family therapy would be helpful except possibly in a supportive way, and the only way of implementing significant change is likely to be some 'shock to the system'. In this context abreaction *[revival of repressed memory]* and hypnotherapy were discussed. ECT was also mentioned, although the majority of people were against this. It is possible that we may recommend separation from her parents, with no visiting for a while, since there is a lot of evidence that contact with them has had a mainly negative effect in the past..."

* * *

Thursday, February 10th: I have just come back from a meeting with the consultant and the registrar at the Unit. Sybil's team now feels that it would be inappropriate and unhelpful for her to return home when discharged. They are going to look for a "placement" for her, possibly at a "therapeutic community" for adolescents. I am as shocked and upset as when they previously told me that she might have to be discharged home regardless of her condition, but the former panic is now replaced by a dull ache in my heart and a feeling of despair: "How tragic our family life has become, our massive pile of attractive, well-stocked family photo albums just a mockery!" Even though the two doctors did not explicitly fault anyone, I am engorged with self-blame. I accept their recommendation about Sybil's future without much dissent, as does Neil, dully, when I call him in Nigeria that evening, just as we once yielded up the infant Sybil to the policies of the Tehran Clinic.

Just about this time I receive a second blow. My therapist, with whom I've developed a very close relationship thanks to the three visits per week, tells me that she will have to discontinue my therapy just before Easter (due to her pregnancy, which I only discover by accident). She has helped me to survive and to develop in strength throughout this extremely challenging period—dealing with Sybil's extraordinary illness and Molly's exaggerated rebellion while Neil is in Africa. I am devastated by her news, but resolve, with her encouragement, to use my freed-up time to visit Sybil more frequently.

Sybil is picking up. In one visit in March, when I arrive bearing a long letter from her friend Purnimi, I find to my delight that she has prepared a Mother's Day card and gift for me, and is so 'up' on this occasion that she writes brief letters to her old Latymer class and her former teacher for me to deliver, overcoming her acute embarrassment. However, she has mixed, indeed confused, feelings about the plans for her future. One day at the end of the month she writes down, "How is Ali-Biba [our cat]?" I answer, "He's just fine!" Poignantly, she writes down, "I wish I were a part of ...", and stops, crossing it out. I am sure she meant to write, "of the family", but I remain silent. Then she writes, "I'm not sure I want to go to a..." and crosses it out, again. I supply, "to a therapeutic community?" No comment. I do my best to present this option in a rational, optimistic light, but I am aching inside. I ask, "How does Natalie [fellow patient] feel about going to a therapeutic community?" and she writes, "She wants to go." "Why?" Sybil writes, "Because when she's with her family, she has OCD."

Lois Chaber

Sybil at this time has a very good relationship with a group of other patients in the Unit and is well-liked, despite her mutism and her other severe handicaps. For the first time in her life she actually feels she 'belongs' to a clique of young people. This, more than anything else, appears to be spurring improvement and buoying her up. The peer group therapy, which is at the heart of the Adolescent Unit's regime, really is working for her! It comes to a climax, as in the previous year, around the time of her birthday, her sixteenth, in mid-May, when once again her usually abysmal self-esteem is boosted by all the attention she receives. Over the phone, the nurses tell me that there's been a birthday party for Sybil during which she has actually *spoken* to one friend, saying "Thank you", and, teased and encouraged by the other young persons, she has actually *eaten* a tiny piece of birthday cake!

A week later I walk into her room and settle into the usual monologue of family 'news', only to be interrupted by Sybil: "I'm talking now, and eating, too!" Even the positive reports I've had from staff haven't prepared me for this, the first sound of my daughter's voice for almost two years. "I fancy James [a fellow patient]," she proclaims to me with naïve pride. A stream of personal feelings gushes forth, feelings she would have normally repressed. I am ecstatic and can hardly wait to return home and phone the good news to Neil. It is near miraculous; earlier in the winter her life was at risk, and there was little hope of recovery.

It's a momentous event even for staff, whose official policy had been to 'play it cool' if and when Sybil started talking. Gwendolyn, now Sybil's key teacher, tells me later:

I remember the first time she spoke, in one of the confidential groups that meet regularly at certain times, with the same adults and peers. She suddenly got up in the group and said

230

"THE THING INSIDE MY HEAD"

"Hello" in this very little voice, and she smiled;
you could see it was a great effort, but
suddenly, it just came out. I didn't make a fuss
about it, because when they talk, especially
when Sybil talked, you're never sure, if you
make a fuss, whether they'll ever talk again.

But Nicola was caught off guard: "I'd been on leave and she
came up to me and put her hands to my ear and she went,
'Hello'. I wanted to be calm and cool and very professional
and go 'hmmm', but I didn't. I screamed and burst out
laughing and then said, 'Oh, that wasn't very good, was it?'"

These few weeks, when Sybil begins to utter words
and take in food and drink, are the high point of her stay at
the Bethlem Royal.

* * *

Over the ensuing months, frightened by the giant
steps she has been taking towards 'normality', Sybil
occasionally goes backward. Moreover, now that her
mutism and food refusal have been largely eliminated, it has
made her obsessive compulsive disorder more marked and
obvious: her ritualistic gestures, her rigid posturing, her
repetitions and hesitations, excessive hand-washing and
fear of contaminating others become at times quite
pronounced, although at other times she is quite lucid,
amiable and functioning well.

Sybil starts taking more interest in her appearance,
in late May getting her *first* haircut at a hairdresser's *in
almost two years*, a move she has consistently resisted
heretofore. She now begins to take a great interest in
information about sex, asking me to bring her the teenage
magazines, *Mizz* and *Just Seventeen* when I come. In fact,
we develop new 'rituals' of interacting, Sybil and I, in this

231

post-birthday period. Every week I bring her one or two of these somewhat sensationalistic magazines and we go through them together, at her insistence, with Sybil absolutely devouring the 'advice' columns, which are mostly about sex. I also bring two gooey, sugary-smelling donuts from the train station, which she devours as hungrily as the teen magazines, her mood almost invariably lifting.

This burgeoning adolescent 'normality' has its downside, however. She confides to me that when she told James she 'fancied' him, he replied that he liked her "only as a friend". This rejection by good-looking young men on whom she has a crush is to become a persistent and frustrating pattern in Sybil's life A male nurse tells me about a distressing incident when Sybil and her crowd were in the lounge one day: When Sybil noticed James chatting up her friend Natalie, she started *screaming,* and soon poor James was crying. The nurses had to intervene.

During Neil's end of April leave, he has taught me the rather circuitous car route down to the Bethlem Royal, a big step for me with my poor sense of direction and my phobia about getting lost. I make this car journey, with great trepidation, every few weeks from here on in because Molly is more willing to come, and it's possible with the car to take Sybil on outings to the cinema, which she is willing to attempt from June onwards. She is eager to see family films like "The Lion King", but it is always tenuous as to whether she's going to be able to get into the car and not get 'stuck' with OCD at the last minute, and on one occasion she spends half the time in the theatre covering her face with her hands.

Another regular outing the three of us start making in the summer is to a Wimpey's in the nearby town of West Wickham. When Sybil does eat, she has a hearty appetite, and it gives me an enormous gratification—perhaps too much, considering our pathological family associations of love with food—to see her consume cheeseburger, chips and pie á la mode after two years of extreme anorexia. But perhaps I have rushed her into these activities; my Tavistock therapist always chided me for pressuring Sybil with too many expectations. At Wimpey's, Sybil stands up and sits down repeatedly, sometimes endlessly, before she can settle into eating, while Molly and I watch on, trying to be patient, but feeling excruciatingly uncomfortable as Sybil becomes the focus of attention for staff and customers. One time, worried about Molly's acute embarrassment, I say to Sybil, somewhat sharply, "Sybil, please stop now; that man behind the counter is just *staring* at you!", and she replies, with an appropriate put-down for me, "That's *his* problem."

* * *

Excerpts from Sybil's Medical Notes—comments on parents:

June 9—[*From the Clinical Review Management Decision Meeting*]: "There have been two meetings with the parents, the last of which incredibly constructive. Mother seems realistic about Sybil and has listened when the consultant suggested that she take an interest in Sybil's sister. They have taken on the plan that Sybil will not go home on discharge. In this visit and visits on the ward, both parents are making great efforts to give Sybil some responsibility and to be more age-appropriate."

* * *

In late June, both staff and Sybil feel enough confidence in her eating to discontinue the use of the feeding tube—the end of an era!

In June, also, Sybil is particularly lucid, writing for the first time to Neil in Nigeria, a Father's Day card with her own drawing of a giant teddy bear carrying a briefcase:

Lois Chaber

To Daddy:

To say that your braveness to work all alone in Nigeria, your diligence and thoughtfulness to phone and write every week, and every time you bounce back from my rejections just to show me more continuing love, and your faith in me, is appreciated.

She also writes a brave letter to her former Latymer classmate Michelle, whom she idolises:

The place I am in is actually a psychiatric hospital. I don't know what the name does to you, but when a doctor first suggested it to me I was shocked and horrified, but no one is mad here; I think I've come to the conclusion that no human being is 'mad' in the way people use the term. People come here if they have emotional problems or mental illnesses and they are unable to live a normal life and receive help in the community or they need very intensive therapy.

I've made friends with some of the young people. In a way, I'm more confident about myself and being with other people now, but in other ways, I have a lower view of myself. I have learnt some important things about myself and about other human beings too.

Neil now has more reason to use the telephone, but there are new difficulties in making a call, he explains—only

"THE THING INSIDE MY HEAD"

one aspect of the increasing political and social turbulence in Nigeria:

> All communication at this time is heavily restricted by strikes and petrol and cash shortages due to the political instability in Nigeria. Mail is not being sorted or forwarded for weeks, the electrical supply, unreliable at best, becomes weak and sporadic, telephone signals can be weak, backup generators for transmitters don't have fuel with which to operate, couriers and operators are not paid. Any of the three ways I telephone might work on the day or might not. But the thrill of hearing Sybil's voice makes the hours spent and the frustrations worth all the effort.

In August, intense negotiations over the funding of Sybil's future placement begin between the hospital and the Department of Social Services in the Borough of Barnet. The Bethlem Royal has been in contact with them since March, only to face constant delays and obfuscations. Nicola, Sybil's nurse, warns me that this funding issue is usually a sticking point for these local bureaucracies, and negotiations may go on for some time. The therapeutic community costs about sixty thousand pounds a year for one adolescent and there is always a hassle over exactly who is going to foot the bill.

We feel that the Bethlem is pushing Sybil and us to accept Jacques Hall, in Essex, as the therapeutic venue, and with the very limited information they provide plus our own ignorance, there seems to be no other choice. Meanwhile, in late September, Barnet Social Services agrees to fund half the costs if Barnet Health Authority will

Lois Chaber

provide the other half. But as the autumn goes on, the hospital's attempts to have Social Services keep their part of the commitment continue to meet with nothing but excuses and passings of the buck from one person or sub-department to another. Sybil and I both are consumed by anxiety over this long drawn-out bureaucratic wrangling. Sybil, feeling ambiguous about leaving the Unit anyway, starts deteriorating due to all the uncertainties. I find myself having nightmares about Sybil literally being thrown out on the streets, not realising that when the hospital sets a 'final discharge date' it is in part a manoeuvre to put pressure on the borough's bureaucracy.

During this period, also, I question the head nurse as to why the Unit is not giving Sybil therapy for her OCD like some of the other adolescents have had and I am told "It would be too intrusive in her fragile condition." Maybe this is true, but I also suspect they are unwilling to start such a programme because they are anxious, if I may put it bluntly, to see the back of Sybil, who has been one of their longest-staying patients, and clearly one of the most difficult. The issue of therapy specifically for her OCD is not to be addressed for almost two years as the therapeutic community will not have the personnel for such treatment.

* * *

Excerpts from Sybil's Medical Notes—Sybil's self-harm

August 11: "... Episode of self-harm last week following a missed session with a nurse—appears to be related to Sybil's high level of anxiety..."

August 15: "Difficult worst episode of self-harm—stuck drawing pin in her wrist and attempted head-banging when Mum visited..."

"THE THING INSIDE MY HEAD"

October 27: "Today absconded from ward and was found on the green verge outside the hospital near road—back to ward—expressed her anxiety about leaving the ward *[for the therapeutic community]* and whether she would feel as safe in another hospital."

October 31: "—Commenced head banging extremely hard in intensely deliberate self-harm on wall of room. Restrained by staff—held. Repeated after approximately 45 minutes—restrained again. Placed on close observation as thought to remain at serious risk of self-harm. Uncertainty about impending discharge and leaving long-term institutional placement."

* * *

Despite the aggravating, drawn-out transfer process and its injurious effect on Sybil, I remain flush with pride and excitement over her general recovery, not comprehending how fragile she still is. I convince a hesitant Sybil and a hesitant Purnimi that the time is ripe for a visit together, which will be the first one in almost two years and Sybil's first contact with a friend her age from the outside world. There are somewhat constrained negotiations with Purnimi's wary family over exactly when Purnimi can come and how long she can stay at the Unit, but it finally happens on Sunday, October 30th.

Purnimi comes dressed to kill in a very formal long skirt, bearing a huge bouquet of white calla lilies, while Sybil is in her usual scruffy trousers and old woolly, sweaty jumper. I want to leave them alone together, but neither of them seems comfortable with that. They seem at a loss after some initial chitchat, so I suggest they look through the latest teen magazines together, which they do, making stilted comments. It soon becomes obvious that Purnimi, who has left the neighbourhood comprehensive school to do her sixth form privately at the City of London School for Girls, has moved far beyond Sybil in educational level and

237

social sophistication. When Sybil asks plaintively, "Do you think I'm like the old Sybil?" Purnimi responds "Yes", but she doesn't sound very convinced. Sybil does some of her standing up, sitting down rituals, but I have prepared Purnimi for that, and on the way home with me the latter remarks that she had noticed Sybil's 'repeating things' as far back as primary school. The visit has definitely been a mistake.

In late November 1994, the funding fiasco still trundles on. The hospital has set several successive 'final' discharge dates for Sybil and has given innumerable deadlines to Social Services, but excuses are still being made. The latest is that they cannot decide whether Sybil, aged 16, is legally a child or an adult, which affects the decision about funding. I am at my wits' end because Jacques Hall has said they can only hold the place there for Sybil until December 12th. The hospital keeps up steady, patient pressure, and I write a desperate but very articulate letter to the Local Government Ombudsman. Something works, for on December 8th I receive a call from the head nurse telling me with great relief that Social Services has finally signed up to the funding agreement.

At last it is Sybil's departure day—December 12th 1994. Both of us are sitting in her room, waiting nervously for a hospital van to become free to take us to Jacques Hall in Essex (I am too fainthearted to venture driving there on my own), both feeling very ambivalent about this upcoming, possibly permanent, separation from the family. The nurses have told me that Sybil handled her recent leave-taking party at the Unit with great aplomb, giving and receiving gifts with dignity. Her time at the Bethlem Royal represents the greatest crisis of her life so far—so close to perishing she came—and thankfully she has emerged, while not fully cured by any means, a very different girl from the mute, pallid creature knotted up in painful contortions who was admitted almost two full years ago.

"THE THING INSIDE MY HEAD"

Her teacher Gwendolyn is among the many members of staff who come to say goodbye to Sybil:

I can see her on that last day when she was leaving, and I came to say goodbye and be with her. She was packing her bag in her room. We were talking about her leaving and her future, when we looked out the window and saw either a fox or a squirrel. I said that the creature must have guessed she was going and had come to say goodbye. She smiled because it was almost within touching distance.

Lois Chaber

Chapter 2: "The Thing inside My Head Which I Thought Was God"—Sybil's Memoir of the Adolescent Unit

I have tyrants ... living in my head. ... They make me think thoughts and do things that I don't know why I do. They are crazy. But I have to do what they want. And I look crazy.

(From a novel for teenagers, *Kissing Doorknobs*, by Terry Spencer Hesser, New York: Bantam Doubleday Dell Books for Young Readers, 1998, p.122.)

The following account, slightly abridged here, was written in 1996-97 by eighteen-year-old Sybil at the suggestion of her Care Coordinator and Community Psychiatric Nurse (CPN), Jane Clark, and was 'confidential' till after her death. It gives *her* view of those same two years (1993-94) described by me in the previous chapter:

* * *

When I first went to the Bethlem, Mrs. Wells, who I had been living with in foster care, drove my mum and I down to the Bethlem. I wasn't eating; I had an ng [nasogastric] tube up my nose. I wasn't talking. I had my head right back as if I was looking up at the ceiling and my eyes rolled right back. I kept my eyes and head like this all the time except for when lying down in bed. I didn't communicate at all except for a sort of smile, which meant agreement or 'yes'. On the second day there my key worker Jane was on shift. That was when I started communicating with ticks, crosses and question marks. Jane suggested it and the thing inside my head which I thought was God said I could do it.

"THE THING INSIDE MY HEAD"

On the first Sunday I was there I wrote for the first time. It was when my mum came to visit that I wrote 'Mummy I love you' with the crayons and paper I'd been using to draw on. When I sat down I always sat in a certain way with my hands holding the tops of my legs. When I stood I had my hands on my stomach. I can't remember why I started doing that but I'm quite sure it was because of the thing inside my head which I thought was God.

I gradually started writing more. I was told by the thing in my head which I thought was God how much I could write. I had already been sort of befriended by and made friends with Kirsty and Fiona, two other teenagers there. I still had my head up. I went to school and was given things I could try to do without being able to see them because of my head. I felt I was enjoying school for the first time in a long time. I know this sounds strange but I was sort of happy. The thing inside my head was letting me do more and more things and after doing nothing but stand there at Hill End [previous Adolescent Unit], it felt good.

I forgot to write that when I first came I wasn't dressing myself or washing myself at all; I wasn't even pulling my trousers and knickers down when I went to the toilet. Other people were doing all these things for me. It is embarrassing writing about that. Eventually the thing in my head let me write as much as I wanted to and was also letting me gradually do small bits in dressing and washing. I used to go out for walks with staff. I used to do painting and cooking. I used to listen to the TV and I was very good at telling the time by what I heard on the TV and what was going on around me.

Things started to go wrong. I had to do a ritual which the thing in my head told me I had to do every morning and night.

I feel a bit depressed now and weird after writing all this. I will continue writing later.

Lois Chaber

The ritual involved visualizing words in my head which were supposed to come from God. I started having trouble visualizing them because of intrusive thoughts.

One morning I hadn't finished doing a ritual when it was school time. Two of the staff carried me over to the school. I felt terrible. I felt so alone. I tried and tried to complete the ritual. In the end I did it and Gwendolyn came down and talked to me (Gwendolyn was my key teacher). They had been reducing my chlorpromazine. I had been talking of voices in my head. I'm not sure whether they were thoughts or voices. I used to go for a run with Debbie (a nurse) when I felt bad.

The intrusive thoughts got worse. I got stuck on my knees because I couldn't finish the ritual and wouldn't do anything else until I'd done it. My knees started getting pressure sores, so a nurse had to lift me up and make me sit down and hold me there for the first 5 minutes every hour, then longer, to a half hour every hour. I sort of gave up on doing the rituals. When they held me down I kept trying to get up. I didn't want to, but I had to. I couldn't even go to the toilet so I was wetting and soiling myself. It is embarrassing writing about it. You may feel disgusted at me, but I didn't want to do it. I thought that the thing inside my head was God and I had to do it. I had to punish myself for not trying hard enough to do what the thing inside my head wanted me to do, and I had to do the punishments it told me to. I ended up doing the opposite of what I wanted.

One day I saw a picture in the air as I was kneeling or posturing in my room. It was a drawing, no colour, of a mouth stretched in pain or screaming or something like that. I wasn't really afraid. After that I started to see more mouths, all over my room, and many different things. Once I saw a mouth with a toothbrush and another time I saw a mouth with a stick of rock [rock candy]. I wasn't afraid. In fact, I quite liked it. It was entertaining and it occupied my mind with something other than trying to hold my posture

242

"THE THING INSIDE MY HEAD"

and think certain thoughts all day long. Then I started seeing faces. They were like in smoke; it's hard to describe them. They sort of melted and the eyes were in the place of the mouth and everything was muddled up. A few times I saw my mum's or dad's face. That did scare me. I think that the other things scared me a bit because one day I really wanted to tell Pat, my primary nurse, about them but the thing in my head had told me that if I ever told anyone about them I would never hear God's voice again. Pat had mentioned something about the pen and paper and I was going to tell her, but the thing inside my head said that I could do it if she brought the pen and paper and couldn't if she didn't. She didn't bring it.

* * *

At this time I was being tube-fed at night. I was connected up to a drip stand and liquid food supplement, 4 litres of it, was dripped into the tube and down into my stomach every night.

Part of my care plan was to be taken into the lounge for half an hour each shift, because otherwise I would be in my room all the time. I wouldn't walk anywhere, so they had to carry me. I didn't want to do this to them at all, but I had no choice; God (or who I thought was God) was telling me to do it. One evening one of the nurses came to take me out. A couple of the friends whom I had made before I went really downhill, came to see me in my room. The nurses suggested they take me by the hand and suddenly I found I could walk. I walked to the lounge. I started communicating with signs. This was sort of one of my 'ups'. During my stay there I kept having 'up' periods and 'down' periods.

At the start of this 'up' period I felt really good. I started playing games, going to school again, talking with signs. I made friends with a new girl called Jenny who had OCD; I had been told at my assessment that I had OCD, but I didn't think I had. I went for walks, I did a lot of things, and

Lois Chaber

I had friends. But the 'up' started to go down again; I couldn't stop it. I went back to doing the same sorts of things that I was doing before. I was doing the opposite of what I wanted, so I ended up doing the opposite of what they wanted. They didn't want to hurt their backs again, so they used a wheelchair. I had to keep getting out of the wheelchair even when they put a belt on it. I didn't want to but I had to.

One day in the summer I was in the kitchen, posturing, and they were peeling apples for apple crumble. I really wanted to join in and I just got up and did. This was the beginning of another 'up' time.

During the 'up' times, I was really friendly and did a lot with my friends. Jenny, Natalie and sometimes Kirsty used to sit in Jenny's room and listen to music and talk and have a laugh. We sat in the dark because Jenny wouldn't turn the light on because of her OCD. She had to undo everything she did. I really feel nostalgic for those times and all the 'up' times. Sometimes I really miss them and I wish I was back there in those times. When I think about it properly I don't want to be back there because I'm so much better now and things were so scary and difficult then. Things are scary and difficult now but they were much more so then. I think what I miss is the friendships and being really good buddies with people my own age. Writing this now I feel sort of empty and lonely; I feel like crying because we had such good friendships and even though I went through some really hellish times I also had really good times. I think what I miss as well is being a teenager and being able to have fun with each other. Now I'm grownup and an adult and can't have fun in the same sort of way. I think I also miss the feeling of soaring from the 'downs' to the 'ups', where I felt' Yippee!' and felt so excited and pleased. I also miss the lovely school.

During this period the voice started turning people into devils and putting me on another planet which looked

244

"THE THING INSIDE MY HEAD"

like earth and the people looked almost exactly the same as the people on earth except they were all devils, pretending to be the people I knew and trying to lead me astray. I told the nurses about this. I also once saw something happen to people. I saw a nurse and another young person's face sort of melt and become all cartoony and turn into a grotesque evil face. I had told the nurses about the voices and the planet and the changing faces. I went downhill again because I realized that the voices and the planet and the devils were true. They increased my chlorpromazine a lot. This was one of my worst 'downs'.

I went home on Christmas day which was good even though I was going downhill. Boxing Day wasn't so good and after that I really deteriorated including when I went home on New Year's Day. I was in one of my 'downs' again, probably the worst one. I had to do things like roly-poly's on the floor in the corridors and lying on the floor in the corridor in people's way and standing in front of the TV when people were watching. You may find it hard to believe that I didn't do these things on purpose, or just to be naughty. I hated it, but God, or who I thought was God, was telling me to do it and it took a lot of courage to do what I thought was God's will. At one point I had to start pulling my n.g. tube out and when they tried to put it in I had to struggle to stop them even though I was weary, hungry and thirsty. At one point I went without food or water for 3 days. Twice I had to be held down by three people while someone else put the tube in. I didn't mind; I was glad in fact because it stopped me from doing all those things I had to do but didn't want to. I came 'up' for one or two days but then had to go back 'down' because it was 'proved' to me that the voice was true by something it said and something in the Bible.

* * *

It was January [1994], my second primary nurse left and I had a new really nice one called Mary, plus a new associate called Nicole who I was scared of. There were

245

Lois Chaber

some new young people and I hated doing such weird things in front of them. I wanted to be with them. I remember someone kept playing the song by 'Metallica' called "Nothing Else Matters"; it seemed to be describing part of how I felt. It may not sound like it, but life was really difficult, lonely and sad. It is hard doing things that you think God wants you to do when it means losing your friends and making people angry, as well as making you feel bored, sad, alone, scared, terrified, trapped and exhausted. It was during this period that I first felt suicidal but couldn't do it because I would go to Hell. I was feeling more and more miserable and I still wasn't meeting up to God's (the voice's) expectations and I was still thinking bad thoughts. So one day I thought, "This isn't getting me anywhere; I'm only thinking more bad thoughts," and I decided to start acting normal again. The voice negotiated some things I had to do first. This was the beginning of my biggest and best 'up'.

When I first started talking I negotiated with the voice. I had to do punishments as a way of earning it. I could only say one word a day. One day I was sitting with my friends in Kirsty's bedroom and they were all chatting and I really wanted to join in, so I negotiated with the voice and earned it. Then I started talking. They were really surprised and pleased. I started drinking that night for the first time in over a year. I had a cup of hot chocolate. I didn't start eating until my 16th birthday. I negotiated with the voice and did something to earn that, too.

I negotiated with God (the voice) this thing called an absolute fresh start, which meant I was forgiven for the sin I had done, and all the punishments I had, things I couldn't do, were stopped. I went out the day after my birthday with my primary nurse Mary to do some shopping. I kept messing up and losing the absolute fresh start, so I kept stopping and starting talking and stopping and starting eating and drinking.

"THE THING INSIDE MY HEAD"

One Saturday, lunchtime came and I just decided I was going to eat something. I did, and I managed to eat at least one meal a day for the next two weeks. Then, on Friday, the same day one of my friends left, I was doing something and my tube caught on something and was pulled out quite a bit. It was out, so for that I pulled the rest of it out. Later on, when I was having one of my sessions with my primary nurse and my associate nurse, they said that since I had been eating so well, they weren't going to put the tube in, at least for a week. So I started eating without the tube!

I don't think words can ever express or convey what that year and 10 months were like for me. It was a very emotional time. I went through terrible times which it took a lot of strength to get through, and some really awful nightmarish, almost hellish times, especially when I was having to do the opposite of what I wanted to do. I can't explain what it was like. It was like having to work your way through a dark tunnel and not even being able to see a light at the end but just having to force yourself to believe there was a light at the end.

I also felt lots of other emotions: happiness, trust, really good friendships, some of the best friendships I've had in my life, excitement and elation at being able to do normal things again. I also had a massive crush on one of my male friends. I told him, but he was really cool about it, and we carried on being good friends. I felt empathy and sympathy for other young people in the unit. The staff and young people became my friends and family and even at times it became like my home.

* * *

During all this time I thought that some other people in the unit were there for the same reason as me, that they had sinned against the Holy Spirit and were being punished like me. I thought that of Daniel because he kept talking to

Lois Chaber

and about Jesus and Satan. I also thought that of Cindy and
of Neil and Simeon [other young persons]. Poor Simeon, I
used to feel bad for him then, but now I know that he wasn't
behaving in that way because God told him to; I wonder
what was really wrong with him. Natalie, Jessie, James and
I used to go and visit him when he was transferred to
Fitzmorcy 2, the Schizophrenic and Psychosis Ward. I
wonder where he is now and if he is better. I feel guilty
because I stopped visiting him.

I feel a bit like giving up trying to write like this. I just
can't convey what it was like for me during that year and 10
months. I'll try and tell you about the Adolescent Unit.

Everyone was woken at ten to eight. Breakfast
wasn't compulsory and lasted till about 8:15. Community
group was at 9:05. School started at 10. There was a
timetable and there were four lessons a day, each one hour
long. Then it was lunch. It was compulsory to go to lunch
and dinner even if you weren't going to eat anything. There
were two more lessons till 4:00. Then we had free time
unless we had a session with our primary or associate
nurse. Dinner or tea or whatever you want to call it was at
6:00. After dinner it was free time again. The night staff
came in at 8:45, had handover, and went on from around
9:00/9:10. At 9:30 they brought drinks and biscuits into the
lounge and at around 10:00 it was medication time and
bedtime.

We had community group on Mondays,
Wednesdays and Fridays. If someone became too
disruptive, they would be made to go or taken out. I used to
try and go out as a punishment and because the voice in my
head that I thought was God told me to. So, a nurse would
stand by the door and stop me from leaving. In community
group we talked about what we wanted from the week,
general comments or complaints, talked about changing
rules, like the rule that boys couldn't go into a girl's bedroom
and vice versa. We went where the conversation led us.

248

"THE THING INSIDE MY HEAD"

There was another group called 'small groups'. In the small groups we shared our problems, gave support and advice, shared experiences. They could be quite good.

Everyone had a primary nurse and 1 or 2 associate nurses which are the same as a key worker and co/associate workers. I had three different primary nurses while I was there. I formed very close relationships and bonds with some of the nurses, especially my primary and associate nurses. After all, they were looking after me and doing very personal things, like washing me, feeding me, trying to help me to feel better, pacifying me, keeping me company and keeping me from hurting myself, counseling me. They became like a second family, second parents, second sisters to me. When I went home today [in 1997], my mum brought out my gold jewelry so that I could choose one or two to take back to Eaglehurst with me. One of them, she reminded me, was from Pat. I felt sad and touched and thought about Pat. My mum said that Pat really wanted me to get better and it was her idea about the force/encouraging feeding thing. My mum said that when that didn't work Pat felt like a bit of a failure. I remember the day that Pat left. She was crying and trying to hug me, but I pulled away and wouldn't let her even though I wanted to because the thing inside my head that I thought was God told me not to as a punishment. I feel so frustrated, sad, helpless and angry when I think about that and how the thing inside my head stopped me from doing that. I wish I could get in touch with her.

* * *

Back to the story. One day, as part of school, Sue and another teacher, I think Thomas, took a group of us to 'Down's House', which was Darwin's old house. I felt a bit weird and I didn't like the atmosphere. I went into a room and there was a really, weird, strange, horrible feeling in there. I went walking in the grounds with the others and I felt strange, like the devil was near. At one point I felt this really scary strong feeling that some bad thing or force was watching me or near me. I told the others about these experiences and at least two of them had felt strange and scary feelings, maybe a presence, in that room that I had, and two of them had felt something near the fireplace, like an odd heavy feeling dropping. I felt really freaked out. I thought everyone had turned to devils or I was on the devils' planet. I went inside.

In a way, I liked this 'adventure', but when I thought about them being devils, I felt guilty and horrible. I felt both scared and excited and I wanted to be in the normal world, but I still wanted to have the excitement and adventure. When we got back I felt these really strong, bad, dirty, but really strong sexual feelings about James. But when I thought that James was the devil, I hated him. I said to him something like, "Sometimes I love you and sometimes I hate you." I feel really embarrassed about saying this now, especially as I now know it was the real James I was talking to, and there was no devil James. I started talking to them [her friends] about what had been going on and asking them if they were devils and stuff like that. I saw them get together talking in low voices and I thought they were the devils, conspiring against me and how to make sure I didn't find out they were the devils. I mentioned this to James, who at this period I didn't know whether he was the real James or not, and he said they were talking like that because they were worried about me. I didn't know whether to believe him or not; I think I didn't really believe him. I tried talking to Sandra (a nurse) about it, but I didn't get anywhere.

I remember one time asking the art teacher about jealousy and whether it was bad or not. I had a lot of respect for Jack (the art teacher). He seemed to be a very nice and good person. He said, in answer to my question, that it depended what you did with it. I asked because I was feeling very jealous of other people in the unit, especially James, because they managed to do something good in school, like a good piece of writing that was put up on the wall, or good art or good poems. After that chat with Jack I started putting more effort and priority on doing things that I could feel good about at school. Soon after, I started writing a poem in the art lesson. It was really good and it expressed what I felt, and I carried it on after the lesson.

* * *

Towards the end of the school year and the holidays we did some fun things. We had a sort of fun, sports day with the Children's Unit and some of the girls from Eating Disorders came too. I saw them and said hello in passing every so often. One of them seemed a really nice person. Sometimes I wished I was in Tyson West 2 (Eating Disorders) with them.

Oh, I forgot to write something down. One day James said to me that he had something to tell me. I thought it was going to be something good but when I went and sat next to him and he told me, it was that he was leaving, being discharged. This made me very sad, because I would miss him. He said it was because he had been there 6 months and hadn't really gotten any better. He had OCD and severe depression. This made me very sad as well. It didn't seem fair. It was horrible. It sort of snowballed inside me and I felt worse and worse that evening and night.

I think I forgot to mention a song which expressed exactly how I was feeling. It was "Runaway Train" by Soul Asylum. The words, "Runaway train, never going back, going down a one way track," were similar to how I felt. I felt like, since I had said something bad about the Holy Spirit, I was on a runaway train and I couldn't go back and change the past. I felt so alone and no one could help me. Everything was so different and sad and painful. The song also said, "I know what no one else can know, I can go where no one else can go," which seemed to be exactly about me or someone in the same situation because I knew

251

the voice or thing inside my head which I thought was God had told me and revealed to me all sorts of secrets—secrets which I couldn't tell anyone about. I had done the terrible sin and it had made an exception. It had revealed to me other people who had done the same thing and were going through or had gone through the same as what I was going through. One of these people was Freddie Mercury from Queen. So many of his songs seemed to express my feelings, situation and thoughts, especially "Bohemian Rhapsody" and "Living on My Own". When the song said, "I can go where no one else can go" it seemed to fit my experience of being put on the other planet with all those devils. Music was very important to me while I was there and there were lots of songs which seemed to express lots of different feelings I felt.

Jenny and Natalie were really good friends. We had a laugh together and even when I was in a terrible state they used to talk to me even though I wouldn't answer back, especially Jenny. Sometimes it was horrible because I could see the staff dragging her places and forcing her to do things when she couldn't or it was very difficult for her because of her OCD. I thought it was wrong and very unfair and I think they might have been abusing their position of power over her or at least they came near to it. Jenny used to say when I was feeling a bit blue or when she passed me in the corridor during some of my bad times, "Think of elephants with pink umbrellas," or something like that. I remember that quite often when she would pass my room at night, when she was doing her bedtime rituals, she would call out, "Good night, sleep tight, don't let the night nurses bite," which I thought was great!

After a while, Jenny started to be naughty and rebellious and started to get out of control. She got really bad, to a point where I didn't want to be friends with her anymore. I wish now that we had stayed friends even if I didn't like her and was angry about her behaviour. Eventually, she had a meeting where she was told that they

"THE THING INSIDE MY HEAD"

couldn't help her with her OCD anymore and she was going to be discharged in two weeks. I think what they said about helping her with her OCD was untrue and they really wanted her to leave because of her bad, out of control behaviour. On the last day or one of the last days she [Jenny] was there, I remember her being very kind to me when I was stuck and going through a bad patch. I didn't say anything because I wasn't allowed to (the thing inside my head made me believe that). I now really regret it.

I forgot to tell you about Kenneth. During one of my bad patches, when a nurse came to pick me up from school in a wheelchair she told me there was someone I knew here. I didn't know who it was but it turned out to be Mr. Jones from Hill End. At Hill End we had to call staff by their surname and Mr. Jones was one of the staff. When I had last been at Hill End, he had been quite horrible (or so I thought), but the time before that, when I was getting better at Barnet General Hospital, he was okay. Anyway, it turned out he was now a new charge nurse at the [Bethlem] Unit and I felt so embarrassed and ashamed and worried that he would see me like this. He turned out to be nice and he was different from when he was working at Hill End. I said this to him once and he said because the different jobs required different things.

* * *

It was the summer holidays. I think it was around this time I was starting to worry about contaminating other people with germs from myself. I started to feel like I was hurting other people or going to. I tried to become like a robot and not have any thoughts or feelings, just controlled actions, because it was when I thought or felt that I hurt someone or could. I was also worried about contaminating people with my conjunctivitis that I had at the time on top of hay fever. I got really worked up about it. I was doing everything so slowly and I wasn't doing much.

Lois Chaber

Around this time I started doubting the voice. There were some things about it or what it said or was saying that contradicted themselves. I was doing the difficult things like not talking and sometimes strange things that God (the voice in my head) told me to do. I started getting confused, going from one end to the other, believing in the voice and obeying it even if it was difficult or embarrassing, to being very doubting of the thing inside my head and occasionally feeling almost convinced that it wasn't really God. I can't remember why and maybe there was no identifiable reason, but I started feeling very depressed. I had thoughts of suicide, at one point they were very strong and I think I came close to planning something.

At about this time I went to Sharon [a nurse] and talked to her. She was okay. I told her I felt suicidal. She seemed surprised but was nice. Later on I went to visit Simeon in Fitzsimmons 2. It was very hard and it took me quite a while to get there and back. I had been getting pains in the chest and other places and spots over my body and I had really bad hay fever, and I felt dizzy and out of it. For some reason I thought I was or might be really ill or dying with a fatal disease. I felt quite upset and really scared. I told Sharon and she said something like, "Earlier you said you wanted to kill yourself and now you are scared and you think you are dying of a disease or something." This made me feel upset and I thought she was saying she didn't believe me and that I was putting on an act. I said something about this to her, but she said that was not the case and she was just trying to get me to think about it, or something like that.

I had set days and times each week where I could meet with my primary nurse or one of my associate nurses for a 1-1 session. Any other time I wasn't allowed to have a 1-1 when I felt upset. They encouraged me or *I had to* (sometimes that's what it felt like) do an activity which would make me feel better, like going for a run outside or a walk or doing art or writing down how I felt for the next session.

"THE THING INSIDE MY HEAD"

Well, on this Tuesday that I talked to Sharon and the Wednesday after, I used this time to hold onto the thought of my session on Thursday. I felt terrible. I felt like I was in a tunnel; the thought of the session was what made me cope and hold on. Thursday came and I found out that I must've misread my timetable because it wasn't on Thursday, and I had missed it. I begged for 1-1 time but they wouldn't give me any.

I was crying and I went into my room and started cutting myself. I think I was using the sharp bit of a can ring opener bit. I don't think I wanted to commit suicide; I felt I couldn't carry on like this. The past few days had been terrible and I was in darkness and the one thing that kept me going and holding on was gone, disappeared into thin air. I stopped because the thing inside my head told me to. I suddenly remembered that the thing inside my head had told me that if I tried to kill myself I would be lost forever (unforgiven, separated from God and not allowed into Heaven). I felt really scared and a dreading feeling came over me. I didn't know what to do. I went over to the window. I felt frightened about what God would do now that I had cut my wrist.

The next day, a woman doctor wanted to have a chat with me. We were in the interview room and she asked me if when I cut myself last night I really wanted to die. I said 'no'. She was usually nice but she seemed horrible and she left; I was stuck in the chair. I remember feeling terrible and alone and abandoned. I cried and hoped someone would hear. I was stuck in the room and it was taking me a long time to do anything. I got off the chair, I don't know how or why. I knelt or sat or squatted on the floor. I cried there. No one came. I felt so awful. I felt a great emotional pain, if not in agony, then almost. You are probably thinking that I'm exaggerating and thinking I've got no reason to feel that bad, but I'm not exaggerating at all. I felt in agony. I tried to numb myself to the pain, which took concentration, but it

255

Lois Chaber

worked. I managed to get myself in a state where I had no, or virtually no feelings.

I was worried about contaminating someone with my eye infection, I was trying to do everything controlled and very slowly and I was trying to do whatever the punishment was I mentioned before. It felt like I was crossing an unstable bridge on my own, in not very much light over rushing torrents and rocks of madness below. That probably sounds over the top, but you have to believe me, that's how it felt.

Mary (my primary nurse) let me have a session with her even though it wasn't written down. I told her how I had been feeling and she said that she thinks in pictures as well. The thing/voice inside my head that I thought was God said I could tell Mary about the terrible sin I'd done, saying something bad about the Holy Spirit. I only had one moment and one chance to tell her, and I wasn't allowed to say anything more about it, but when I did, all she said was that she thought I was taking the Bible too literally, Subject Closed. I felt very disappointed and let down and alone.

* * *

Around the time she was working on this memoir, Sybil confided to me that when she had been doing Bible studies in her early adolescence, she had read the passage in the Bible—Mark 3: 28-29—about the unforgivable sin

Verily I say unto you, all sins shall be forgiven unto the sons of men, and blasphemies wherewith soever they shall blaspheme.

But he that shall blaspheme against the Holy Ghost hath never forgiveness, but is in danger of eternal damnation.

256

"THE THING INSIDE MY HEAD"

She at once became convinced, she told me, that she had committed this sin because of her blasphemous thoughts.

* * *

Around this time, 3 new people came to the unit: Emma, Tony and Lisa. I felt a bit scared/nervous of them and what they would think of me. Some or most of my friends had left. I also kept thinking that people were talking about me. I got a really strong feeling that they were. Mary said that I was just feeling a bit paranoid at the moment.

I was really worried about hurting people at this time. It felt at one point like I was in a living nightmare. I was in the toilet and negotiating with the voice about cutting my wrists. I wanted to die. In the end I couldn't; I can't remember why. The next day I felt the same and was working and screwing my way up to it all morning when my mum came, or just before the time I could finally do it. I started cutting myself on my wrist; I think it was with a drawing pin. My mum got upset and called a nurse who had to take me down to the flat area [the seclusion room]. It must have been awful for mum and I was selfish, but life just seemed like a nightmare I couldn't wake up from and it was one of my only chances to kill myself, but I shouldn't have done it then; maybe I shouldn't have done it at all; I don't know.

It was the first and only time I was in the flat. They had me lying on my tummy on the mattress, with my arms behind my back, but not roughly, quite gently. I could have moved if I tried. They had called the duty doctor and he came and checked my wrists and said they weren't that bad or dangerous. Then, soon after that, the nurses let me sit up. I did. I struggled a bit sometimes, to scratch or cut more with my fingernails and to maybe bang my head. They kept trying to stop me. My mum left sometime during all this. She must have felt absolutely terrible. I felt a little bit guilty.

257

Lois Chaber

Candace (one of the nurses) and I went for a walk. I had been feeling suicidal. I was allowed by the voice to phone the Samaritans the next morning. Phoned Samaritans. The lady just said I should talk to the nurses. I just hung up on her. The reason I phoned the Samaritans was because I couldn't talk to the nurses. They wouldn't take me seriously. They would just say I was doing it for attention.

After small groups I asked Sandra if I could have some of my money and go to the hospital shop to get some lozenges because I had a sore throat. I said that as an excuse but really I was going to get more tablets. I went out of the grounds as quickly as I could and up to Boots. In Boots I looked at the pain killers. One of them said 'Disprin'. Since the ones I had taken yesterday were called 'Disprol', I thought 'Disprin' was the adult version. I bought it and walked down to a shop and bought a milkshake to swallow them down with. I realized I couldn't go back to the hospital now that I had been out for so long. I went into a side street and started to swallow them. It was hard and the milkshake ran out quite quickly. Some kids stopped and looked at me. Then a woman came up and asked if I was alright. I can't remember if I answered or not. I had the packet in my arms and some tablets were showing. I think she noticed. I took some more when she had gone. A police car drew up and two policemen walked out. The woman came and talked to them. I think she must've phoned them. She was very nice. When I was taking the pills, part of me was weakening and hoping I wouldn't die, so I didn't take the whole packet. I only took about 10 or 12. I should have taken all of them. Sometimes I wish I had achieved what I was trying to do.

The policeman said, "Are you popping pills?" I couldn't answer him. The lady said she thought I was from the hospital. They phoned for a female person. Then they phoned an ambulance. They walked me to the ambulance. I didn't struggle very much, which I am ashamed of. I had given in; I was foolish. They took the packet from me. I

"THE THING INSIDE MY HEAD"

cooperated. I was pathetic. They took me to casualty. A doctor came in and took my blood. She asked me how many I had taken. Oh, I forgot to mention that when I was taking the tablets I read the packet a bit and to my dismay I found that I had made yet another mistake. It was aspirin, not paracetamol. I hoped that it would still work.

In casualty, I guess they must've phoned up the hospital and the unit because I heard someone say that I had an obsessive disorder. That was the first time they had said that about me for ages and it surprised me. After the doctor I think someone came in once, but after that then I was in that room on that bed, alone and not knowing what was going on for eight hours! You might be thinking, "Well, she jolly well deserved it, too." I hadn't spoken much or at all as far as I can remember and I felt worried and scared about going out and asking where the toilet was although I needed it. I wet myself really badly. At about 8:00 or 8:30 some people came to take me back. There were two men and they stared at me. I was standing there with soaking wet trousers. It was obvious that I had wet myself, but for some reason I seemed to bear it quite well. Then a kind ambulance lady came in and spoke to me as if I was normal, which I was glad of. She took me back. I was feeling sick and she gave me a bowl. That was the first time I had been sick since I took both sets of tablets. She was really nice to me.

When I got back I went straight to my room. After that I was on 5 minute checks. I had been waiting so I could bang my head again. I banged it, smashed it against the wall. Again, I saw a bit of blood on the wall. I banged it 4 times, but the nurses in the office next door heard me. The thing inside my head which I thought was God didn't let me bang my head anywhere except that wall that was next to the office. I just hoped I would achieve my aim before they got to me.

Lois Chaber

About 4 nurses rushed in and before I knew it I was on the floor. They got me lying face down with my arms behind my back in a restraint. They didn't put my legs up. Mary had her hands on my behind, but gently. Them doing that made me want to struggle. It was humiliating, but it showed they cared. Nicole was there and she said about me something like, "She always needs to take control because the people who were meant to be in control couldn't; look, she can't even let us take control now." She wasn't being horrible; she was being nice.

* * *

Meanwhile, all the sorting of where I was going to go was going on. They had given me some booklets and information about 2 different places. One of them was called Jacques Hall, and the other was called Sea Meadows. Since my 16th birthday, I had a social worker who came to see me about once a month. She was called Rosemary and was very nice. There were all these battles going on about funding. We had to get social services to fund me to get to go to a place. My mum was worried and was working very hard for this all to get sorted out for me. She wrote letter after letter, met with people and made phone calls. She worked so hard for me. Then my social worker suggested a place in Barnet. I found out that it wasn't a therapeutic community but another hospital. I felt betrayed by her. I thought the point was to get out of hospital.

Terry Lee, the principal from Jacques Hall, came to see me. I was so nervous. I remember waiting in the office, so nervous, waiting for them to call me in. I remember that Terry unsettled me; he seemed to laugh at me or something. Afterwards, Nicole said that's just him, and he's just jolly, or something like that. He said that people sometimes smashed windows and cut themselves there, and I told him it happened here. I had cut myself, but I didn't tell him that. Nicole said he just wanted me to know the amount and sort of acting out that happened at Jacques Hall. Smashing

"THE THING INSIDE MY HEAD"

windows and cutting yourself didn't seem like much, but he didn't tell me the real amount of acting out, which was much worse, which I found out afterwards. Now I had to wait for his answer.

I can't remember much except that later I started banging my head on the wall near my door. Nicole and I think someone else came and they didn't restrain me but Nicole told me that if I was going to 'indulge' (that word indulge made me feel angry) in head banging, she would cancel the visit to Jacques Hall and going there at all and I would go to an adult ward, which was what I really did not want. I stopped banging my head then. I felt so alone. I stayed in my room and it got darker for hours. Then Meg came in. She saved me; she was so kind and caring. She comforted me and got me to sit down on the bed with her. She said she would help me to iron my clothes for tomorrow. It was as if she had turned the light of hope on.

* * *

We went along country lanes and at last we got there [Jacques Hall]. Then we went into the office of the man who had picked us up who was called Tim Rodwell and who was one of the managers, and he asked questions and I think we might have asked some questions. Tim Rodwell told me that one of the girls, Korreana, had offered to show me around. She was pretty and seemed like an intelligent, nice person. She showed me her room and she showed me some of her art work. She asked me if I liked 'Mizz' Magazine and I said 'Yes.' She seemed really, really nice. I asked about bullying and she said it does happen quite a bit. She warned me about the boys, that I shouldn't go out with them if they asked me. Tim Rodwell came into her room while we were in there and said that the girls' group and relationships in it were quite complicated and difficult at the moment. I felt a bit more relaxed now that I had been to Jacques Hall.

Lois Chaber

I can't remember how long it was before I talked to my primary and associate nurses. When I did, I felt quite pressured because they said some things which were putting pressure on me to hurry up with my decision and, I think, choose Jacques Hall. I thought about the bullying there. I just wanted to get the decision, which was hanging over me, over and done with. I said "Jacques Hall" even though I didn't feel quite right. Before I had gone to visit Jacques Hall, the brochure had said that there was a 1-week trial. After one of my suicide attempts I was in the interview room with Nicole. She said that if it was moving to Jacques Hall that was bothering me, she could arrange it so that I went there slowly, like one or two days at first. But when we went to visit Jacques Hall, they said that the initial assessment period was one month. Nicole now said that I would go straight into the month, and if it didn't work out, I wouldn't be coming back to the Unit to find another place. I think this was very different to what she had said before, and I felt angry about it.

* * *

Sometimes I still felt rather desperate to die. I had to do things that the thing inside my head told me to do so that I could kill myself with a good chance of not being sent to Hell. I took the metal hook off one of the coat hangers in my wardrobe. I bent the end of it straight and put it in the plug socket, pushing it right to the back. All I had to do was click the switch. I got to this point a couple of times. After a while I suddenly thought or realized that if I electrocuted myself and someone came in and saw me and touched me, they would probably get electrocuted too. I know this sounds stupid, but I thought of putting a sign on the outside of my door as a warning so no one would touch me, but I thought that they might not read it and touch me anyway. So, I realized I couldn't electrocute myself.

Around this time I realized a pattern of thoughts and feelings that led me to feeling suicidal and trying to kill

262

"THE THING INSIDE MY HEAD"

myself. Once I got to a certain stage, past asking for help, I truly believed that suicide was the best or only option. So I decided that when I got to an earlier stage, before I felt really suicidal, I needed to ask for help then. So I talked about this with my nursing team and they made it so I was allocated a nurse every hour, and if I felt my thoughts or feelings getting to that earlier stage, I would go to my nurse and ask if they could spend some time doing something with me or just a lighthearted chat (not about my feelings or problems) to distract myself and so break the pattern.

I was feeling bored on the Unit, and during my spare time I had read a book for the first time in about 1 ½ to 2 years. It was a very simple book about the elephant man but it was a big achievement for me. Then I started on some very simplified, shortened, abridged versions of *Wuthering Heights* and *Jane Eyre*. I read them quite quickly and it was a big achievement for me. I remember in school doing a project on cats. I was really getting into it.

Lesley [Sybil's ex-dancing teacher, who came for a visit] brought up the question of why I couldn't stay here longer as I wasn't really better. When she said it, it occurred to me that she had a point. I had only felt it vaguely before. I felt a little bit angry, but I accepted (I had to) that I was going to move on.

Purnimi had always been faithful to me while I was in hospital. She had written regularly, often long letters. She used to be my best friend and in a way still was, but I felt distanced from her a bit and I had my new, really great friends here. I was still friends with Purnimi, though. On one weekend my mum brought her down with me. She told me about her new school. She had left Ashmole and was going to the sixth form at, I think it was, City of London Girls' School. I felt a bit jealous of her. We didn't seem to 'click' like we used to, and we both were different people than we used to be when I was at home and well. I could really sense during and after that visit that the 'spark' in our friendship had gone and we had grown quite apart.

All my friends at the Bethlem had left and I felt a bit lost. Things seemed a bit empty for me there. I felt that the staff didn't really want me there anymore. I didn't feel that they really cared for me anymore, even Mary. I knew I had been a lot of trouble and hard work, and I felt that they just didn't want me anymore. I had been living in the Unit for such a long time and it had become a sort of home. I had gone through so much there: trauma, despair, unhappiness and also excitement, vitality, happiness I had made good friends and my stay there had been a very emotionally intense part of my life.

* * *

Lisa still kept trying to kill herself, and staff had to be with her all the time. Then the staff decided to stop Lisa's treatment at the Bethlem and transfer her to a horrible adult unit. It was too awful. It was like they were throwing her away as rubbish. They were abandoning her. I hadn't gotten on with Lisa during most of her stay because she and some others bullied Frank and me a bit, were always putting the Unit down, whispering and giggling and creating a bad atmosphere. But sometime before the staff decided to transfer her, I started caring about her and getting on with her. She wasn't happy and kept saying she would be dead by the time she was sixteen. I felt angry that they were treating Lisa this way. She was so ill, and they were sending her to a horrible hospital. She and Tony used to be friends, but just before she left, they fell out. Tony said she had taken £10 from his room to get something to kill herself with. I can understand Tony being angry, and I would have been quite angry too, but it shows how desperate and unhappy and ill she was.

One afternoon, I think it was a Wednesday, I came back into the Unit from school, and Nicole told me that the

"THE THING INSIDE MY HEAD"

funding and everything had finally been sorted out, and I was going to move into Jacques Hall on Monday. I felt relieved and excited and nervous. I felt very nervous because I had the next five days to get through without doing anything wrong, because if I did, God might punish me and ruin things in some way.

Then I had my leaving party on Friday. The leaving and birthday parties were usually very nice. All the young people, all the staff and teachers that were on that day came and one of the young people had made a card and got everybody to sign it. There were small presents at the leaving party and there were also crisps, cakes, pops and stuff at the parties. I had thought up a speech for my leaving party and felt quite positive and good about it. I felt nervous and self-conscious, I think, but I can't really remember, when Nicole, I think, said, "You had that all ready and prepared" (or something like that) about my speech. I felt embarrassed and that I had made a fool of myself with that speech and that it was stupid.

I was still looking forward to and a bit excited about my goodbye parting thing I was going to have with Mary, my primary nurse. I used to really like her and feel close to her and like she was on *my* side, but gradually she changed. I think she just got fed up with me. I felt like there was no one left who I felt safe with and close to and like they were on my side; they had all gotten fed up or tired of me or had enough of me. I feel sad and a little bit like crying as I write this now. I felt very lonely there; plus all my real friends had left. Anyway, I was still looking forward to the leaving do with Mary. I so much wanted her to like me and care about me, even love me a bit. I wanted to find or extract as much affection from her as possible, and I was sort of fooling myself about her.

After the video, Mary wanted to spend a little time with me alone to say goodbye because, although it was only Friday and I was leaving on Monday, she was going to be

Lois Chaber

off-duty, and I wouldn't be seeing her again. I felt a bit like she was a big sister and I wished she could stay by my bed until I fell asleep. I think I said this to her sort of jokingly. She smiled. I felt a little bit panicky. This couldn't be the end; it couldn't end like this. It didn't seem real, but it was. She and I said goodbye for the last time and I went to bed.

* * *

I didn't mention earlier that I had started masturbating, and I think they found out because I stayed in my room a lot and on my bed, and one or two times I fell asleep while I was doing it, and I think someone may have come in and seen something (although it wasn't obvious), which revealed that I had been masturbating. I was on checks, and they started checking on me without opening the door, which I was sure was because they had found out. I also just sensed that they knew; they seemed to be behaving differently towards me and talking about me. I was convinced. It felt like a nightmare to me.

Some of the times I was incontinent was because I was fed up with holding it in, and I thought, well, if it doesn't come out sooner it will come out later, and so I let it out. Sometimes I let it out on purpose to get attention and help from the staff because I felt so alone and was posturing and doing all sorts of strange, difficult things, and when they changed me or put me in the wheel chair, it was like a kind of rest or comfort. I know it sounds disgusting and pathetic and sick, but if you had been in my position where you had lost almost everything, you couldn't speak or eat, walk where you wanted to go or do anything that you or anyone else wanted you to do or dress or wash yourself or even take yourself to the toilet, and you had lost your dignity and thought that people around you were devils a lot of the time and felt so alone and frightened and isolated, you might well have done the same. Even so, a part of me is ashamed of it.

"THE THING INSIDE MY HEAD"

Sunday night and Monday morning I was incredibly anxious. It was *so important* that I mustn't get put on the unreal world or have the nurses replaced by devils or me not be able to say goodbye or give my goodbye cards or presents to the real nurses or arrive and be welcomed at Jacques Hall by devils.

Mum came at about 8:00, I think. She was nervous as well as me. We packed final things and made sure we were completely ready. An ambulance car or hospital car or something like that was meant to take us. I was so nervous and I was just edging on and hanging on till nine. Then they were a bit late, or so we thought. Mum was very anxious as I was in such a state and finding it so difficult. At eleven they still weren't here. In the end, it was about 1 or 1:30. Meg (the nurse) was coming with us, so I really wanted the journey to be quick and over soon, but it was such a long journey; it seemed incredibly, or unbearably, or almost unbearably long to me.

It was cloudy and gray and I think it was raining when we arrived at the main building. There were teenagers playing around. I remember saying goodbye to Meg, thinking that this was the last time I'd see her and I felt both sad and happy but my thoughts were mostly caught up with the new place and the nervousness and excitement I was feeling.

* * *

These final thoughts were added at the end by Sybil:

How I had any, let alone so many friends at the Bethlem, still amazes me. They were people with wonderful qualities. They could see past the outer appearance and behaviour to the person inside and they could value that person and see them as equals. At least I think they saw me as an equal. They had so much compassion. They were such good friends. I wish I was still in touch with more of them.

My family stuck by me in a way that can't be described in words. I don't know how they did it. They had so much patience, love and comfort to give to me though I was giving nothing but pain and frustration back to them. It must've been terrible for them to see me like I was then. And they had faith in me, that I was still 'Sybil' inside and that I could get better.

Until nearer the end of my stay, when I could sense that the nurses had had enough of me, the nurses, or most of them, were so good to me. I could hardly believe so much goodness and care and kindness around me. I had great primary nurses. My key teacher, Gwendolyn, stood by me so much, even when other staff were so fed up with me. I can't remember her ever being horrible to or really angry at me or really hurting me.

I remember one of the teachers, Valerie, was pregnant. I was refusing to walk at the time and the nurses were having to carry or drag me. I remember them using her to try and move me because if I put my weight on her I could seriously damage her baby. Valerie didn't appear to be angry when I walked for her and not the others, but I remember when one day Debbie (a nurse) was going with Valerie and me and she was quite angry, and after Valerie had said something, I can't remember what, like, "Thank you for walking for me, Sybil," Debbie said angrily something like, "I just wish Sybil had more consideration for our backs."

I can see now that she had good reason to say that.

My mum came to visit me every Sunday. The first few times were good. We used to walk and she would hold my arm or hand. We had some nice walks. She would sing sometimes. I remember her singing "Wouldn't It Be Loverly" and "I'm Getting Married in the Morning!" from *My Fair Lady*.

"THE THING INSIDE MY HEAD"

I wrote and drew pictures I think and she used to read to me. I remember her reading me a book about an orphan and the different ways her life went. At one time she [the orphan] even ended up in a psychiatric hospital.

But this isn't how it always was, and several weeks after I had been at the Adolescent Unit, I started going downhill, and the visits were hard and distressing for her and me, though she struggled to hide her distress and tried to help me, and I couldn't communicate my distress; eventually I couldn't communicate anything. During the worst times her visits brought some change and relief from the thoughts I was thinking and that were going on in my head all day and every day. But I also found them very difficult because I didn't want her to be taken away and the devil in disguise put in her place; sometimes that did happen, and it was very difficult trying to hate and pay no attention to her even though she looked and sounded like my mother and brought a small relief to my weeks and showed me love and comfort and affection and patience and understanding, which I so desperately needed.

Sometimes mum would bring Molly. Molly didn't, I suppose she couldn't, say much to me. It must've been a very confusing experience for her to see me like that. Even though I and my mind were caught up with doing and thinking strange things all the time, I was still Sybil inside, and I thought normal things as well, for instance, wondering what Molly was thinking of me. I felt embarrassed and ashamed to be doing the things I was doing in front of her.

My dad wrote to me [from Nigeria] roughly twice a week, usually on postcards. I looked forward to and relished his postcards, but sometimes God (the voice in my head) would take them away and put a fake one in its place to punish me. I felt really disappointed when this happened, but I treasured the ones that I were sure were from him. Eventually, as I became more and more stuck alone in my room and doing and thinking the same things every day, I

Lois Chaber

looked forward to and liked the fake postcards. Dad came home about every three months.

Sybil's account breaks off at this point. The following is on a separate, final page:

I started to make a card for Molly's birthday. I took ages drawing it and colouring each bit in with pastels and painting. Sometimes when I did art, I disobeyed the voice in my head that I thought was God, and I had to throw the picture away or make myself stop liking or feeling proud of it, or sometimes it was sort of cursed. But when I did this card for Molly, I painstakingly obeyed the voice so that it would be alright and it would get to the real Molly, not to a devil and so she wouldn't be hurt. It took me quite a while. When it was finished, I felt quite a big sense of achievement, but I also felt a bit scared and sad inside because I knew that if I hadn't obeyed the voice, and I didn't like the fear the voice brought with it, I would have been punished, and it was that feeling of always having the fear of the voice (and I really wished and hoped that it wasn't God, but lots of times things happened that proved to me that it was, though years later I now know different) and what would have happened if I didn't obey it, which followed me and coated me with fear.

When Molly got the card, she said that it was beautiful.

* * *

A few years after Sybil's lengthy residence at the Bethlem Royal, I was introduced to an eye-opening book, *The Boy Who Couldn't Stop Washing His Hands,* by Dr. Judith Rapoport. Not only was Rapoports's book one of the very first on OCD for the general public (1989), but the first to include an in-depth discussion of religious morbidity as one of the typical manifestations of this disorder. Rapoport's chapter offers several case histories bearing remarkable resemblances to Sybil's: the conviction of having 'sinned',

"THE THING INSIDE MY HEAD"

the ritual penances or self-punishments to ward off a greater punishment by God, the complex rules for what God will and will not 'permit' the sufferer to do, and even the belief in devils and their personalised agency. Rapoport names this aspect of OCD "scrupulosity" after the term used by the Roman Catholic Church for excessive, self-punitive religiosity, recognised and treated by the Church since the twelfth century.

Reading Rapoport, I was jubilant:. So, my daughter had not been 'crazy' after all!! Her disturbing behaviour was a recognised syndrome, shared by many others! This knowledge would help Sybil, I assumed, to shed any remnants of the 'voice' and all the baggage that went with it. "Sybie," I said, eagerly, next time we sliced vegetables together for a family salad in my kitchen, "you must read this book!! It shows that what you thought and did when you were in the Bethlem is actually a common symptom of OCD, and many young people who have felt exactly the same way as you have been treated by this doctor!" But Sybil's initial response was denial, and, unbeknown to me, she wrote this account of our discussion:

...I said that it wasn't scrupulosity, which is a form of OCD, because I was really guilty while people who had scrupulosity in OCD just felt they were guilty or thought they were guilty and had to repeat or they worried that they might be guilty and so had to repeat just in case. Then Mum said because I was me I saw myself as really being guilty and them not, while they saw themselves as actually being guilty of something as well. I asked what kind of things they thought they were guilty of and she said that it was things like me, i.e. blasphemy, impure thoughts and I remembered that extract [in Rapoport's book] from John Bunyan as having blasphemous thoughts, so I sort of partly accepted Mum's theory.

Six years after Rapoport's ground-breaking book, one focussing entirely on scrupulosity was published: *The Doubting Disease: Help for Scrupulosity and Religious Compulsions,* by Joseph Ciarrocchi. Personally, I am sceptical of the Roman Catholic Ciarrocchi's insistence that "Religion does not cause scrupulosity any more than teaching someone French history causes him to believe he is Napoleon." However, Ciarrocchi does astutely point out that scrupulosity generally afflicts persons with "an overly sensitive moral conscience". His book reveals that not only Bunyan, but Ignatius Loyola and Martin Luther were at various times victims of scrupulosity. Bunyan believed, like Sybil, that he had sinned against the Holy Spirit, and when he confided his 'guilt' to a friend, the latter admitted harbouring the same conviction! Both Bunyan and Loyola, moreover, were driven by their scrupulosity to contemplate suicide.

One particular case history of Rapoport's provoked me to rethink Sybil's overall behaviour during these two fraught years: In it, a young man, Daniel, describes "how hundreds of times each day he would 'get a feeling' that he had 'done something wrong' and that it displeased God." Like Sybil, to avoid eternal punishment, he would punish himself. Significantly, these "punishments", among other things, included denying himself pleasurable activities and making himself appear foolish before others. Daniel's story suggested to me that the majority of Sybil's extreme symptoms—her food refusal, her muteness, her grotesque posturing, and so on—may have been interconnected, a single constellation of behaviours stemming from 'guilt', that is, from OCD scrupulosity.

"THE THING INSIDE MY HEAD"

The Adolescent Unit consultants had increasingly viewed Sybil's beliefs as psychotic, but the cautionary statement in *Obsessive Compulsive Disorder: A Guide*, by John Greist, from the Dean Foundation for Health, Research and Education in Wisconsin, USA, is particularly relevant in the case of Sybil's scrupulosity: "[B]ecause obsessions can be so strange (even bizarre) they are sometimes mistaken as hallucinatory or delusional symptoms of psychosis." One wonders what difference it might have made to her treatment had Sybil's often-puzzled team taken on board Rapoport's findings, published in the UK two years earlier.

Chapter 3: 'Moving On'

> Were there any lessons about how young people's
> safety while in care settings could be maximized?...
> more thought is needed at the time of placement
> about the match between the needs of the child to
> be placed and others already in the setting, and the
> risks which each will pose to the other.
>
> (From Elaine Farmer and Sue Pollock, *Sexually
> Abused and Abusing Children in Substitute Care*, John
> Wiley & Sons, 1998, p. 234.)

"Sybil's not quite ready, yet." Nicky, Sybil's
"personal tutor" at Jacques Hall, the therapeutic community
to which she has been transferred, conveys this message for
about the third time as we huddle nervously in the reception
room on Christmas Day, 1994. Neil, just arrived home on
leave from Nigeria, burning with eagerness to see his
beloved daughter, and Molly and I, keen to celebrate
Christmas all together as a family, have been dismayed to
find that Sybil is apparently so anxious about this family
gathering that she won't give us permission to enter her
room. We put it down to the recentness of her move to this
new institutional environment on top of her usual difficulties
adjusting to her father's comings and goings from Africa and
her longstanding hyper-excitement over Christmas
festivities. It's all too much for her. Nicky, the personable
twenty-something-year-old counsellor—short, slight, brown-
haired and bonny-faced, an 'English rose'—with whom Sybil
has already closely bonded in the fortnight she's been at
Jacques Hall, is at present the only one allowed into her
inner sanctum.

Despite mounting frustration, we wait patiently, and,
eventually, after what seems *endless* although it is about an
hour, we are cautiously ushered into Sybil's small utilitarian
room, awkwardly juggling bundles of gifts in our arms. The

"THE THING INSIDE MY HEAD"

situation sadly reminds us that Sybil, although she has been deemed well enough to 'move on' from the Bethlem Royal Adolescent Unit, is still far from fully recovered. All too aware of her fragility, we slowly progress through the annual family ritual of exchanging gifts, with Nicky having to "help" Sybil, physically and emotionally, to open her presents, a replay of her fifteenth birthday at the Adolescent Unit.

The ice broken, Sybil gradually relaxes more, and we are able to make the transition, near lunchtime, of transporting her from Essex to the Borough of Barnet. Not ready to face having Christmas dinner at her erstwhile family home, Sybil has agreed in advance to a meal together at a restaurant near our home—one of the very few open on Christmas day and prepared to serve a vegetarian option, stipulated by our conscientious daughters. As talk begins to flow more readily, in cheerful if mundane channels, Neil and I begin to glow with hopes for the future. Neil exclaims with appreciative wonder: "How terrific it is to be sitting here having a conversation with my two grown-up daughters!"

But we overstep the boundaries. After dinner, Sybil very tentatively suggests she might like to stop in briefly at our home to see Ali-Biba, our family cat. We all eagerly second the idea and make for our home ten minutes away. But as Sybil walks over the threshold into the darkened, quiet house and spies Ali asleep in his little bed, she is hit by a surge of painful and difficult memories and all at once begins sobbing violently, unable to stay a minute longer in her old home. We bundle her back into the car and begin the long night time journey back to Jacques Hall, our Christmas spirits dampened.

Sybil recovers from this mini-trauma but doesn't want to discuss it with us. To Nicky, she confides that "she negatively associates her family home with the past events which led to her initial breakdown" (Jacques Hall's "Four Week Assessment"). Midway through Neil's Christmas break, Sybil is well enough to participate in a planned

Lois Chaber

excursion to a West End musical, our first all-family cultural outing in many years, but it is a mixed success. Overly taken up with my own preferences, I have chosen *Phantom of the Opera* for the family. Sybil is stimulated and impressed by this spectacular gothic show, but also unnerved and a bit frightened. It is Bad Jelly the Witch from our New Zealand holiday all over again!

All too soon it is time for Neil to return to Port Harcourt, Nigeria. His enquiries after other positions during the previous year having led nowhere despite some improvement in the UK economy, he has no choice but to continue this work abroad that supports the family financially while at the same time de-stabilising it emotionally. Even his position there is precarious:

The current military rulers under General Saani Abacha have undermined an already shaky economy by fixing the exchange rate and siphoning off billions to Swiss bank accounts for themselves, friends and rivals whose acquiescence has to be paid for. Due to the consequent shortage of funds, the government has not been paying the oil companies in full, including Shell, where I work. The oil companies refuse now to bring in their own funds to make up their budget requirements, and, as a result, development and other activities have been heavily cut back. Cutbacks, of course, mean reduced personnel needs, and expatriate contract staff such as myself are first in line to go. On top of these uncertainties, the project that I work on, the new office buildings for Shell in Port Harcourt, is currently at a standstill due to a major dispute between Shell and its French building contractor. So far I have survived all the

276

"THE THING INSIDE MY HEAD"

reductions and have been told that I am needed at least until June, but there is soon to be another review, and who knows what will happen?

      With Neil soldiering on in Nigeria, I settle into a routine of weekly visits to Sybil not unlike those of previous years to the Bethlem Royal. Nerve-wracked by my usual dread of getting lost, I heave a sigh of relief these winter days after having negotiated the long route to the little signpost on a lonely country road that marks the turnoff to Jacques Hall. I slowly bump my way along a muddy dirt road past assorted decrepit farm buildings and reeking, cow-filled barns belonging to a neighbouring farmer, till I come to the entrance to the sixteen-acre, privately run therapeutic community. A handsome red-brick Victorian mansion in quasi-Jacobean style in a picturesque setting near the Stour Estuary on the north-eastern coast of Essex, the main building of Jacques Hall has a welcoming exterior. But going inside is always a bit of a 'downer' since the refurbished interior is somewhat cheerless and shabby and the furniture occasionally in disrepair owing to the boisterous young inhabitants.

      Although I don't usually arrive there until late morning or early afternoon, Sybil is invariably not dressed and unwilling for me to see her in pyjamas. My arrival is announced to her by a member of staff, and then I'm told she'll get dressed presently, but this hardly ever happens. Time goes by, and eventually I start complaining. Someone goes to find Nicky, to "help" Sybil get dressed. Her inability to do things for herself and "getting stuck" is part of her current disorder, but I feel sure this paralysis is intensified by, not so much an outright reluctance to see me, as a formidable anxiety. Nicky, in her "Four Week Assessment", observes:

Lois Chaber

Sybil has expressed mixed feelings in terms of family contact. Her reaction has become fairly ritualised, she experiences anxiety and her mannerisms notably increase, leading up to her parents arriving at Jacques Hall. Once they have arrived the initial contact is often very difficult for Sybil to cope with, although she then relaxes and appears to enjoy these visits and trips out.

Although actually off-duty, Nicky, good-natured as she is, intuits so well how much these weekly visits mean to me that she comes to both our rescue and proceeds to wheedle and chivvy Sybil into her clothes, a process that can take anywhere from fifteen minutes up to another hour and a half. I muse about how Sybil's institutionalisation has created such formal barriers between us; on the one hand, it has forced me to acknowledge her right to privacy; on the other, it has made it difficult to relate to her in a casual and motherly way. At home, I would think nothing of walking in on Sybil in her night clothes to chat, or urging her myself to get dressed.

When Sybil finally emerges into the reception area, she is reticent and sheepish, shrinking from me if I try to embrace her too warmly (as my own emotional needs provoke me to do), but eventually we make hesitant conversation, which chugs along, stopping and starting for the next couple of hours. Sometimes there is a change of pace for both of us when Sybil makes her way into the community kitchen and nervously and self-consciously puts together a cheese sandwich for herself. Eating my own packed lunch, I hang on every crumb that she consumes, relishing her current normality in eating. When I feel I can

"THE THING INSIDE MY HEAD"

depart into the darkening late winter afternoon in good conscience, she gives me a tentative hug goodbye.

* * *

What are very apparent now at Jacques Hall are Sybil's classic symptoms of OCD, particularly the intermittent frozen postures and the excessive hesitation and repetition in walking and in doing most ordinary things. In contrast to the Adolescent Unit, there are no other young people in Jacques Hall with OCD or any similar disorder. Jane Lee, an attractive and pleasant woman of about forty who is the Admissions and Marketing Officer of Jacques Hall and the wife of Terry Lee, the institution's Director, comments on Sybil's uniqueness in the community:

> It was always a job for us to try to get the other young people to understand obsessive-compulsive disorder. To try and relate that to other young people was very difficult, but it was a task that, as a group, we took on. Some of the group would empathise with Sybil, but for other members of the group it was harder; they had come to know Sybil, her warmth and her fun, and then the Sybil who was unwell was so different from that, that they could become quite frightened. And Sybil herself was almost embarrassed by it, and very conscious that at the time she was the only one with that illness.

From our point of view, Sybil's situation here is more akin to that at Hill End than at the Bethlem Royal. The Jacques Hall Foundation's official brochure in 1995 describes their client adolescents as "'casualties of the 90s'"—that is, sexually and physically abused young people.

279

Lois Chaber

According to the informal booklet for the residents, they are "young people who display a range of challenging and often anti-social behaviour." Sybil is introverted, passive, ultra-sensitive, and very naïve, disabled by an extreme anxiety disorder, while her companions here are extroverted, mostly aggressive, and clearly street-wise despite being younger than she. The few older girls who join Jacques Hall during Sybil's stay are far more socially experienced and on a different wave length; as Molly bluntly pronounces when she accompanies me: "They dress like tarts." Sybil is unable to make the kind of friends she had in the Adolescent Unit, who meant so much to her. Whenever we are sitting in the living room, all around us there is an atmosphere of barely-controlled mayhem, with noise, scuffling, loud arguing going on and youngsters occasionally intruding directly upon us. Jane Lee readily admits that the atmosphere at Jacques Hall is "quite robust, loud and noisy," but goes on to say, "We were always worried that the atmosphere would be too robust for Sybil; however, she always managed to cope with it."

However, Neil's Cousin Edna, who continues to visit Sybil when she is at Jacques Hall, finds the situation there very disconcerting:

> The children there were rather unfriendly and rowdy, and, as a result, Sybil stopped wanting to go out. The staff members at this place were mostly unhelpful; when we tried to talk to them about the unruly behaviour, they chose to ignore it, their attitude being that 'it was nothing to do with us'.

Neil and I, though we certainly do not share Edna's feelings about the staff, increasingly come to feel that Sybil is *not*

280

"THE THING INSIDE MY HEAD"

always able to cope with the rowdiness. Nicky, although generally as optimistic as Jane, has some disarming details to convey in her May 1995 "Review":

> There have been several occasions where conflict has occurred between Sybil and other students, for example, Sybil has been the victim of teasing, as other students recognise that she gets annoyed by this. On one occasion, a snakeskin was thrust into Sybil [sic] face in order to see her reaction, and at other times Sybil has experienced verbal bullying from the girls [sic] group. She handles such situations fairly well, though, and stands her ground. Sybil has expressed to me how unhappy she is amongst her peers at Jacques Hall, stating that she doesn't feel comfortable around them, and as a result, she doesn't tend to spend much time with them.

Although we think it is highly appropriate and socially beneficial to provide a therapeutic community for the kind of disturbed and disruptive adolescents who twenty or thirty years earlier would have been written off as 'juvenile delinquents', we don't think it's the right place for Sybil. The official Jacques Hall brochure states that "[Jacques Hall] is about creating an environment and an atmosphere which is safe." This may be true for most of the young residents coming from dubious care situations or abusive homes, but Sybil does not seem to feel "safe" within her peer environment here. In a "Students' Review Form" she fills out after her first six weeks there (dated 25/1/95), her answer to the question, "Is there anything you don't like about it [Jacques Hall]?" is as follows: "Bullying, intimidating, stealing, not being able to trust people, feeling frightened sometimes." As the year goes on, Neil and I feel we were let down by the Adolescent Unit, which manoeuvred Sybil into Jacques Hall without offering her or us a wider range of alternatives. And she is locked into her residence here by the elaborate funding setup from the Borough of Barnet that was so very difficult to put into place.

* * *

However, some aspects of the community are clearly pleasing and beneficial to Sybil. On the same review sheet, her answer to "What are the best things about being here?" is: "going out, being in the country, working with Nicky, Dr. Berry." In evenings and on weekends, the young people are taken to Rollerworld, to the cinema or on shopping excursions, which Sybil seems very much to enjoy, despite some embarrassment about her ritualistic behaviour in public at times. Dr. Rowland Berry is the community's Consultant Psychiatrist, an elderly, kindly man with whom Sybil does feel safe, whom she sees roughly once a week, but he is not an expert in OCD. Moreover, Sybil is clearly deriving much pleasure and support from her relationship with Nicky, who is in charge of coordinating all aspects of Sybil's care in Jacques Hall and, even more importantly, as the young people's booklet explains, is there to "help, guide, advise, support and above all listen". With this personal tutor, young enough to be a kind of surrogate older sister as well as role model for her, Sybil has formed an extremely intense relationship—perhaps too intense, perhaps in lieu of a friend her own age.

Sybil is asked at one point to enumerate, as therapeutic "homework", the ways in which she "uses" Jacques Hall care workers. The resulting list implies a high level of kindly responsiveness on the part of the staff but also reveals Sybil's ongoing emotional neediness:

"THE THING INSIDE MY HEAD"

Being with them, talking to them and listening to them helps distract my thoughts and feelings.
They cheer me up or make me laugh.
For a feeling of safety
To feel looked after
To help me sort out or resolve things on my mind
For help doing things I can't or feel I can't do on my own
For a hug, comfort
For a way of venting my feelings by talking about them [the feelings]
When I feel suicidal, talking to staff usually helps a bit.

Members of staff here, moreover, unlike those at the Bethlem Royal, who found Sybil's often disturbingly uncooperative behaviour a major inconvenience, have unambiguously positive feelings about Sybil, thanks to her overall improvement. Nicky speaks for most of them when she describes Sybil on a Barnet "Review of Child Looked After Form": "She is a quiet & mature member of the Community, who is pleasant to be around & has a helpful and positive relationship with staff... She has a lovely personality, & is transformed when she relaxes and laughs. Sybil is a cooperative, genuinely caring & honest member of the community."

The school sessions that Sybil attends are, as in the Adolescent Unit, quite truncated, nothing like a 'normal' secondary school regime for a girl close to seventeen, but they certainly fulfil the brochure's promise of being child-centred and individually programmed. Her main teacher, Mr. Blacker, has Sybil bring to class the postcards that her dad sends her from Nigeria and constructs a geography lesson around them, and her other enthusiastic teachers seem to be aiding her character development: "Sybil can be an articulate contributor to group discussions and a sympathetic

Lois Chaber

and constructive listener. She asks appropriate questions and interjects in a polite but firm manner," according to her school report. Of course, the syllabus is primarily remedial, going back over ground she would have covered years earlier at Latymer and then again at the Bethlem Royal, one of the many repercussions of being on the mental illness treadmill. Sybil comments under "School" on the September Borough of Barnet review form: "What is frustrating is having to relearn things I've already done, because I've forgotten them & gone backwards."

What Jacques Hall uniquely offers to Sybil is its setting—unlike her previous venues—in an authentic, working countryside environment, and the opportunity this provides for the young people to relate to animals as well as people, a major component in what the brochure boasts is its "holistic approach to living". At the time Sybil is here, the resident farm animals are a small group of chickens and ducks, two large Vietnamese pot-bellied pigs, and a group of about seven attractive brown and white goats. She soon takes on the confidence-building role of the most dependable and willing young helper with the animals, feeding them regularly and helping to 'muck out' when her OCD phobias about dirt are in abeyance. Sybil has always loved animals, and this opportunity to work with them, as well as frequent trips with groups from Jacques Hall to the Mistley Environmental Centre in nearby Manningtree, a sanctuary that rescues animals from harm or neglect, helps to mitigate her loneliness amidst her uncongenial peer group.

Jane Lee, whom Sybil gets to know mainly through their mutual work in the farmyard, relates an incident epitomising Sybil's very special relationship with the animals at Jacques Hall.

"THE THING INSIDE MY HEAD"

One of the goats had a bad foot. Sybil was very distressed that it was poorly. She accompanied me and the goat to the vet, with her in the back and the goat in the hatchback. The goat travelled with its head on Sybil's shoulder and didn't bleat once. It was quite content being with Sybil all the way to the vet's, about a half hour trip. It was just her ability to be so wonderful with an animal; the goat felt so safe with her. I know it's only a goat, but goats are a very special clever animal. And then there was her joy when the vet said it was something simple.

The animals also facilitate *my* relationship with Sybil. (It seems I always need something external to mediate between Sybil and me—a book, a magazine, animals or food....) Our visits improve greatly when winter gives way to spring and Sybil and I can spend time together feeding the goats, petting and admiring them, and generally tramping around outside. When Neil, home on leave for Easter, and I propose taking Sybil out on some excursions in the surrounding Essex villages, animals, again, are the incentive. Sybil is delighted when we take her to some animal shelters and farms, feeding and touching sheep and other farm animals, her face wreathed in smiles.

She is less ecstatic but still quite interested when we take in some landmarks of Constable country, but we are puzzled by her absolute refusal, with no explanation, to enter any of the lovely old churches that Neil and I want to explore and photograph. There have been no signs this year, as far as we can see, of the religious obsessions and scrupulosity that plagued her at the Bethlem Royal; is she now entirely averse to religion? Or frightened of triggering the obsessions again? Discussing Sybil's inner world with her is taboo. Later on, in September, filling in a Borough of Barnet

285

review form, under the heading of "religion," she writes: "Christian (a bit)".

It is still quite difficult to get Molly to accompany me on my Sunday visits to Sybil when Neil is not here. She has problems getting up in the morning and cherishes her Sunday lie-in so much that getting ready in good time to drive up to Essex is a major sticking point between us, one issue among many that makes my relationship with her this year quite volatile. But the real problem is that the girls' lives are growing more and more apart, with Molly's educational and social experiences vastly overtaking Sybil's. Studying now for the GCSE exams that Sybil has never taken, going on a Russian exchange visit to Belarus two years in a row, visiting my sister and brother-in-law in California for three successive summers, playing in four different instrumental organisations during the year, and travelling to Austria with one of them, attending co-ed parties regularly, Molly has an expanding life-style, while Sybil's institutionalised one is extremely limited. Getting the girls together becomes an incentive for me to learn the route from Jacques Hall into Colchester, where I manage, precariously, to get the three of us to a few plays and films, crowned by feasts in Pizza Hut.

My own psychic work at the Tavistock has resumed in February, with a new psychiatrist, and while it has been comforting to have this support with Neil still so far away and so many family problems, the sessions have been less fruitful than before. I am unable to form a genuine therapeutic rapport with my new therapist, whose psychiatric methodology I find rigid and uncongenial.

But as the summer comes on, my mental state is buoyed up by the tentatively widening horizons for Sybil within her institutional confines. My visits with her have now expanded to include fairly regular trips into Manningtree, the nearby town. We stop just outside the town at a small sanctuary for swans along the shore, and, with mutual delight and much laughter, we feed these very spoiled

"THE THING INSIDE MY HEAD"

creatures a whole loaf of bread, always amazed at their boldness in coming up to us to grab large pieces and their just-barely contained aggression as they fight for the largest share. These swan-visits are among my happiest moments with her. From there we head into the town itself to have as gargantuan a meal as we can manage at an Indian restaurant. Feeding Sybil up is still a profound need for me, harking all the way back from her underweight 'preemie' days to her recent extreme anorexia; of course, in circular fashion, it keeps 'eating' on the agenda of fraught issues for her.

Sybil takes even more exciting expeditions under the auspices of Jacques Hall this marvellous summer of '95. The Community owns a yacht moored near Ipswich, and Nicky, a keen sailor, is allowed to take Sybil and a few other girls to a variety of destinations—out to sea, into the River Stour, and to Walton backwaters, returning to the marina at day's end. According to Jane Lee, Sybil really takes to sailing, deriving immense pleasure from these "girlie days out". These excursions help to prepare Sybil physically and mentally for what is an annual event at Jacques Hall, an early August adventure holiday for the young people in Embrun, in the French Alps. Neil and I are thrilled when Sybil's behaviour is deemed stable enough to qualify her for inclusion on this exciting trip abroad, despite her fluctuating OCD and occasional lapses into near-anorexia. We are told afterwards that she has thrived on the week of strenuous walking, sailing and white water rafting, and was able to weather the long coach journey and ferry trip both ways.

* * *

During this period of stimulating activities, however, there is the inevitable pressure on Sybil to 'move on' and 'grow up'. Understandably, the ultimate goal of Jacques Hall is to prepare its inhabitants for an independent life outside the institution, as the informal booklet for the young people explains:

287

Lois Chaber

We feel preparation for leaving Jacques
Hall is very important and make every effort to
help students move on in a planned and
positive way. Where rehabilitation to families is
not possible, we are able to offer facilities in the
main house and also a cottage in the grounds
for the purpose of semi-independent training.
For those students who feel ready to join
society, the next step is our Outreach Project...
Our Outreach worker continues with the life
skills programme begun at Jacques Hall and is
able to offer ongoing support and guidance
within the bed-sit situation in the local
community.

To this end, Sybil, who at over seventeen is just
about the oldest teenager in the community, is moved from
the main building into 'The Cottage' in late May, with two
other, slightly younger girls, to begin independence training.
It starts out well; the three girls proudly invite Jane and Terry
Lee and a few other staff members to a modest little dinner
at 'The Cottage'. However, Sybil has little in common with
the other two teenagers, and it all ends in tears. In early
June, as some kind of a 'joke', the two girls lock Sybil up in
the cupboard and ignore her tearful pleas to come out. Sybil
completely crashes and cuts her hand with glass that same
evening, though only superficially. To Nicky, she confides
that her intention was "to get herself admitted to hospital and
away from Jacques Hall" (September "Review"). "This
independence was something we all wanted for Sybil," Jane
Lee admits, but "we decided it was a step she was not ready
to take." Jane sees it as a shared problem, speaking of
Sybil's "inability to manage the other girls' behaviour" and
their "inability to empathise with her sensitivity". She is
moved back to the main house to a room of her own.

"THE THING INSIDE MY HEAD"

Sybil tries cutting herself a couple of other times, but again without serious damage. Although she has been experimenting with self-harming since Bethlem Royal days, this behaviour is reinforced, I am sorry to say, by her stay at Jacques Hall, where, we find out later, it is endemic. Only a short time after her arrival at Jacques Hall, Sybil's roommate at the time, a slim blonde girl of about fourteen or fifteen, tries to slash herself and Jane Lee admits that some of the children actually have to be taken to hospital after incidents of self-harming. In *Reviving Ophelia*, Mary Pipher claims self-harming is another wide-spread trend of the 1990s among adolescent girls. And even in 2005, in an article in *The Guardian Weekly*, June 3-9—"Olympic star Kelly Holmes reveals her hidden scars"—the chief executive of Sane, a mental health charity, declares: "We believe that self-harm has become almost an epidemic, particularly among young people, who are damaging themselves in increasingly disturbing ways." Pipher sees it as a response, in lieu of other coping strategies, to intense stress: a cry for help, a way of calming down, and an attempt to regain control. She warns that with repetition it becomes ingrained, which we see happening with Sybil.

From the end of the summer onward, things begin to look bleaker for Sybil at Jacques Hall, or maybe the basic problems have just been quietly simmering under the surface all along. Jane Lee describes Sybil's positive interaction with the Community—"through her gentleness, Sybil was always able, at Community meetings, to offer so much support to children who were really struggling"—but that is not the same as actually forging close individual friendships. Sybil's enuresis, her bedwetting, is still haunting her, a symptom of emotional disturbance, and she eventually has to take medication to control it.

Most important of all, her OCD has not really been improving, but rather comes and goes, with varying intensity. She is not receiving any specialised therapy for it, although we have started pressing for this and have had some vague

Lois Chaber

promises from staff that they will look into obtaining for her some cognitive behavioural therapy (CBT), now a recommended treatment for OCD sufferers. In the second half of the year she has started obsessively washing her hands, splashing a lot of water onto herself and the floor, mopping it all up with large amounts of toilet paper, and generally making a mess in the washroom. She also takes ninety-minute showers. One day, we are told, she gets so "stuck" washing her hands repeatedly before a Community meal, that she misses dinner entirely, and even then, Nicky has to come, finally, to turn the water off and take Sybil away.

Jane maintains that Sybil's personal tutor relationship, a keystone of the therapeutic philosophy of Jacques Hall, has benefited her disorder: "When Sybil was really overcome with OCD, that opening, through Nicky, made it possible for it not to become intolerable for her." Jacques Hall's therapeutic philosophy, she explains, is based on "psychodynamic practice." As described in a "Philosophy Paper" by her husband, Terry Lee, this consists primarily of encouraging the young people to "act out" their feelings, sometimes recreating their early experiences and family situations, with both adults and peers within the Community.

But this system, by autumn, does not seem to us to be working all that well for Sybil. Although in later times she is often to feel quite nostalgic about people and events at Jacques Hall, some time after leaving she confides to paper some angry criticism of the Community, tempered by profound compassion for the other adolescents:

> At Jacques Hall they used punishment and reward. If you went to school, for example, you could go out on ents. [entertainment] in the evening. If you didn't go to school, you

couldn't. That's just one example, but for me, that's mostly how the place worked, or didn't work. The kids had reasons for behaving the way they did and sometimes these reasons or emotions were stronger and harder to deal with than the punishments. The kids there were very traumatised. They had had terrible, awful things happen in their short lives. Some of them had been physically abused; some of them had been sexually abused. Some of them had been raped by their own fathers. Some of them had been in care since they were a baby [sic] and had been abused while they were in care in foster homes. If you just try and imagine how this terrible abuse could have affected them and still affects them now, you can see why they do some of the things they do. They may do naughty or sometimes bad things, but they are hurting inside. Even when they harmed themselves, they got into trouble.

It seemed like at Jacques Hall no one acknowledged the abuse and pain very much. They expected them to just get on with their lives. There wasn't nearly enough proper therapy which they could use. I got more time than any of them and it still wasn't enough. That was because I didn't have the same kinds of problems they had. I could recognise some of my feelings and what caused them and ask for help. I didn't have the terrible burdens, dark secrets, shame and guilt as an obstacle to getting help, but they did. And when they were kicked out, abandoned, on top of it, they were made to again feel worthless, hated, unwanted, uncared for and guilty. They needed love and therapy to help them work through and relieve them of the guilt, shame and pain. They didn't deserve guilt; it is the people who did this to

*them that did. I feel like crying and screaming
when I think of those poor kids. I would like to
do something to help them.*

The degree of accuracy in Sybil's strictures is not for
us to say as we did not experience Jacques Hall on a daily
basis. They may reflect just one subsequent mood of hers.
Nevertheless, the poems that Sybil writes sometime during
the latter part of her residence there, though not technically
proficient, reveal considerable pain:

*It's like my outer body is a mask
to the messed up ugly Sybil inside,
Bleeding and scarred.
Will I heal?
I don't know how.*

. . . .

*My heart screams inside me
but my outside is quiet.
The creature of me, for that is what
I feel it is, is trapped inside. . . .*

. . . .

*There's no one who can share the
burden of my pain. I wish I could
just disappear or self-destruct.*

* * *

Neil and I, meanwhile, ignorant of the depths of
Sybil's unhappiness, welcome the news that the Community
has been recently accredited to teach GCSE courses. In
May, Sybil had been given the opportunity to take AEB
(Associated Examination Board) exams in a few of her basic
subjects, thereby gaining some sense of achievement, but
these exams do not play a role within the official secondary

school curriculum. Clinging to our hope that Sybil will at some point become a 'normal' student again, we exude enthusiasm over her enrolment in this new GCSE programme. This is not the first or the last time we inadvertently pressure Sybil with our expectations.

Sybil has not been at her best in recent weeks, but Jacques Hall decides anyway in mid-September to make another attempt to move her on to greater independence, setting her up in 'The 'Gatehouse', a tiny building situated (symbolically) at the outermost edge of the Jacques Hall estate where it joins up with the muddy path leading out onto the main country road. She occupies it jointly with two other girls (different ones), but has a room of her own, provided, significantly, with a lock and a safe for valuables. The staff also hopes to arrange some weekend work experience for Sybil at the Mistley Environmental Centre.

In this same month, September—both before and after the move—Sybil makes a shaky attempt to begin a diary, written sporadically and messily on an A4 pad, but it fizzles out, discontinued in the ensuing months. However, her scattering of entries [excerpted below] suggest that the move to The Gatehouse may not have been appropriate for her at this time: not only are the same old Jacques Hall issues still agitating her, but her mental stability appears to be ebbing:

[Here and in subsequent chapters, I have refrained from using ellipsis dots (…) for material that I have edited out of her diary entries (none of which alters the basic meaning), for the sake of readability.]

10 September: Mum and Dad came today. They gave me some pictures of Ali [our cat]. It makes me feel [a word crossed out, illegibly] to know that he probably doesn't remember me. I'm not part of his life now.

Lois Chaber

Korreanna [a resident] came back she gave me a post card for my postcard collection and a stick of rock [candy] which was really sweet and nice of her. I was touched. Friendship for me is difficult.

13 September: I feel sort of low and grey. I hate my period but its got to come some time. I'm really dreading when I'm next on. I always feel sort of threatened, defensive, wary, nervous with things to do with the cottage. I wish I had a real, good friend here who I knew and trusted and knew she was on my side and who was strong and believed in important things I believed in.

15 September: I'm not in a good way. I wished I was normal then I remembered the pressures Id have then. I don't feel too good. I'm worried I'm in the gatehouse now. ~~I hope~~

I'm sure my feelings from my life the bad things and a lot for the year 91/92 are still inside me and I need to get them out. I think they may be partly why I have problems. **I want to get them out**

HELP

They need to come out.

25 September: Its my review tomorrow, I'm anxious. I hope I don't miss it.

I am worried about what going to be said about future stuff.

I feel unstable in relationship with Vicky and Jo [with whom she shares The Gatehouse].

Review: *[Sybil summarises the issues she brought up, followed by possible solutions suggested by staff]:*

"THE THING INSIDE MY HEAD"

No-one understands what its like to have my problems—Find out address of Phobic Action [a charity for sufferers] and contact them. Keep in touch with Natalie [from the Adolescent Unit].

Bullying—talk to staff I think it would be good to talk to about

Nastiness—Talk to staff I can trust write down how I feel and what happened

Not feeling stable—

Not being able to trust people—

Loneliness—Keep in touch with friends outside here. Phone family, write to family.

Feel in a mess—Write diary, keep in contact with people, talk to Nicky, write this

26: September: I am upset, I've had a difficult day and people have been horrible to me and I haven't got it off my chest because I couldn't talk to most of the staff and Maggie [staff member] has just come back from being exhausted and maybe stressed and I didn't want to stress her and Colin [staff member] wasn't much help when I talked to him and thought people might think I was moaning and making a big thing of it and I shouldn't be telling them

People don't understand how sensitive I am to little things, I have tried a bit to stop letting it affect me but I don't think I can. They really do have a big effect on me and I don't know if anyone understands I feel guilty for thinking that I'm having a hard time.

* * *

Back in Nigeria in late September of 1995, Neil continues trying to find other employment on the quiet, assuming that his return to England will greatly benefit Sybil. He is fed up with his insecure life in Nigeria: "Regarding my job situation, throughout most of the year, several options have been mooted at any one time, and, depending on the level of stability about government funding, company policy on staffing and ever-changing budgets, my contract has been on, off, renewed and/or extended several times." Prospects for other positions emerge from time to time, are chased up by both of us but eventually fizzle out one way or another. In Port Harcourt, there is ever-present local danger due to the high incidence of armed robberies, both on the road and in the compounds. In November, Port Harcourt is also the scene of the shocking government execution of Ken Saro Wiwa, much-respected writer and civil rights and environmental activist, along with eight of his compatriots. The political and economic turmoil of Nigeria is rapidly escalating, and I lie awake at nights worrying about Neil.

Neil is not home on leave again till late December, and we collect Sybil from The Gatehouse on the 24th to take her back to Southgate for the real family at-home Christmas that she has agreed to beforehand. But what starts out as a happy Christmas Day eventually turns into a disaster. Sybil is supposed to be returned to Jacques Hall on the eve of the 25th after a 24-hour stay, but she winds up being stuck with us through the 28th due to an unforeseen chain of unlucky events that make the long trip up to Essex impossible: running out of petrol on Christmas night—with no stations open; an impassable blizzard, a broken car-heater in freezing weather, and so on. Sybil's enforced stay in this house of many memories compounds recent aggravations at the Community—including the theft of some belongings from The Gatehouse, despite locks, and the recent withdrawal of her medication, the OCD drug Clomipramine. Her behaviour at home becomes increasingly bizarre, anti-social and dysfunctional, a throwback to the worst days at the Bethlem Adolescent Unit. The pressure of beginning the GCSE course at the community, given Sybil's ever-present "fear of failure", may also, as Jane Lee suggests, have contributed to this shocking regression.

When we are finally able to return her to Jacques Hall, she regresses further, refusing to see any of her family, becoming severely anorexic, neglecting her personal care,

"THE THING INSIDE MY HEAD"

curling up into a foetal position for hours on end. This throws the Community into crisis, as they do not have the kind and amount of staff to deal with such extreme behaviour. After much distressed communication back and forth involving Jacques Hall, Neil and me, various mental health and social services authorities both in Essex and in Barnet, the decision is taken in late January to hospitalise Sybil in Peter Bruff, the adult mental health ward at the main hospital in Clacton, a nearby seaside town. Sometime in February, she is returned to Jacques Hall to try again, but it doesn't work; she breaks down again and is sent back to Clacton Hospital. According to Jane Lee, some of the young people from the Community visit Sybil in hospital, "but there is no emotional bond," and Sybil spends all her time going back and forth to the washroom, scrubbing her hands.

Meanwhile, before and after Sybil's catastrophic Christmas visit, Neil suddenly finds that the construction industry in England is starting to rally, and he is able to drum up thirteen interviews over the holiday period. As a consequence, early in the New Year he gets the offer of a position as Senior Project Manager for a management company working on the projected Terminal Five for Heathrow Airport. He never returns to Nigeria. It is grimly ironic that, just at this terrible new low point for Sybil and the diminution of our hopes for her recovery, Neil has a breakthrough at last and is able to 'move on'.

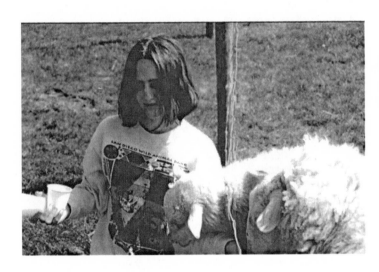

Sybil at an animal farm, 1995.

"THE THING INSIDE MY HEAD"

Chapter 4: Rehabilitation

Principle [sic] aim of rehabilitation is to enable the individual to attain his [or her] maximum level of independence, psychologically, socially, physically and economically.

> (From a handout on "Rehabilitation in Mental Health," given to Sybil in Clacton Hospital.)

Behavioural treatments have lasting results. They do not explore fantasies or hidden meanings.

> (From Sybil's notes on Isaac Mark's *Living with Fear: Understanding and Coping with Anxiety*, New York and London: McGraw-Hill, Inc, 1980, p. 92.)

Sybil, now settled into the Peter Bruff Acute Mental Health Ward in Clacton Hospital, is still averse to seeing Neil and me. We learn that she is barely able to do anything practical for herself, but, encouraged by staff, she manages to articulate her latest OCD handicaps:

There are lots of different aspects to my OCD, but they all centre around one fear: a fear of harming someone. A terrible thought that I might harm someone is in my head. This is terrifying for me but hard for other people to understand, as they know I'm not the sort of person to hurt anyone, but the persistent thought in my head that I might is so strong, real and persistent.

I am scared of getting dirty because once I am dirty I might transmit diseases or contaminate other people and make them really ill even so that they might die. I am scared of being guilty.

I am also scared of getting dirty because then I have to wash it off and I hate going into the toilet and I hate the whole procedure.

I am scared of electric things because I get them wet and then someone else touches them and gets electrocuted or I get electrocuted and then someone touches me and gets electrocuted or damage[s] it.

I am scared of sharp things because I am frightened I will hurt someone with them.

Her goal, she writes, is to overcome these fears and be able to do "normal things" like make tea and shave her legs.

Staff members, trying to assuage the anguish we feel over our disallowed visits, explain that Sybil is particularly afraid of contaminating and harming her parents. Even when she eventually grants us permission for a short visit, a couple of weeks later, we are only allowed, she indicates, to come up to the threshold of her room. She is hovering inside, a few metres away, like a wounded bird trying desperately to take flight, bedraggled-looking and tense. She barely manages to greet us, in a tiny hesitant voice. We speak to her gently and patiently, trying to calm her fears, but she won't allow us to enter ("Everything is dirty"), much less to hug her as we long to do. Soon, we are 'encouraged' by staff to leave. My own amateur psychoanalytic musing leads me to wonder whether all this is rooted in repressed desires to hurt us, but (thankfully) this is not the approach Sybil's carers are to take.

"THE THING INSIDE MY HEAD"

During this stressful period, I discover the newly-founded charity "Obsessive Action" (now called "OCD Action"), dedicated to supporting and informing OCD sufferers and their families, and begin gradually finding out more and more about this insidious and multi-faceted disorder that affects roughly 3% of the population, the most prevalent mental health problem next to depression. I come to realise that, in a smaller way, I share some of these classic OCD obsessions, compulsions and phobias—excessive list-making, magical thoughts (if I do *x* it will jinx *y*), counting rituals (splashing my face with water exactly seven times every morning), excessive requests for reassurance, my driving phobias, and so on—and so does Molly, to an even lesser extent, with her phobias about insects, her excessive fears of embarrassment, and her compulsive hoarding of items in her fly tip room. It seems clear that the predisposition to anxiety disorders in their varying forms and strengths in Sybil and Molly have been inherited from me. Nevertheless, it should be noted that, as Neil Hopkins, writing in the *Obsessive Action Newsletter* on "OCD and Mental Health Categorisation" maintains, obsessions and compulsions on a very minor scale are common to almost everyone, and the diagnosis of OCD is just a point on a "psychological continuum" where the symptoms seriously interfere with the person's life.

* * *

Sybil is at first very dependent on the briskly cheerful nurses of Peter Bruff Ward for all her personal care, and, once again, it is easy for her to form close therapeutic relationships with nursing staff. Not so with Dr. Smith, the Consultant Psychiatrist for the region, who has ultimate authority over Sybil's case. She fears and dislikes him from the first, as do we. (At the interview Sybil is to have later with the Maudsley Trust, Sybil tells her interlocutor that with "some nurses, [she] feels safe," and she identifies "people [she] doesn't trust / powerful, i.e. psychiatrists".) *Our personal impression* is that Dr. Smith, although obviously

301

highly qualified and very intelligent, is also cold, formal, autocratic, and not as sensitive to our daughter's plight as we would wish. There is never to be, as far as we can perceive, any real rapport between him and Sybil, and difficult relations with him on our part are to complicate our efforts to obtain the best care possible for her from the NHS.

The major problem is that Peter Bruff is an acute ward that provides only short-term stays for patients, and it is obvious that Sybil needs extended care. What to do with her becomes the dominant issue of her stay in this ward. To our minds, from the very beginning, Dr. Smith is muttering darkly about lack of funding available for Sybil, and often, disturbingly, in her presence. It seems to us an almost reflex response on his part whenever Sybil is mentioned—despite the fact that the final decisions on financial matters are not entirely within his remit. He is urging that Sybil be returned to the Borough of Barnet, which has been handling her funding up to now. We understand that he is quite naturally concerned about the limited financial resources of his own region; however, we also know that such a move would be traumatic for Sybil—not only because she has already been moved around so much—but for the reasons that we articulate in one of the many letters we write on this issue:

> In her present condition, placement in or near our home is extremely antipathetic to [Sybil]. Her belief that she contaminates people and may harm them is particularly acute in relation to her parents. We also intuit that Sybil experiences distress near her home because of its associations with the very unhappy and traumatic events leading up to her breakdown in 1992.

"THE THING INSIDE MY HEAD"

We also make the case that Sybil has been living in northeast Essex for over a year now and should qualify as a local resident.

These contested issues of Sybil's funding and placement are to draw in a large number of medical and social officials from both boroughs, besides Dr. Smith, and their discussion back and forth drags out over several months. Neil and I go into battle mode, making endless telephone calls, writing impassioned argumentative letters, attending numerous tense meetings, in order to secure what we feel is the right care for Sybil, in the right place. Our efforts are supported by Heather, manager of the nearby Tendring Advocacy Service run by MIND, the mental health charity, who has befriended Sybil, is monitoring her case, and sits in on many of her hospital review meetings where the problems are discussed.

For the family of a sufferer, it is intensely frustrating to come up against the considerable gap between their loved one's acute medical requirements and the rigid workings of NHS and local government bureaucracies. Like two disturbed tectonic plates, human needs and material resources relentlessly grind and abrade one another, rarely sliding into a smooth fit. Of course we know that nurses have to be paid, that bed space is limited, that medications are expensive, and that there are even more adolescents out there getting less treatment; however, when your child is suffering, your only instinct, surely a primeval one, is to fight for *her* needs.

I put aside my tentative plans to return to teaching for the time being in order to engage with 'the system', yet again, while Neil is heavily preoccupied with establishing his role in the Heathrow Terminal Five Project, not easy for someone who has been away from the British building industry for three and a half years. For almost three months I drive up to Clacton every Friday to attend Sybil's weekly review meetings, where major and minor decisions about her are made, in order to ensure that she is not railroaded out of the ward. As time goes on, many members of the Clacton staff move onto our side, but Dr. Smith remains opposed to the Regional Trust taking on Sybil's care. At these uncomfortable reviews, Sybil is extremely anxious, frequently popping up and down from her seat, one of her typical OCD behaviours; she says little but is occasionally quite bluntly outspoken to Dr. Smith, contradicting statements he makes about her.

* * *

Notwithstanding the funding dispute, we have no quarrel at this point with Dr. Smith's medical treatment of Sybil, and we respect his professional expertise. He diagnoses Sybil as severely depressed, a condition quite commonly associated with OCD (called "comorbid depression"), and recommends a course of ECT, electroconvulsive therapy, for her. Sybil, of course, with her fear of electricity, is horrified at the prospect, and, to be sure, this 'shock treatment' is still quite controversial. However, having experienced it myself to good effect under Dr. Shirbini in Qatar, and having heard recently of its beneficial effects on the thirty-something daughter of a good friend, I feel strongly in favour of ECT for Sybil, as does Neil. The "Client Information Booklet" from the North East Essex Mental Health Trust that Sybil is given to read, confirms that ECT has come a long way from the cruder methods of decades ago—that schlock cinematic stereotype—in its reassuring account of what the treatment consists of:

> The treatment... only takes a few minutes... The anaesthetist will ask you to hold out your hand so you can be given an anaesthetic injection. It will make you go to sleep and cause your muscles to relax completely. You will be given some oxygen to breathe as you go

off to sleep. Once you are fast asleep a small electric current is passed across your head and this causes a mild modified seizure in your brain. The muscles tense and relax although there is little movement of the body because of the relaxant injection that the anaesthetist gives... Once you are wide awake you will be offered a cup of tea.

This booklet, along with one from MIND discussing the pros and cons, plus our encouragement, eventually persuades Sybil to consent to six sessions of ECT over several weeks. Although we are aware that ECT is no panacea and often has only short-term effects, Sybil and we are very pleased with the result. Her mood lifts considerably, enabling her to function better with everyday tasks and opening up the possibilities of other therapies.

Sybil now allows us to have some more or less 'normal' visits with her in the large, open visiting area of the ward. When we first walk into the cafeteria-style room and see her, still quite unkempt, with sloping shoulders, outgrown lank hair in no particular style, and unsightly crooked teeth (without the braces she had to relinquish during her long mental ordeal, her teeth have reverted to a worse condition), I am pained and even somewhat repelled: "Is this the beautiful child I once had?" Almost immediately overcome by shame and compassion, I greet her with as cheerful a face as I can muster. I don't confide these feelings to Neil, who is more charitable. The usual exchange of little bits of news take place, but the climax of the visit is when Sybil offers to make tea for us, proudly playing the polite hostess and demonstrating that she has now mastered at least some of her fears.

Meanwhile, the funding saga goes on. In response to our great concern, the Peter Bruff Ward Manager sets up a 'case conference' for April 23rd, at which members of the different interest groups, including a representative from MIND and a new participant, Jane Clark, a CPN (Community Psychiatric Nurse) from the North East Essex Community Mental Health Team, along with ourselves, will discuss Sybil's future. It is yet another tense meeting, where everybody speaks his or her mind, sometimes at cross purposes. Dr. Smith proclaims that Sybil's depression has lifted, but Sybil, perhaps just to cross him, insists she is still feeling very low; of course she still has major problems to deal with and these are getting to her, but in this case we agree more with her psychiatrist. We have been lobbying all along for specific OCD treatment for Sybil, something she's not yet ever had, and, finally, in response to this, Dr. Smith has agreed to formally refer Sybil to the highly-regarded Maudsley Behavioural Psychotherapy Unit, a residential, high-intensity programme for sufferers of OCD and other anxiety disorders, located on the grounds of the Bethlem Royal Hospital (also the site of Sybil's former adolescent unit).

However, as there is a long waiting list, even if Sybil is accepted, the issue of where she will stay in the interim period is up for discussion at this "case conference". Heather from MIND has strongly recommended Eaglehurst, a rehabilitation centre in Clacton, but Dr. Smith claims that Sybil is not independent enough to cope with this. His favoured proposal now, in order to remove her from Essex, is the Northgate Clinic in Barnet, which, however, is only open on weekdays and only takes adolescents from thirteen to eighteen (Sybil will be eighteen next month!).

The issue is left unresolved by the conference, to be explored further, and Sybil is to try out a four-week programme at the hospital with Allen Brown, a behavioural therapist. We are assured by the ward manager that funding matters will be handled solely by the contracts department, not by Dr. Smith, but the latter continues to resist Sybil's entry into the infra-structure of the Trust. As late as the fifth

"THE THING INSIDE MY HEAD"

of May, Sybil's social worker from Barnet, who has been conscientiously keeping in close contact with Sybil and with the hospital throughout this controversy, has an alarming conversation with Dr. Smith: He is still pushing for Sybil to go to the Northgate Clinic, even though the social worker insists it is not an appropriate venue for her, and he expresses irritation that this Essex region is still funding our daughter. Fortunately, from our point of view, Sybil ends up staying on Peter Bruff Ward for another two months, more or less by default.

* * *

Meanwhile, Sybil is taken under the wing of Allen, the behavioural therapist, who, though somewhat austere and humourless, is well disposed towards Sybil and enthusiastically agrees to be a co-therapist for the programme at the Maudsley Unit, whenever that takes place. Behaviour therapy, and the related Cognitive Behaviour Therapy, are by now known to be the preferred methods of treating OCD, a disorder apparently not well suited to psychoanalysis, and I obtain a very lucid description of the first from the "Obsessive Action" charity:

> Behaviour therapy involves learning self-restraint in the face of the situations which would ordinarily provoke compulsive actions. The components of the treatment are exposure and response prevention. The sufferer is encouraged to enter situations or undertake activities that are feared (exposure), but to refrain from the ritual that they would normally undertake (response prevention). Sufferers learn to resist the compulsion and to tolerate the discomfort they experience as a result.

Lois Chaber

According to *OCD: A Guide*, by Greist, roughly between 60 and 90 percent of patients achieve good results from behaviour therapy, with their symptoms reducing about 50 to 80 percent.

The first symptom Allen tackles is Sybil's "reassurance seeking," a habit, I confess, not that transparent to me, because I do it myself! Both Sybil and we (as well as the ward manager on behalf of the staff and Allen himself) have to sign written "contracts" devised by Allen, not to give Sybil the reassurance she craves when she constantly asks if people are angry with her, laughing at her, and so on, or questions related to her obsessive contamination concerns, like, "If I touch my eyes with my hands, will they have bad germs on them?"

The notes Sybil later dutifully takes on *Living with Fear*, by Isaac Mark (quoted in the epigraph), the self-help book for anxiety disorders that the Maudsley Unit has instructed Sybil to read, point out that "The addiction for reassurance is like other addictions and treatment means withholding reassurance" and, sure enough, Sybil experiences painful 'withdrawal symptoms'. She writes, as part of a prescribed exercise in *Living with Fear*, "My anxiety when I want to ask someone a reassurance question but know that I can't fluctuates somewhere between 25 and 50" [out of 100]. It is equally hard for us, especially for me, to remember to respond to Sybil in the quasi-mechanical way our 'contract' has mandated—"Sybil, I believe that is a reassurance seeking question and as per our contract I am not allowed to answer it." Her therapy thus becomes a learning process for the whole family.

But the big one to tackle is the classic OCD obsessional hand-washing that currently dominates Sybil's rituals. She is instructed to write out a "cue card" that will take her through a 'normal' hand wash step by step, with the hope of eventually eliminating the prolonged and obsessive version of this mundane activity: "Go to sink/ Turn tap on/

308

"THE THING INSIDE MY HEAD"

Wet both hands/Pick up soap/Wet soap/" and so on, up to "Leave the room and say well done." Sybil has to work at modifying the frequency as well as the duration of her hand washing routine; to this end she is issued a sheaf of neatly printed self-monitoring charts, with columns for putting down dates, times, ticks, etc. when she washes her hands. She continues with this highly empirical programme, with varying success from day to day, throughout the rest of her stay on the ward.

* * *

Sybil's appointment to be assessed by the Maudsley Unit for their Behavioural Programme takes place on June 20th, 1996. Much to everybody's relief, she is accepted; however, the bad news is that the waiting time is currently a year! There is still no clear decision on where she will be able to stay in the interim, but she is apparently not being pushed out of Peter Bruff Ward for the time being. Hence, Neil and I, drained by the long struggle to obtain suitable care for Sybil, decide to take a long-overdue fortnight's holiday in the US at the end of June. The hospital has promised not to finalise any decision about Sybil or change her abode until we return from the US, but when we call Sybil from the States in early July, we find that she is about to be moved to the Eaglehurst Rehabilitation Centre (the venue recommended by MIND), at another location in Clacton. We are upset at the broken promise, but because we had been anyway lobbying for Sybil to go to this facility—initially ruled out by Dr. Smith—we bite our tongues.

Eaglehurst, situated in a large but quite ordinary mock-Tudor residence, houses only six adult patients, with a high staff ratio of nurses, housekeeper, and occupational therapist, and is dedicated to empowering improved mental patients to the point where they are capable of living on their own and re-integrating into the community. Just as soon as we return to the UK, we attend a review meeting there for Sybil. Of course, the first thing they let us know is that Sybil will have to 'move on' some time in January, as clients' time at this facility is limited to six months, and we naturally start worrying whether she, the youngest one there, will be robust enough to move to a bed-sit situation in that time.

We learn also that Dr. Smith has recently put Sybil on Prozac (Fluoxetine), one of the four relatively new SSRI (selective serotonin re-uptake inhibitor) psychotropic drugs, the others being Fluvoxamene (US: Luvox, UK: Faverin), Paroxetine (US: Paxil, UK: Seroxat) and Sertraline (US: Zoloft, UK: Lustral). These medications have been prescribed since the 1980s for depression but only lately, since1991, have they come into use for OCD, which, like depression, has been linked to low levels in the brain of the feel-good chemical serotonin. Like the earlier Clomipramine, they facilitate the release of serotonin, but with fewer side effects since they *selectively* target that neuro-chemical only.

Although the beneficial effects of this drug have not yet begun to kick in for Sybil, we support this new treatment as it is in line with what we have just found out from my psychologist cousin during our Stateside visit. I, in particular, still very dependent on psychotropic medication myself, have no qualms about Sybil receiving drug therapy (which she has been getting off and on, anyway), despite my awareness that there is a segment of the mental health community that strongly disapproves of the "pill-for-every-ill" approach. Actually, drug therapy *in combination with* behaviour therapy (usually referred to as ERP, or Exposure and Response Prevention) and/or Cognitive Behaviour Therapy (CBT) is now coming to be recognised as the optimal treatment for severe OCD—like Sybil's—by the mushrooming field of experts in the mid-to-late 1990s. However, not until November 2005 does NICE, The National Institute for Health and Clinical Excellence, publish, for NHS personnel and the general public, definitive descriptions of OCD and its related disorders along with guidelines for treatment that include these three types of therapy for varying degrees of severity.

"THE THING INSIDE MY HEAD"

* * *

With Sybil having recently turned eighteen and now legally considered an 'adult', a good part of the funding problem, particularly her room and board at Eaglehurst, is dispelled, since she is now eligible for social benefits such as income support and disability allowance. However, new issues for us, Sybil's parents, have emerged. Sadly, Sybil is quite immature for her age, a result not only of her having missed out on the social, educational, and emotional experiences of a 'normal' adolescence (she is piercingly aware, for instance, that her sister Molly has taken her GCSEs this past summer and has achieved brilliant results), but also of her ongoing resistance to leaving childhood behind. Sybil's difficulty in 'growing up' was well recognised at Peter Bruff, where the care plans regularly included 'reinforcing Sybil's adult status' as part of her therapy there. Nevertheless, she is now legally entitled to 'confidentiality' and, as such, signs a routine agreement with the staff of Eaglehurst, which includes a specific request not to pass on details of her health to her parents without her consent.

This situation restricts our participation in her care, inhibiting our continuing efforts from this point on as her loyal advocates, as well as distorting, in some ways, our relationship with her. A mentally well young woman of that age would most likely still be living at home and, in the normal course of things, would be regularly interacting with her parents on health issues and events. We realise that confidentiality for young adults with concerned parents is a sticking point in medical ethics, and that 'confidential' treatment for Sybil will make her feel more 'adult'. However, perhaps it should have been taken into consideration that with all the many different institutions and different carers' hands that Sybil has passed through in these years—from the Sunshine Ward through Eagleton—we, her parents, notwithstanding our deficiencies and mistakes, have remained her only *constant* supporters. Years afterward, we are to learn that Sybil had taken an overdose sometime late in her stay at Clacton Hospital but she had specifically requested that staff not inform us, whether out of distrust, or anxiety about hurting us, we do not know. At some point during her stay at Eaglehurst, there is another such incident, and a "Risk Management * Suicide" alert is put on her care plan, none of which we then learn about. The debatable practice of keeping us in ignorance of Sybil's self-harming is to continue.

* * *

Only the positive elements of Sybil's residence at Eaglehurst are apparent to us at the time. She is assigned Brian, a very able male nurse, as her key worker, but, as usual, she bonds more closely with her female associate worker, Roberta, another of those lovely, kind young women that Sybil takes to so easily. Her behavioural programme under Allen's supervision continues, with the nurses daily checking her hand washing and Sybil self-monitoring with ever-proliferating charts, and she is now also working on her fear of "sharps"—scissors, knives, etc.—through regular "cutting" sessions with staff members, part of the 'exposure and response prevention' method. Starting in August, moreover, she has begun working with Jane Clark, the CPN from the Community Mental Health Team mentioned earlier, in a simultaneous programme of cognitive behavioural therapy (CBT), which entails verbally working through Sybil's issues, feelings, and memories in order to identify the mistaken beliefs—like guilt—that she holds and to encourage her to try out new, positive thinking strategies. Unlike psychoanalysis, CBT does not dwell on the deep past or attempt to delve into the sufferer's subconscious. Concurrently, she is receiving independence training from the Eaglehurst staff—laundry, shopping, cleaning, self-care, etc.—more successful here than at Jacques Hall, perhaps because carried out under medical supervision.

Sybil is also immersed in a busy programme of pleasurable therapeutic activities, thanks to the extensive

"THE THING INSIDE MY HEAD"

mental health infrastructure of North East Essex. A special extension of Clacton Hospital, called Martello Court, is the venue for a supportive programme of community meetings for mental patients on the mend, as well as for various group activities in games, art, music, literature and so on, in several of which Sybil participates. There is also the Mayfield Day Centre, located in an old office block near the Clacton railroad station, for more advanced patients, which Sybil starts attending. The Centre offers informal courses, drop-in facilities and, best of all for Sybil, a social group where she begins to meet a few people her own age, although she is still dogged by difficulties in forming close relationships with peers. Swimming lengths at the local leisure centre is now also a regular form of relaxation. She begins intermittently attending church, while apparently avoiding her former scrupulosity. For all of these activities, she is encouraged to find her own way about town, walking and, eventually, riding the buses (she has been devastatingly deprived of mundane experiences all these years!). Last but not least, she is gradually coached—within strict safeguards—in how to handle her own medication, essential if she is to be 'independent' in January.

Nothing is being done about her formal education at this point, however, and of course that worries us. Nevertheless, from what we see, from autumn onwards, Sybil is making remarkable progress in conquering her problems and becoming whole, and, to us, her mood, buoyed up by the Prozac regime, seems very positive. We are highly gratified and grateful indeed to the very committed Eaglehurst staff and to the Clacton mental health community.

* * *

What makes us even happier is that later in the autumn, Sybil actually feels well enough to come home to Southgate for one or two days on the weekend—and these visits not only take place without trauma but also promote

313

Lois Chaber

positive family interaction, as this excerpt from a letter Sybil writes to her former Jacques Hall tutor, Nicky (now working in Bournemouth), indicates:

> I am home right now; my dad is teaching me how to use the computer. I stayed overnight. I have had a really good time. I helped my mum make a cake and I helped her with dinner. I also did some glass painting. My sister showed me how to do it. After dinner we (my mum, dad and I) watched a film. My sister was out working.

It is particularly pleasing that Sybil is able to spend some quality time alone with Molly on these weekends, since their previous times together, given Molly's infrequent and largely obligatory visits to Sybil's institutional residences, have been brief and stilted. They are becoming 'sisters' again, although it must be painful for Sybil to witness Molly frequently flying out of the house to parties and other teenage activities with her close school chums.

The only drawback to this otherwise very happy arrangement is that, given Sybil's inexperience with public transport and her general lack of confidence, one of us has to ferry her back and forth from Eaglehurst in the family car, which entails a three hour round trip from Southgate to collect her, and likewise for her return. But even this difficulty has its silver lining. The long run in the car provides an excellent opportunity for each of us to have one-on-one long talks with Sybil, who, as the week's progress, becomes increasingly communicative. For me, particularly, it is a chance to grow considerably closer to Sybil than I have been in a long time; we find ourselves gradually opening our hearts and minds to one another, and mutually 'confessing' past feelings and beliefs during the prolonged journey. One

"THE THING INSIDE MY HEAD"

weekend Sybil and I watch a video, "The Joy Luck Club", whose theme is Chinese mother and daughter relationships. At one climax in the succession of stories, Sybil and I, feeling tearful, hug each other. I tell her, "I found you through your illness," and she replies, "I found you too."

* * *

As it turns out, Eaglehurst does not push Sybil out the door in January but allows her to take her time looking into various accommodation possibilities, with the guidance of her team. She chooses, with some anxiety and difficulty, an establishment at 'Woodland Lodge' described as supported accommodation, with a small non-medical staff, run by a private organization, Granta Housing Association, and is officially discharged from Eaglehurst on March 17, 1997. Despite the troubling undercurrents of suicidal thoughts and attempts that we know nothing about at the time, Sybil has achieved a monumental rehabilitation from the sorry state in which she entered Clacton Hospital a little over a year ago, a rehabilitation she is encouraged to set down in writing for her own satisfaction:

At Eaglehurst I managed to reduce my hand washing and do it at more appropriate times.

I did a behavioural programme about using sharp things and I can now use them and with much less anxiety.

I challenged the idea that everything happened because of the bad thing I did, and that the voice that told me to do those things was God. I went to the church and talked to the Minister about it. He said that I could be forgiven and that God would never punish me like that so I managed to dispel that idea.

I resolved in my heart and mind things that had happened at home.

I wrote a lot about my experiences at the Bethlem when I was very ill.

I [went] from cooking nothing to cooking for myself each day. I reduced the amount of time it took me to do the washing up.

I cooked for others.

I went home again.

I went home overnight.

I went home for a few days.

My bad thoughts became less.

I gained a lot of confidence.

I gained more self esteem.

I cleaned my room, including the toilet.

I got over my depression.

I became more assertive.

I became less anxious and dealt with it better.

I reduced the amount of time it took me to get up. I reduced the amount of time it took me to take a bath or shower.

"THE THING INSIDE MY HEAD"

I worked on my feelings of guilt and I felt less guilty about things.

I cleaned the budgie's cage out.

I went back to Jacques Hall [for visits].

But this is Sybil's public face; the diaries she begins keeping more regularly during her stay at Peter Bruff Ward reveal her private self and a more mixed experience.

Lois Chaber

Chapter 5: Finding [a] Home

Excerpts from Sybil's Diaries
June '96—March '97

> The whole mental health system here is a bit weird. Its patronising and insulting to us. We come in very distressed then they try and get us moulded to a bit more normal behaviour in whatever means, not really caring about the original problem and they try to mould you and get you out as quick as they can without really dealing with the problem so you go out still feeling bad but *behaving* a bit more normal. They don't care about our *suffering*. They just want to change our behaviour so we *fit into society more well*.

* * *

> I feel guilty for faking happiness a little bit.

(From Sybil's diary.)

Sybil began to keep a regular diary late in her stay on Peter Bruff Acute Mental Health Ward in Clacton Hospital, inspired by her sister's gift of a jaunty, black and white striped diary book with bright red corners. Although this first diary is undated, it appears to run from some time in June '96 through the early part of her stay at Eaglehurst Rehabilitation Centre in July. A new diary, dated, begins in September 1996 and her diary-writing carries on consistently from there. Excerpts in this chapter go up to the day she moves into the Granta Housing supported accommodation and correspond roughly with the period covered by me in the previous chapter. It seems Sybil showed her second diary or parts of it to her Community Psychiatric Nurse, Jane, and it is unclear if and when that stopped later. Sybil's

"THE THING INSIDE MY HEAD"

punctuation, grammar and spelling errors, kept intact here and in successive chapters, often correlate with her state of mind.

* * *

[June] I'm not sure what to write. I'm in pain if anyone reads this they will think I'm feeling sorry for myself but I am ~~Im in pain~~ Im not quite sure why

I don't know whether life is always going to be this bad or is it just because of my problems. I feel so insecure and alone. ~~My family loves me but they can't make me feel se[cure?]~~

I want to feel safe.

I wonder if I should try to overdose again.

In some ways I wish I had never said those things to Korreana and Sharon [young persons from Jacques Hall] but in some ways it did me good because I was able to see things more in perspective. I had got them distorted and I am ashamed to say exaggerated purposely, I wanted what I said to be true maybe because I wished we [Molly and herself] had been abused or that what we had gone through was abuse. I still wish that what we had gone through does fit into abuse. I think it might be borderline or near borderline; now I'm worried that the way I saw it was just me. I'm worried about going to the Bethlem [the Maudsley Behavioural Psychotherapy Unit at the Bethlem Royal Hospital], I partly don't want to go. I'm worried about where I'm going to go in between; sometimes I wish that I was at Jacques Hall and had never gone downhill everything is so complicated now, Im in hospital again and I don't know exactly where I'm going.

I read some more of [*Living with Fear*]

Lois Chaber

It said you still tend to get depressive spells which makes me feel bad Is life any better after treatment life seems horrible. I think I am depressed I feel suicidal. No-one else thinks I am depressed

I don't know what to do. I think I will talk to Erica [a nurse] and maybe about the past. This behavioural treatment seems hopeless I want to feel better. I don't know whether to talk about the past or not.

I feel alone even though lots of people do things for me Why?

I wanted to be free but its worse now

I feel like crying but I cant even be free when I do that. I wish Erica could hold me. I wish she was more than a nurse. Shes so nice.

Top of the Pops is on. Can I do it I feel like I cant, like I'd better kill myself everyone would be better off without me but then again it would hurt some people too much. This song is making me feel sad 'Lucky you' or something like that. I hope Nick [a patient] likes me. It was 'Lucky you'. Life is hard. It's a test a battle for everyone. I hope I can watch Top of the Pops I feel trapped I don't particularly like myself. I am worried about the next review and the assessment. I don't know why they stopped my Desmopressin [drug for enuresis, or bed wetting]. I don't think Erica took me seriously but maybe its good I don't dwell on it too much I wish things were like they used to be. I hate periods I feel low, I don't know why, I feel sort of fat.

I think I'm insecure and I think I need cognative therapy as well and I wish someone could be understanding about how bad it was at home. Is there a root cause or is it just OCD I wish I wasn't like this and I wish I didn't have OCD The book and the letter [from the Maudsley

"THE THING INSIDE MY HEAD"

Behavioural Unit] make it sound as if I'll never be completely free.

Everyone at Jacques Hall is in so much pain I feel like really cutting myself I wish someone could mother me and not be angry at me and make me feel better and worthwhile I feel so terrible I'm not a very nice person.

I wish I could kill myself

IM SO ANGRY

I feel like they are whispering about me I feel like taking an overdose tomorrow.

I want to kill myself but I can't for my sisters sake. My life is so painfull because of everything to do with not hurting people and I cant even escape from that because of the same thing.

I am trapped in a nightmare. I'm angry at the Nurses and Valerie. I want to get out of this for once and all but I cant.

HELP, PLEES ERICA HELP

.
No-one can help me This will probably
~~I wish I could take some~~

VALERIE I HAVE TO TALK TO YOU

I NEED A SHOULDER TO CRY ON, Please.

I've had my assessment

I can hardly believe

Lois Chaber

I felt happy with what the lady said. They've [The Maudsley Behavioural Unit] accepted me, I didn't expect to feel so happy but I do. I still think of suicide but I don't want to as much.

Tomorrow I'm going to help walk the dog, I don't think I'll kill myself tomorrow but in a way life seems harder not knowing that there is going to be an end soon.

I wouldn't mind death if it didn't hurt anyone or make anyone angry or let down or think badly of me in fact I'd sort of almost, like it.

I hope I get to sleep tonight, I feel like my adrenalin is still really high and I haven't wound down. I'm glad that it is sorted.

I don't want to read a Mills and Boon [pulp romance] ever again I wish I'd never read one. I've got a bad reputation now for reading them. I suppose in a way it is a bit sad but in a way there is also nothing to be ashamed of. Though I feel people are laughing at me because I read them. I'm glad when I cry because I quite often want to cry but can't. Marjory [a patient] recommended the book but it made me feel worse. It made me feel more lonely and it was a bit sick. A lot of them are a bit sick. If these things happened in real life it would be sexual assault, abuse and rape. And its just weird. They aren't my type of fantasy.

I did it.
I wonder if anyone noticed.
I feel sad and empty.
I'm having a few second thoughts but I'm going through with it for now. . . .

I'm in emotional pain and if anyone ever reads this my diary, if you think I'm self-pitying stuff you!

"THE THING INSIDE MY HEAD"

It's true and I've got to have somewhere to write it down I can't say it to anyone. I want to die but my parents are coming Im a bit scared.

I want to cry uncontrollably and scream I want to be hystericall and hurting myself and then be restrained and people caring not angry.

[This is followed by four crude pictures of a figure standing at a crossroads. Then there are many successive entries of large, barely coherent, very repetitive writing scrawled across the pages, of which the following is a small excerpt]

I DON'T WANT TO BE SCARED OF HURTING ANYONE   I WANT TO DIE NOW BEFORE I HURT ANYONE I THOUGHT THAT FEAR WOULD END I FEEL QUITE ALONE. THERE'S NO-ONE I CAN TELL THERE'S NO-ONE WHO CAN TAKE MY PAIN AWAY IN A WAY I DON'T WANT TO DIE I JUST WANT THE PAIN AND FEAR AND HORRIBLE FEELINGS AND THOUGHTS TO END. NOW I FEEL A BIT GUILTY THERE'S A SONG SAYING DON'T STOP MOVING.

Dr. Smith's review was bad. No-one is acknowledging the fact of how I feel. They've told Cindy [a nurse] to stop I can tell. I wish Cindy was my Godmother or something. I went shopping with her today I saw Allen [her behavioural therapist] and it went alright. These reviews are stupid They talk for ages before you go in then you go in. They ask some fairly useless questions and then make you leave without telling you anything, then they have another chat and then they don't really tell you much of what they said It's a farce. We should be treated with more rights and respect. I think Dr. fucking Smith likes being in a position of power. He gets a kick out of treating as though hes above the patient and in control. The whole mental health system here is a bit weird. Its patronising and insulting to us. We come in very distressed then they try and get us moulded to a bit more normal behaviour in whatever means, not really caring about the original problem and they try to mould you and get you out as quick as they can Without really dealing with the problem so you go out still feeling bad but *behaving* a bit more normal.

They don't care about our *suffering* They just want to change our *behaviour* so we *fit into society more well*.

I feel a lot like killing myself again and I think I will attempt to on Friday or tomorrow even if its just to make them wake up to my suffering. It seems so hopeless. If only Dr. Smith was like the one in Jacques Hall who cared about feelings and the individual.

I hate myself

God please help me get back I'm scared of God, I'm scared of Christianity. It used to bring me comfort and help and happy.

I feel a lot better much better than I've felt for maybe a week at least. I feel brighter like I can do anything I cant wait to get my clothing money and buy some new clothes. I feel almost happy.

"THE THING INSIDE MY HEAD"

There is quite a bit of sadness in me. I feel like I haven't got any close friends I've lost contact with a lot of people. I feel a bit like Ive lost my family and they've lost me. I've failed.

I haven't got a boyfriend.
I don't know anyone in this area.
But I've got Eaglehurst.
I haven't lost my family They are so good to me.
But the missing link is me

I'm getting more depressed so I'll write some good things

I've got Music group and Martello [Court—see previous chapter] on Thursdays but I'm anxious about that.
I've been feeling better so I hope tommorrow I will feel better.
I did a lot of ironing. I went to Martello but I think I may have made a fool of myself in the Karaoke.

I watched *Home and Away*. And this other program about beds. It had a honeymoon suite. I cant wait till I have a serious partner and we make love for the first time. I wish I had a boyfriend. I wonder when I will or if I ever will find someone that fancies me and who I fancy. Sometimes I think there must be something wrong with someone if they fancy me. I wish that they would realise I'm still depressed.

I hope I don't look silly with lipstick on. I'll be happy or shall I say happier when I have smooth, hairless legs. I hope to do it tommorrow.

I'm anxious. I've got my assessment at Eaglehurst tommorrow at 4:30 or 4:15. I really want them to accept me. I don't know whether to go to the pub or not. I'm scared of drinking alcohol and that someone will spike my drink.

I've had a wonderful day.

Lois Chaber

[July '96; at Eaglehurst Rehabilitation Centre]

I wish I could bang my head here but I can't. Food used to be a good helper when I felt bad but now I can't eat as much because I've got a certain amount of money to spend [her social benefits]. I wish I could be somewhere where they could mother me. I feel scared. I do miss Peter Bruff and some of the nurses, maybe all of them.

The nurses here are nice. I don't want to be scared anymore but its not going to disappear overnight. I want to be free! I can't get away from dirt I can't feel very comfortable in here because of it. I hope my bin is emptied soon but by then there will probably be something else.

I wish I was like Mariah Carey or Shannon [Campbell]. Sometimes I fantasize about being a singer with a really good voice, or a dancer or a gymnast. I've forgotten so much of what I learned at school. I used to be good at school. I'll never go to university but I might not want to. I fantasize about being married, about working for the R.S.P.C.A. and starting a rescue home myself. I would have a big house and big garden and I would take in unwanted cats and dogs and maybe other animals.

I feel in pain. I want to die and sleep peacefully I miss times and feelings I miss the Bethlem, I miss Jacques Hall, I miss Peter Bruff and I miss home. Home. I feel like I don't have a home I want to be somewhere where I feel at home and secure.

I'm trying to get through to meds [medication] time its 9:20. It's hard. Why do people have to make a fuss about me watching so many soaps, its not that unusual. I feel bad when they make an issue of it I enjoy them, I need them almost some of the best times of the day are spent watching them. I feel a failure. I haven't got GCSEs I can't socialize with people I've forgotten dancing and how to read

"THE THING INSIDE MY HEAD"

music and be an unselfish person and relaxed and... Oh, I wish time would pass quickly its only 9:25.

Yesterday and the day before I was so upset because I miss being at home and being with my family but I can't because I wouldn't be able to cope and I get so worried about hurting my family. I can't enjoy being with them because of that its so frustrating.

I've had quite a good day today in some cases a really good day. I am still worried I hope I get to sleep quickly. Everyone has been so nice today. Carole [a nurse] gave me a hug. Oh, life can maybe be worth living. I'm just waiting to get my tablets so I can go to bed. Goodnight! [End of Sybil's first diary.]

[Second diary, after an unclear time gap.]

3 September 1996: Brian [her keyworker] is really jokey to me and he is really trying to do things which will help me get on with him better and I feel a funny feeling about this. I feel bad, I feel powerful even though I didn't do anything wrong.

I had a shower and it leaked. I don't think it was my fault. They said it wasn't my fault. Annabel gave me a comforting hug which I indulged in I feel a bit guilty about that. I love getting hugs, but I don't think Allen [the behavioural therapist] would be pleased.

6 September: I had my session with Jane. We talked about how many times 'feeling guilty' had come up in my diary. We talked about me moving on and she reminded me that if people say I'm better they aren't going to chuck me out on the streets. She said she is thinking of somewhere like the Ling Trust [potential supported accommodation]. She asked me to carry on but when I've written in the diary to put it down make a drink, then come

327

back and look at the times when I wrote about feeling guilty or bad, and think about and rationalize them

6 September [her 2nd entry for this day]: I phoned them [her family] and then Molly phoned back It was painful and Mum found it painful too. I told her how much I miss home. I feel in pain, now, sad, I wonder if I should've said so much to her. I spoke to Sura [a care worker] about it and I asked if she could play a game of cards with me. She did. I wonder if I was rude or selfish to ask that. I feel guilty about Kelly [a nurse] helping me so much, but I didn't really do anything wrong. I feel bad about leaving the washing outside for so long and she brought it in even though it wasn't that late; I was going to do it. I'm go[ing] to get a drink now.

I think I shouldn't feel guilty about saying too much [to mum] then, that's asking too much from myself. I suppose it wasn't that bad to ask for a game of cards. After all they are here to help us and I was being sensible.

I don't need to feel guilty about Kelly helping me so much.

I don't need to feel that guilty about the washing. Maybe I don't need to feel guilty at all about it.

11 September: I got up. I had my session with Allen. He was about 35 minutes late and I was angry at him. I thought I had a right to be angry with him. I felt a bit unsure and maybe guilty about thinking and feeling that. He had a quick word with me about how the staff are going to work more closely with me and he is just going to give advice. This made me feel angry and scared, like they were going to gang up on me. A whole staff team of 'Allens' seemed scary and horrible.

12 September: Brian told me they were going to have a budgie. I feel guilty for not being grateful or happy

"THE THING INSIDE MY HEAD"

enough and even not wanting it. I feel guilty for faking happiness a little bit.

25 September: Lorna [occupational therapist] asked me if I wanted to go to the social group. I wasn't sure. I went in the end and Lorna stayed with me. We played the 'Brit Quiz'. I couldn't answer almost all the questions. I felt stupid. Then someone on my team had to do a forfeit, the Highland Fling. They didn't want to do it so I said I would. I didn't do it very well in fact terrible, dancing wise, but it seemed to do the job.

9 October: I did the animals. Then I sat in the smoking room and had a nice chat with everyone. I laughed a bit. I like laughing.

29 October [Sybil's first regular visit home, not overnight]: It was about 10 to 11. I was really nervous. I sat down in the smoking room. The doorbell rang. It was my dad. I was a bit relieved but still very anxious. When we got home, he showed me things in the garden. Then I spent time with my mum as she was making lunch. I helped her a bit by doing little things, which I feel good about. I talked to my sister. I fed our cat. He remembered me because he let me tickle his tummy and normally he runs away at the sight of strangers. That made me feel good. We had a lovely lunch. After lunch, my mum and I walked to get a video. We saw someone we both [k]new in the shop. I felt a bit embarrassed and worried what she would think about me.

On the way back we popped in to see the next door neighbours who are always asking how I am and who I haven't seen in 4 ½ years. They were so nice.

We watched the video. It was really good. It was touching and interesting and at the end I felt like crying, not in a bad way though.

Lois Chaber

My dad showed me how to send an e-mail to my uncle. I was in my room which felt sad and weird. During the whole visit I felt pain inside me, even though some times I felt really good in different ways. I felt sad, helpless, that I couldn't change the circumstances, that I could live there, that I felt so much pain when I visited. That I couldn't change the past and bad memories. My parents made it a really good visit though.

I feel guilty for complaining about feeling pained but its completely true.

30 October [picnicking with Neil's cousins, Eddie and Edna, and their grandchildren]: I felt jealous of their grandchildren for being their grandchildren and being that much closer to them. I felt jealous of them for being young teenagers because I've missed out on my teenage years and I can't get them back. I'm 18 and I have to go on to be an adult even though I think I haven't gone through the process of adolescence enough.

I felt jealous of them. Ever since I was seven I've had problems which have restricted my happiness. I feel a little guilty for writing that 'cause I've had lots of good times too. I feel jealous of them for going to school.

I'm glad for Eddie and Edna's love though.

5 November: I had a shower, did my hair. Then I went to Jacques Hall [her former therapeutic community]. I had been feeling nervous all day about it and excited but I was more so now.

It went really well. I saw quite a few kids I knew and quite a few staff and got hugs from both, which felt good. I was still feeling quite nervous. My legs shook for a little while.

"THE THING INSIDE MY HEAD"

I was anxious to see Maggie [former counselor]. I talked to Maggie and we hugged each other. I said I missed her and she said they missed me. That pulled some heartstrings. I feel full of emotion now we left. I miss Maggie a lot. I feel like crying now. I miss Jacques Hall. I feel mixed up and sort of sad but at the same time I sort of know I'm happier here than I would be there.

6 November: I was going to do some studying with some of the science GCSE books Molly had given me but I felt so horrible. The reason I wanted to do some studying is because I think that my brain is not getting much stimulation and exercise at all, which is why I feel so restless, bored and agitated and have a short concentration span. I think it makes my OCD worse.

I feel so angry and frustrated about what these years of illness have done to me. I can't even write properly anymore; I've forgotten quite a bit of grammer so that will limit me in a job. I probably won't ever get to where I want to because there's so much I've forgotten. I've forgotten Maths, English every subject. I can't dance anymore. I've missed out on 4 years at home and now its leaving home age and I might not be able to cope there, well I wouldn't be able to cope there, and they wouldn't be able to cope with me. I've missed out on 5 years of childhood or teenage years whatever you call them. I'm behind my peers in social aspects, life experience, education, independence. I can't even use a bus on my own. *I feel so horrible.*

I'm going to get a drink [cocoa] and watch Coronation [Street].

22 November: I went with Jane and Brian to see Penfold Lodge [potential accommodation]. I felt really nervous and shy, and a bit clumsy. It was very [word crossed out illegibly]. I'm not sure what to think of it. Its good in some ways but in other ways it isn't quite as independent as I'd hoped. Maybe that's a good thing.

Lois Chaber

24 November: I worry myself that I'm going to become bulimic or a compulsive eater. I think I'm on my way to becoming one. I often eat because I'm bored or anxious or feeling horrible. I want to be thinner but Im not doing too well.

26 November: I watched Brookside and it made me feel a bit better. But it is frustrating. Fred [a resident] says 'Why do you watch it if it winds you up' and the answer is I don't know but it just takes my mind off things and sometimes its easier thinking about the problems on the program than my own problems.

[Next diary]

28 November: I'm getting used to using buses but I'm still really nervous about going to Martello on them because I haven't done that before I got back. I went shopping with Beryl [a care worker]. Beryl was nice and chatty. I wrote some more on the Bethlem Experience [See Pt. 2, Ch. 2]. Its hard. I did the cutting [behaviour therapy]. They (the staff) all waited for me so I could eat with them which was really nice. The table was full. It was really nice. I had a good laugh. Its times like that that its worth holding on for.

29 November: I'm scared. I'm scared of being completely well. I know that sounds wimpish and stupid. I'm scared of being fully responsible for myself. I've always been scared of growing up.

1 December: My mum came. We left. I talked quite a lot for quite a while. We talked about OCD and anorexia and the past. I told her that the reason I had rejected her was because I thought that she had been taken away and it was the devil pretending to be her. I'm not sure if I did the right thing by telling her. She seemed to take it well. When we came home my dad greeted me with a big hug which

was nice. We all had lunch. We talked and shared ideas about the poem Molly had to analise. Then I spent a little time talking to Molly about it. I felt hurt because she didn't seem to write down any of my ideas. Then I had one idea she really liked.

3 December: The group [at Martello] made me feel sad. We had to pass a piece of paper round which had a Christmas tree on it. We each had to draw something which came to mind when we thought of Christmas. I drew a stressed face and a sad face because when I think of Christmas I think of stress. I feel flat and cold and empty. This is partly because I don't have a good relationship with God and I used to. It's also because I feel like a bad person. That sparkle and magic seems to have gone. Christmas makes me feel sad and bad and horrible.

I went with Carole to the shops. That nice girl was on the checkout next to ours and we looked at each other and smiled. I wish we could be friends.

5 December: I went to Sommerfields. I saw that nice girl again. I wanted to go to her checkout but I thought that I would make a fool of myself if I did that so I didn't. The girl on the checkout where I went said hello to me. Maybe the other nice girl is just being polite. I hope she isn't.

19 December: I went to Sommerfields. That nice girl is there and she was nice to me but the way she spoke finally made me realise that we can't be friends and maybe I was silly to think we could.

20 December [home]: I want relief and an end to my pain. I want to kill myself. I can't understand my feelings or why I'm having them. I feel guilty for feeling like I want to kill myself. You may be asking why I should feel like this at home. *But I do!* I want to starve myself to death. I want to self mutilate I feel such pain! I feel like crying but I can't

unless someone hears me. I want to cry in a nurses arms but I can't. I feel like I'm going mad. God help me

25 December: It is Christmas Day.

We got an E-mail or two E-mails from Aunt Mady and Uncle Steve [Lois's family in California]. They said 'keep up the good work' to me. I feel scared. I hope I do. I feel scared of responsibility. We had a lovely day. I hope my watch [a Christmas present] doesn't get water on it. I'm worried about dad because of his bad cold. Im worried about Mum as well. Im not quite sure why. Im worried about Molly 'cause she said that the lead person in 'Prodigy' was her role model, which is a bit disturbing. We had a lovely day. I've probably gotten a bit fat!

27 December: We went to see 'Blood Brothers' [West End musical]. It was Brilliant. At one point I put my arm around her [Molly] and asked if she was really okay. She got a bit annoyed which hurt but I realized I might have gone over the top a bit. Im always jealous of Molly but she's suffered a lot too. She's been through a really bad patch and she's seen me when I was in a terrible state and when I wouldn't have anything to do with my family. She must see the special attention I get and I dont have to go to school and she might miss me not being there at home. I love her. Its so complicated. I feel so hurt but she must be hurt too. I feel jealous of her but she is probably jealous of me. I'm worried about her. She distances herself from the family. I think she is a hurt, angry, little girl inside at least partly or a bit. I don't want anything to come between us ever. I love them all.

8 January 1997: I went to see Ling Trust with Brian. It didn't seem as good as last time. There wouldn't be so many staff on and you didn't seem to get as much support. We went back. I felt scared and like crying. I decided to starve myself until I went home at the weekend. I wanted to see if I could still do it and get the pride from being able to

"THE THING INSIDE MY HEAD"

achieve it. It was a way of coping with my feelings. It went really well for an hour or two. Marjory was here. I offered everyone chocolate and flapjacks but didn't have any. The thought of starving myself made me feel elated and happy. Marjory had taken another overdose and was in hospital again. I felt very sad for her. I had to occupy myself so as not to eat. I didn't feel the horrible, painful feelings anymore. It was as if by deciding not to eat, I had made a space for and put my feelings in my stomach. I was still carrying them around with me but I didn't feel them anymore.

14 January: I'm 18 years old but I'm not 18 years old mentally. Because of my illness and being preoccupied with all that I haven't gone through all the processes teenagers go through in their mind to become an adult and form their personality. Now because I am suddenly a lot better I'm bombarded with all these feelings and questions teenagers have gone through.

15 January: I talked [to an Eaglehurst nurse] about my fears and about how I didn't want to leave and how I felt I was going to be so lonely. She said that almost everyone who had been in Eaglehurst was the same.

30 January: I had a long [phone] chat with Molly. I'm quite worried about her. She isn't well and she feels exhausted, plus she has her sleeping problems. I started telling her about my feelings of my talents having gone/going down the drain. I told her how hard it would be for me to get qualifications and trained. She consoled me. At least I know she thinks good of me. I feel guilty for talking about those things. I hope nothing bad happens because of it.

31 January: Jane came. She said that she didn't think that Ling Trust was the right place for me. I did suspect that she might say that. I felt sort of shocked, disappointed and flat, sort of empty. She was very nice. I am very grateful to her for all the hard work she has put in for me.

Lois Chaber

8 February [home]: I went through a file of certificates and other things of mine with dad. With them were some pictures, black and white. They were of desperate agonized faces with the words 'Help me' and 'Please' written below them. Dad said that I had done them when I was at home before I went to hospital, when mum was in hospital [Lois's breakdown, Feb. 1992] and I was very distressed. I couldn't remember doing them at all. But the style and I think memory makes me think that Molly did them. She was very distressed that year as well... but dad said I had done them. The pictures and words were very powerfull. I can't get them out of my mind.

9 February: I had a really big dinner. Dad said it was bigger than his. I get the feeling that mum is trying to fatten me up or she's giving me loads (because she always gives me loads) because she's frightened of me stopping eating and getting very underweight again. This makes me feel uncomfortable and I'm not sure how to deal with it.

12 February: I'd forgotten that we were going to Granta [Housing] at 10. I was both nervous and excited but when we got there I felt really nervous. Diane [care worker] was the one seeing us. I had hoped that it wouldn't be her. When we sat down and she said 'So, you've changed your mind Sybil; you want to come and live with us' I felt bad. I thought she was angry at me and maybe mocking me a bit. It got better though. She seemed nice so I have hope.

15 February: I feel like crying my heart out. [Molly's] two friends were from Latymer [Sybil's former school]. Oh why couldn't I be part of that, why couldn't I be a sixth former like the rest. I felt sad then anger then helpless passive calm. The what could have been seems so good but I cannot get it. The future looks so hard. Can I still have a good life like I would have been able to. I must *make* my future. I must make it good. I can and I will. I am writing to make myself believe it.

19 February: I did my careplans with Brian. We discontinued the suicide one which feels like a big step for me.

28 February: I opened Michelle's [former Latymer classmate who has kept in touch through the years] letter and read it. I had really been looking forward to hearing from her, and hoping for a good response from my letters so I could ask her if she wanted to come and visit me one of the weekends I was at home at Easter. After the last letter when she was upset and asking for my advice it brought her down a bit. I had always looked up to her so much and it brought her down to more of my size. Now all that is gone. She is way above me, she is so different from me and living such a different life from me. I feel now that I will never be able to mix in with my old peers or anyone who hasn't been ill.

Why did I have to have a nervous breakdown. She's [Michelle] spouting French in her letter and I've forgotten all my French. My mum knows I'll never be a normal Sybil or the Sybil that I want to be. She [Michelle] is probably only writing out of pity. She doesn't want or need me as a friend, and I need and want her to be my friend so much. There is no-one to talk to about this. When I had the breakdown I did all those things for God and to be saved. I gave up my whole life for him and now I don't even have God, because I've lost my faith and love for him. And now I've got no life for the future. I gave it all up. Why did this have to happen to me

It feels like this letter has brought me the reality that my whole life is ruined I'll always be disabled by my problems and inexperience of life and I'll always be a weirdo or a freak.

I WANT TO BE NORMAL

Lois Chaber

On the way home [with her dad] I talked about today which included how I felt after reading the letter from Michelle. He said that I have had a very different experience these past 4 or 5 years from them and it has affected me in different ways and that as I get out and about more I will be reminded and in conflict more and it will take a lot of strength to cope with that. But he says that he knows I can do it. At first I felt angry and depressed and pressure on me, but then I saw how right he could be and how helpful his saying those things has been. I started to see that I may never be like them or like the old Sybil but I can be a good, happy new Sybil. At the moment as I write this I'm in two minds about that a part of me doesn't want to give up hope for being like my friends and sister.

5 March: Ronald [a patient] walked most of the way back [with] me. We talked quite a bit, considering we've never had a conversation with each other before. It made me feel more confident and glad and hopeful but it also made me feel suspicious again. I really hope that they aren't all laughing at me and making fun of me. I've had a long chat with Molly about Patty [a patient] and Ronald and my suspicions. She helped me to quell them and gave me lots of good advice.

10 of March [move to Granta Housing]: I dislike packing. It was really hard. I realised that I could be myself and be accepted for who I was at Eaglehurst and I felt worried and a little sad because I was leaving. We went. Kim and Diane [Granta staff] were so nice to me. I unpacked most eventually. I felt anxious here. Roberta [nurse from Eaglehurst] came and brought me a present with a card which I wasn't expecting. I think she sees me as as [a] friend which is great.

I hope I sleep well tonight. I'm worried about dad driving in this fog. Its terrible. I am lucky.

338

Chapter 6: Sybil's Annus Mirabilis

> SYBIL:
> Happy—always joins in activities.
> CONCIESCIOUS[sic]   KEEN TO PLEASE.
> *You have a lovely laugh and smile.*   SWEET☐
> SENSIBLE AND INTELLIGENT.   *WARM SMILE*
> **EXTREMELY GOOD-NATURED**.   Happy
> GOOD AT THINKING THROUGH THINGS.

> (From a group exercise at Martello Court. Participants
> were asked to pass around pieces of paper and write
> their impressions of each other, each in turn.)

"I want a white wedding," Sybil asserts, with startling optimism—she doesn't even have a boyfriend. This is her riposte to my snide remarks about the conventional syrupy nuptial photos displayed in the photographer's studio where our family is waiting its turn. It is late February, 1998, and to celebrate Sybil's rehabilitation and reunion, emotionally, with our family, Neil and I have decided to have some professional photos taken of the four of us, perhaps an attempt to freeze-frame this happy moment in time. Our confidence arises from the succession of achievements that Sybil has racked up over the past year, impressing and gladdening everyone within the radius of her daily life.

* * *

At Easter time, 1997, shortly after her move to the Granta residence on March 10th, Sybil accompanies Neil, Molly and me on our first holiday abroad together in many years, a week's trip to Bruges and other cities in Belgium—and it is a resounding success. She is again in great form at the August Bank Holiday, when she, Neil and I take a five-day sightseeing trip to Warwickshire, where she enjoys the historical sights, as well as the animal feeding farms we visit, as much as we do. Moreover, in the course of the year, she gradually takes on the journey from Clacton to London by public transport—in gradual stages: first travelling by train with Diane, her key worker at Granta, and met by me at Liverpool Street Station, then alone on the train and met by me; then, coping with the busy underground system with the help of my written directions, she at last comes home completely independently, lifting a great burden from Neil and me. Finally, at the close of 1997, she finds herself able to spend eight quite happy days at home during Christmas week.

She has also settled well into her home away from home, the Granta residence in Clacton, Woodland Lodge, with its communal setup, putting into practise the life skills she had been learning at Eaglehurst. Not only does she have to care for herself, her room, her laundry, but also do her share, on a rota, of general housecleaning in the residence and preparation of communal meals. She continues to participate in the programmes at Martello Court and Mayfield Centre, but over the course of the year she is considered so 'well' that she is discharged from first the one, then the other, and fills up the space with many other activities, such as swimming, weekly aerobics, the Mayfield-sponsored Youth Group, extensive letter-writing, mostly to old friends, relatives, and adult pen pals, as well as correspondence with and for several charities such as Amnesty International.

Her behavioural therapy programme is now carried on by the staff at Granta, while she continues to have weekly sessions with her CPN Jane, eventually replaced by Hazel, a much younger woman whom Sybil eventually comes to worship fervently, as well as informal talks with her new Granta key worker, Diane, a feisty middle-aged woman and very experienced social worker. Her new life is also punctuated by get-togethers and little dates with friends within the mental health services—both other clients (these relationships are a bit wobbly) and past carers—May and Roberta from Eaglehurst and Sue from Jacques Hall. Kim,

"THE THING INSIDE MY HEAD"

an attractive twenty-something blonde on the Granta staff, who is not officially assigned to Sybil, nevertheless takes my daughter under her wing, acting as a role-model and older-sister figure, to improve Sybil's social confidence and savoir-faire: taking her out to the local pubs, teaching her about makeup, doing her hair and lending her clothes.

Once settled into Granta, moreover, Sybil begins attending to her much-interrupted education, taking a remedial class in English during the summer '97 term at the nearby Tendring Adult Community College and adding on a Maths class in the autumn, hoping these will enable her to start GCSE work in the autumn of 1998. Similarly looking to the future, social services advise Sybil to take on some voluntary work in order to gain useful experience and test the waters for a potential career. She declares she is interested in helping either animals or people, so in June '97 she begins working once a week at Crescent Cat Rescue, a small one-woman, privately run operation. There, she regularly suppresses her obsessional horror of dirt and germs to perform the full gamut of necessary menial chores at such a place, while relishing the opportunity to handle cats and kittens. In October, she supplements that by starting to work as an 'escort' once a week on a "Dial-A-Ride" minibus service for the elderly and infirm. For this volunteer work she has to overcome her OCD fears of harming vulnerable people as well as a life-long physical awkwardness under stress.

All this mentioned above, as well as coming home to us on weekends, makes for a very full and busy life for Sybil, as Tracey, another Granta member of staff, attests: "I remember when Sybil was always rushing around. On a Wednesday, when we had the [Granta community] meeting, it'd get just three o'clock, and you'd see Sybil, running down the road from swimming, 'sorry for being late' (she wouldn't have been late; she'd have been on time). She just seemed to have so much to fill her day."

Lois Chaber

The overall picture for this period is one of a young woman moving steadily from introverted timidity to increasing confidence, epitomised in these two following accounts of her. One is from Sue Patch, Sybil's English and Maths tutor:

When Sybil first came to English and Maths, she was very shy and quiet. Over a period of time, it was lovely to see her personality emerging as she made friends. She soon felt at ease and would be happy to join in class discussions, expressing her opinions eloquently and with a great deal of insight.

There was one very special moment. We had a reading and achievement evening at the college when students and staff were gathered to acknowledge and celebrate the work of the students during the year. Quite a few people opted to have their tutors reading for them, including Sybil, who had written a lovely piece about cats.

When we arrived that evening, there was a very large gathering which included all the special needs and basic skills classes at the college, plus staff and volunteer helpers. As you might imagine, reading aloud in a large room to a big audience was rather nerve-wracking. We watched other people reading and the atmosphere was wonderful as each student was applauded. When it came to the time for Sybil's piece to be read, she came up to me and told me that she had changed her mind and would read aloud herself. She took her work from me, and in a clear strong voice, with her head held high, read out her work.

"THE THING INSIDE MY HEAD"

She received an enthusiastic round of applause and stood there with a beaming smile. To overcome her fears and stand up in front of all those people must have taken so much courage.

Theresa Coyne, the Dial-a-Ride administrator with whom Sybil had her first, informal interview for the escort duties, describes a similar progression:

At that time she was shy and had very little to say. I placed Sybil under the supervision of our longest serving and experienced driver, John Ruffell. Under John's wing, Sybil's confidence grew, and she became a valued member of our team. We watched her confidence grow as we involved her in the day to day activities of this organisation.

One thing that sticks in our minds is the day that we were huddled around the answer phone machine trying to understand the message left there by a passenger who gave her name—which we could not understand. Seven of us in turn listened over and over to the message but could not get the passenger's name. Sybil came in with a cup of tea in her hand and immediately said "That's Mrs..." Needless to say, we were all very impressed, and showered her with praise. What we learned from the incident was that Sybil not only helped our passengers, she remembered their names, their disabilities and recognised their voices.

Lois Chaber

Sybil seems so much on the right track, moving towards wholeness and independence, that I feel secure enough in the summer of 1997 to apply for teaching positions, and obtain one in August as a lecturer at a branch of a small, private institution, the American College in London, where I will teach a Composition and Rhetoric class, part-time, in the Liberal Arts Programme.

* * *

This is not to say that there are no setbacks during this period. The worst one occurs in May '97, when Sybil is due to have her reassessment interview by the Maudsley Behavioural Unit prior to joining their programme, finally, in June. Neil and I are worried but only because we fear they will decide that Sybil is too 'well' to profit from the programme. On the day of the interview, however, much to our surprise, we receive a call from Sybil, who confesses, in an anxious and miserable voice, that she has declined her place in the Unit, having declared she "can't cope" with the rigours of the programme. We are very disappointed, but work hard to suppress our feelings and give her comfort and support at home during the rest of the weekend.

As part of the fallout from her decision, Allen Brown, the supervisor of her local behavioural programme, declares he won't work with Sybil anymore, abruptly severing his relationship with her. Although ourselves inwardly chagrined at Sybil's faintheartedness, we believe the important thing is for her to keep up her spirits and persevere with battling against her OCD symptoms, so we are angry and disturbed at Allen's behaviour, which we perceive as unprofessional and irrational. Sybil, naturally, is also very upset and Diane suggests to her that she write, but not send, a hypothetical letter to Allen venting her anger:

"THE THING INSIDE MY HEAD"

To Mr. Allen Brown:

I got your letter. Is that the real reason you don't want to carry on working with me, because I've declined the Bethlem? Or is it because you think I'm a loser and youre not going to waste your time with me? Or are you just so angry, because I declined it, that you cant deal with it and so you're stopping working with me is the only way you can deal with it?

I think you are being very unfair and that you have just "dropped" me. I think you are snooty and weird. It's unfair because you never said that you were seeing me just for the Bethlem. Did you 'pretend' to help me at Peter Bruff [Ward] by getting me to stop doing the things that annoyed the nurses, and that was your main function, to stop me from being a nuisance until you could just pack me off to the Bethlem? And you started being funny to me at Eaglehurst which really angered and hurt me.

I think you expect me to be perfect just because you think you are.

You've let me down!

But in a way, I'm glad I'm not working with you anymore because you are very depressing and you really made feel depressed and crushed.

SO PISS OFF!

Allen has claimed that Sybil can only make progress at this point by participating in the intensive Maudsley programme, as a reason for severing his connection with her. However, Sybil had been successfully overcoming her OCD on a gradual basis, fully cooperating in her weekly behavioural sessions. According to A. J. Allen, Director, Paediatric OCD and Tic Disorders Clinic at the Institute for Juvenile Research at the University of Illinois, behaviour therapy can be carried out equally well in weekly sessions or on an intensive basis, though the former takes longer ("Afterward," *Kissing Doorknobs*). Had Allen been more compassionate, more tolerant, Sybil could have continued to profit from weekly sessions; instead, she is to go without any specifically OCD therapy for the next year, a significant setback. And, as her key worker Diane has pointed out to us, the Maudsley Unit is also to be faulted for simply saying "That's it", rather than giving her the option of another interview in six months, when she would have been more settled into life at Granta.

Not all of Sybil's other undertakings prove successful, either. Everyone involved professionally with Sybil, as well as we, her family, is keen to see her make informal contacts with the world beyond the mental health services, with the hope that this will more profoundly normalise her life. But this is not to be. She tries during the latter part of this period to join a troop of Venture Scouts since she had enjoyed the Girl Guide movement so much as a youngster, but a couple of meetings put her off so much that she cannot even talk about the experience. Yearning so much to resume her beloved 'dancing', she enrols in a class of modern dance (ballet is not available for adults) at the Tiffany Dance School, only to become totally discouraged after a few sessions because she can't keep up, and the teacher seems unsympathetic to her needs. She calls me one day in the early part of '98 to say, in a voice husky with sadness, "I'm past it." She is also contacted by a newly formed group of young people who have previously been 'in care' in our borough, Barnet, who call themselves VIBE (Voices in Barnet etc!). She goes hopefully to one meeting with some of the young organisers, only to be dropped without explanation by them shortly afterwards.

Nor does Sybil have success in the 'romance' department. She develops crushes on a series of young men in her various therapeutic groups, but none of them reciprocate her affections. Particularly devastating is the occasion of her nineteenth birthday in May '97, when she musters all her courage to invite one of these young men, Brett, to a birthday party on which she has built high hopes, only to find that he brings along his kid brother, and then leaves the party abruptly and precipitately. (Some years later Tracey finds out from Brett that he was totally unaware Sybil had asked him as her date, unaware she was sweet on him, and had left early only because another resident, Ken, was teasing him inordinately). She becomes equally upset when young men she doesn't fancy pursue her romantically, which happens twice this year. Diane, Sybil's key worker, discusses Sybil's distress:

> She was worried, because [a young man] had asked her to go out for a cup of coffee. I said "Well, go!" She said, "I like him but I don't fancy him." "Well, why won't you go for a cup of coffee with him?" "He might get the wrong idea." And I said, "But, Sybil, he's asking you for a cup of coffee; he's not asking you to get married!" She was that naïve that she couldn't work out that it was OK to go for coffee with somebody without it having any meaning. A lot of things that children do and learn along the way, Sybil was having to learn at a later age, and it was very difficult.

Lois Chaber

As the year goes on, moreover, cracks in the communal harmony of Sybil's Granta 'home' appear. She is increasingly bothered by the frequently loutish behaviour of two male clients on her side of the two-unit residential home, Ken and Alex. Ken, in particular, is creating serious tensions because of his recently discovered drug addiction and the disruptive, anti-social, and uncooperative behaviour to which it leads. Staff, having tried to help him without success, are fed up and want him to leave the Granta project, which he refuses to do.

Similarly, at our home, there are some tensions and conflicts, primarily between Molly on the one hand, and Neil and me on the other, which we do not manage to keep under control during Sybil's weekend visits. We no longer inflict physical punishment on Molly for what we perceive as her rebellious and stroppy behaviour, but there are a lot of harsh rows and shouting on both sides, and, it seems, we are so focused on Sybil's illness that we don't think to explore whether Molly's behaviour indicates underlying problems of her own. At the same time, Neil is under great stress in his job on the Heathrow Project. Overworked, and with his position under threat from political intrigues within the project, his occasionally tetchy moods do not lighten the atmosphere in our home.

My own psychic recovery, moreover, suffers a setback when my second therapist declares out of the blue that my therapy is to end at Easter '97, refusing to give me any explanation whatsoever, in line with what appears to be a (disconcerting) Tavistock policy. If, perhaps, she had said, "I am dismissing you as my patient because our relationship doesn't seem to be working out in a positive therapeutic way, but you are welcome to reapply and try working with another therapist", I might have persevered. But she is blankly noncommittal, and, discouraged, I give up on therapy. Eventually, I begin to backslide, unable to suppress the old symptoms of anxiety and depression, particularly as I haven't taught classes for eleven years and my new job, with

"THE THING INSIDE MY HEAD"

its labour-intensive essay marking, has created new stresses. These increase when, later that year, desiring a chance to teach literature and a bit more income, I take on a second part time teaching job with the Workers Educational Association, a community-based, informal adult education service. What with these intermittently unpleasant episodes at home, Sybil decides, encouraged by her Granta care workers, to come home only every second week in the latter half of this period.

All during this time, Neil and I feel the strain of our ambiguous relationship with Sybil, who has so many other, more influential and officially sanctioned mentors in her life. We are compelled to tread delicately, hesitantly, in the limited and very part-time parental role we have been allotted. For me, especially, it feels as if most of Sybil's life I have been *'a mother and not a mother'*.

* * *

Despite these ongoing problems, Neil and I still enjoy many uplifting times with Sybil, watching films and TV programmes together, taking walks, and going on outings to museums and the like. She is occasionally taken out separately by Molly, who also spends a fair amount of time chatting intimately with her at home, and a comradely Sunday swim with me at the local leisure centre becomes a regular feature of her weekends. More importantly, her busy life in Clacton continues to promote her personal growth, as does her interaction with the various care workers in the Granta residence. Diane describes how Sybil develops emotionally during this period and the nurturing techniques she employed to this end:

> *The week she moved in, I really wanted to be Sybil's key worker. I remember seeing her when she came; she was this little insecure*

349

Lois Chaber

waif. She had all the hallmarks of having come through an institutionalised system. She was just waiting for me to tell her what to do . I remember going up to ask Sybil down for a cup of tea and she was standing there, in the middle of the room, and there was all this stuff around her, and she started to apologise to me for the mess. And I just looked at her and I said, "Well, the mess isn't important—you've only just moved in and that will be absorbed in a couple of days." And she really didn't think she could come down and have a cup of tea with me until she tidied her room up. And that's when I realised I had got somebody who was very institutionalised on my hands, somebody who'd been told. "Do this or you can't have that; you have to do this or you can't do that," and I think that's what made me decide I was never ever going to do that with Sybil.

Another time, I sat in the office, and there was this little noise behind me with just a little shuffle, and I looked through the door and there was Sybil; it was about 9:00 at night. I said hello and she put her head down, and she mumbled something and I said, "What's the matter?" She said, "I'm tired; is it OK if I go to bed?" I remember getting up and going to her, and I put my hands on her shoulder, and I said, "Sybil, why did you ask me that?" She said, "Because I had to at Eaglehurst." And I said, "Sybil, this is your home; you get up, you go to bed, you go out, you come in. You don't have to ask me or any other member of staff." And the only thing I asked her to do was, if she left the building, just to come and say "cheerio, I'm off now," so that we knew for fire safety reasons, and go. It took a while for me to get that through to Sybil.

"THE THING INSIDE MY HEAD"

At the next staff meeting, I asked other members of staff, "Look, you know, please stand back from Sybil." It would be so easy just to take over doing everything for her. And what we had to do was get some independence and confidence. The only way she could do that was to find it herself, but with knowing that we were there if she needed it. And somebody said to me, "Oh, you're going to be a bit like a mother," and I got really angry at that. And I said, "No, Sybil has a mother; I have been a mother; Sybil doesn't need another mother; she just needs a friend, and that's what we have to be—not a mother, not a guardian, but her friend."

Sometimes I felt I was being a bit hard on Sybil because I stood back and made her do things. At first she didn't think she could go shopping with us, but I gave her the list and sent her off down one aisle, and I went down the other. I played on the fact that the tendons at the back of my legs were hurting—I really played upon that! So Sybil ended up doing a lot of things without realising she was doing them. And then she would suddenly realise afterwards that she'd accomplished things.

I don't think that the psychiatrist [Dr. Smith] approved of me very much. I remember the first meeting I went to with him and Sybil: I said to Sybil: "I'm not talking for you tomorrow; you have to." And she said, "I can't!" And I said, "You can, and you will. I'm not going to say anything. I'll help you, but you must do it." We got in there, and he started to talk to me, and I said, "Sybil is here; please speak to Sybil. She can speak for herself." I don't think the man

Lois Chaber

was very amused by that at all. And then Sybil
started talking, and she wouldn't shut up
talking. She talked and she talked and she
talked. When we left, the psychiatrist said, "I've
never heard her like this before!" I said, "Well, it
could be because no one's ever given her the
chance to before." And after that, Sybil spoke
for herself, and if she got into difficulties we
would help her out. What she needed was a
safe place to blossom, to grow and to just
stand. That's what I tried to give her.

Actually, she got very cheeky, which was
nice. I encouraged it. Tracey [Granta staff
member] and I were two Northerners.
Northerners have a lot of banter going between
them—not nastily insulting—but they will snipe
at each other. And at first Sybil couldn't
understand it. She used to sit very quiet, but,
gradually, she got into it, and if Tracey and I
were quiet, she would start us off. She would
say something to Tracey or to me which would
set us off again, and she would actually join in,
and she was getting very confident at holding
her own in this two-way conversation, which
suddenly became three-way, between three
women. Sometimes it would be Tracey and
Sybil ganging up on me, and sometimes it
would be Sybil and I ganging up on Tracey. But
it was always good fun. She'd come up to the
bungalow where I was living with Tracey on a
Monday morning so that we could go shopping,
and she'd shout through the letter box: "It's
Sybil. C'mon you lazy madams, it's time you
were up!" Three months before, she wouldn't
have even knocked on my door! She could
enjoy life; she just needed to know that it was
safe to do it, and I'd like to think she was
beginning to get that.

"THE THING INSIDE MY HEAD"

We had bad days, but I also pointed out to Sybil that everybody had bad days. She came to me one day and said that it was awful, that she didn't seem to be going forward. I said, "Is it like walking through treacle?" And she said, "Yes". I said, "Oh, it's a treacle day today then." So after that, it became the password between Sybil and me. She would come to me and say, "It's a bad day today; it's a treacle day." Or if I was not feeling too bright, she'd say, "Is it a treacle day today?" "Yes, it is, Sybil." Then she'd say, "What would a cup of tea do?"

When Sybil had been with us for a few months, I remember talking with Michael [Granta staff member], *saying I was so pleased with how Sybil had progressed, but I was also worried because she was moving a bit faster than I'd anticipated. I was glad that she was going out to do things, and that she wanted to go back and re-start her education and do various other things, but I also wanted her to slow down a bit because I felt she was taking on too much and not giving herself any time to relax at all. It seemed to me as if Sybil had got something on every morning, every afternoon, and most evenings, and then she was coming home every weekend. I was getting quite concerned because we all need to just sit around sometimes. I didn't want to say "Don't," in case it stopped her doing everything else. So what I did do was to work out a programme where I knew she'd got one afternoon and one evening where she was set to do absolutely nothing. She could clean her room, she could play music, she could write letters, but she was to do something for herself.*

Lois Chaber

Most of the time, if Sybil wanted to make a decision, I would say, "Well, what do you want?" "I don't know." I'd say, "If you don't know, there's no point discussing it then." So, I would make her tell me what it was she wanted. A couple of times she actually said, "Can't you decide for me?" And I said, "No, no". But what I had used to do with her was, we'd sit down and look at all the various options that she had. But I would make her identify the options. I wouldn't do things for her. That sounds terribly hard, but Sybil had come through a lot of institutions where everything had been done for her, and all decisions had been made on her behalf.

I felt that I had to give Sybil a door through which she had to go to become the young woman that I knew she could be. I could see this quiet, intelligent, and very, very beautiful young woman trying to come through but being held back by lack of confidence. And I just felt that I had to get that confidence into her, one way or another.

Enormous achievement, growing confidence, a blossoming personality—this is how not only Diane but ALL of us more or less perceive Sybil during this extended 'year', from early 1997 mid-way through 1998; however, her diary entries are prolific at this time, and we need to see the same year from her perspective, without necessarily taking that as the ultimate 'truth' either.

"THE THING INSIDE MY HEAD"

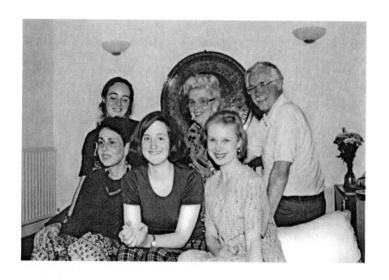

Sybil's 19th birthday. Back: Molly, June Keyte (pen-pal), Christopher Keyte; Front: Lois, Sybil, Lesley (dancing teacher)

Lois Chaber

Chapter 7: Taking Responsibility

Excerpts from Sybil's Diaries
March '97—late May '98

I'm an adult now, I'm the one responsible for me and how I get on.

* * *

I feel its my responsibility to keep [Molly] on the right path.

* * *

I feel confused as regards responsibility, worry and concern about my family.

(From Sybil's diary)

Individuals with OCD have an inflated sense of responsibility.

(David Veale and Rob Willson, *Overcoming Obsessive Compulsive Disorder*, Constable & Robinson Ltd, 2005 p. 54.)

Throughout this period (roughly equivalent to my time-frame in Chapter 6), Sybil is based at Woodland Lodge in Clacton, run by Granta Housing, and she goes from nineteen to twenty years old.

* * *

19 March: I feel a bit like crying and screaming and I feel this really insecure feeling which I didn't get so much at Eaglehurst and if I did I knew I could tell the staff I was feeling 'horrible'.

"THE THING INSIDE MY HEAD"

I feel alone. I'm an adult now, I'm the one responsible for me and how I get on, whether I overcome my problems or not. I feel a bit better while I'm writing this.

23 March: [Mum] asked me how I was getting on with the [Granta] staff and I said that there had been times when I wanted to talk to someone but I didn't feel I could talk to them. She said I must try. Then she started saying that I could always talk to her and dad and to phone them up if I felt lonely and stuff. She said that she wants to listen to me and that she wants to be my friend. Then she lay her head on my shoulder. I felt a bit upset by all this because she seemed sad and she was offering me so much, too much for them to take on.

24 March: I don't think that Jane [her CPN] realizes that things are still very difficult for me. I still always worry about hurting someone and have to do things and feel terrified. I know I don't usually feel as bad as I did today but I do get depressed and am not always as happy and calm inside as I may look. I'm still sad and angry about my illness having had such an affect on my life, which is one of the reasons I think about the past and what could have been so much. I think another part of it is that I'm very anxious and scared about the future. I've got to go through the Bethlem course [the Maudsley Behavioural Unit] start going home on my own, do voluntary work which I am really worried about and get some education and qualifications which is going to be very painful, frustrating and difficult for me, and I'm scared of all the hard work that is coming up in the next year or 6 months at least.

28 March [family holiday in Bruges]: Breakfast was lovely. Dad was being very witty which started me off in hysterics of laughter. I was laughing so much. I hope Molly didn't think it was stupid. The man who owns the house was going to take us on a guided tour of this area. Molly had to work (school) so we (mum, dad and I) went. When dad told the man about Molly I felt jealous that I wasn't studying or a

Lois Chaber

student. I wondered if the man looked down on me because I wasn't. The walk was lovely. I've had such a brilliant day, you almost can't describe it. Sometimes it felt or at least reminded me of the old times when we were on holiday doing those sort of things but not all the time.

What Jane would say: Do you think you were disgusting and stupid when you were laughing? I (Jane) think she [Molly] would probably find it funny as well and it sounds like you would both be having a lot of fun together. Laughter is good and it shows that maybe you are more relaxed with your family than you used to be.

About the school work, would you really be jealous of having to work on holiday? Think what you would feel like if you were in her shoes, you would probably be feeling jealous then!

Why would that man think you are stupid or look down on you for not studying? Would you look down on someone if they weren't or hadn't been studying? Anyway, what does it matter what he thinks, he's just the owner of the bed and breakfast.

I'm glad you had such a good time.

10 April: I've got so many strong emotions in me, it is hard to sort them out. I feel so touched by Michelle's [former Latymer classmate] letter. She offered to go to the cinema with me this weekend to see Romeo and Juliet. Molly has seen it and she says it was brilliant and I'd like to see it, but I still feel too self conscious. I'm crying with joy, and fear and sadness and really touched(ness). She said I could phone her "but hey don't feel pressured, love Shell" I don't know how to deal with these emotions.

16 April: I don't think I'll be able to do the Maudsley thing [the behavioural programme]. It's so, so much harder than the other stuff I've done, and they say you can't

"THE THING INSIDE MY HEAD"

reassure yourself, but I reassure myself all the time and I've tried to practise for the Maudsley but I can't do it. Mum and Dad and everyone is expecting me to do it and I feel like I'm doing it under pressure and maybe for them more than myself.

I heard a song on the radio which really brings back strong memories and feelings from my time at the Bethlem [Adolescent Unit]. It makes a part of me feel like I want to go back there. But when I think of how much harder and scarier life was for me then I don't want to go, but I feel a strong pull or connection from there like a cord holding us, like an artificial umbilical cord.

17 April: We went to Wimpy's where I had my dinner and Patty and Marjory, which was good for Marjory. On the way there Patty mentioned that Marjory had been thinking of taking an overdose. I said some things to Marjory which I hoped would help her not to take one. I'm a bit worried that I might have said the wrong thing. Anyway at Wimpy's Marjory said she was glad she had come which was good.

22 April: We watched the end of "Children's Hospital". I felt very nostalgic about being in General hospitals and on drugs and having nurses look after you. I felt a bit that I wanted to go back to that, I'm not sure why. Part of it is the security of knowing someone else is taking care of you and is responsible for you and being looked after like a child and babied a little bit. I don't know why I feel like this.

26-27 April [home]: I felt suicidal a couple of times today. Its just that I never or hardly ever feel safe in myself. I'm always struggling with something and I'm never at peace in myself. I wish I could feel better towards God.

[next morning] After breakfast this morning I was playing with Ali [our cat] and listening to the music coming

359

from the kitchen. I felt so at peace and happy it was really good. I hope I get that again.

Mum's leg is still really bad which I am worried about and she has been muttering a lot which she does when she is upset. She has gone back to her old and higher dose of medication. I'm really quite worried about her. I'm also quite worried about her memory loss. It could be to do with her anxiety and depression. I feel really [unreadable] and anxious I can't write anymore.

30 April: I felt really anxious about going to college. And being well is very scary as well as being ill being scary. My life is my responsibility and I don't like responsibility; it scares me and always has done. The thing I trust least is myself. I'm so worried about the Bethlem [Maudsley Behavioural Unit]. On one hand, I want them to say I'm too well, cause then I wouldn't have to go through that hell, but on the other, if they do say that I'll feel lost because I'll have to get better on my own, which may not be so bad, but what if it means I can't improve much and I'll never be able to do things like drive a car and stuff.

And then there are all those 'growing up' questions inside, like what do I want from Brett, how do I really feel about him, what do I want to do about it.

And I really want a boyfriend. I've got to lose weight.

[Undated; after the Maudsley interview, probably 2nd May]: I am so scared, what have I done. Not only have I to face everyone and their disappointment and anger but have lost a chance of getting better. What will they think of me (my family) if I kill myself. They have been more than wonderful. They don't deserve it, but it's my life. I really wish that I could do it without them being hurt or thinking bad of me. I wish I could still go to the Bethlem and that I had said 'Yes, I could cope' but I wouldn't have been able to do it. I'm thinking of getting the train back to Clacton while mum is out and leaving a note and taking some paracetamol when I get back. I don't care (well I do) what anyone else thinks. It's not their life. I never asked to be born.

[One day later]: There is no one I can really talk to about how I really feel. I certainly can't talk to my family and I can't talk to Jane and I feel like I can't even talk to the Samaritans. I'm a coward. Jane please understand, I beg you I beg you. I feel this awful feeling inside me. I want to cry but I can't even do that. It's a sort of dreading feeling but worse, closing in on me. I feel a bit better now. I can't see hope but I can imagine that its there and ~~my family are too~~

[Undated, probably a few days later, at Granta]: I think Molly was right when she said that I was the one who was really upset at not going and who had built it up to be a big thing, not my team. I thought it would help me to drive a car and go to college and be a vetenary nurse and I was going to be so much better after the summer. I think I made the right decision.

7 May: I'm confused. The voices and messages I get now seem the same as the ones I used to get that I thought were God but weren't. I feel scared. I feel scared of the responsibility I have to take over my life.

10 May: Mum, dad and I watched the end of a film called 'Fanny and Alexander'. It was really good. It was a bit scary at times. At one point the evil stepfather was beating the boy and this made me feel very uncomfortable because I was wondering what dad was thinking because I think he was brought up in a very hard way with plenty of beatings. I think it is disgusting. I also felt uncomfortable, upset, angry and thinking "what is dad thinking" because he beat Molly once [Neil hit her with a belt on her thighs on one occasion]. Just writing about it makes me feel angry and uncomfortable and my skin crawl.

Lois Chaber

I was going to take the train from Liverpool St. to Clacton on my own. After Mum left I stood waiting for the platform number to show up on the board. I worried that people would think me odd standing there and that they were looking at me and I looked a state (thoughts). The platform number came up. I felt tense (feelings) I worried that I might have misread the sign or read the wrong one (thoughts). I checked it a few times (behaviour). I walked to the platform and the train had just come in, people were coming out. I looked to see if anyone was going in yet because I wanted to board the train as soon as possible. I was worried that something might go wrong or I'd be too late or look silly in the station if I didn't (thoughts). I walked up the platform (behaviour). I couldn't see anyone going in. I walked back. I saw some inspectors looking at me and talking "Oh no! they think I'm trying to board without a ticket" (thoughts). I sat at some tables I kept looking at my watch and going to the platform to see if anyone was getting on. Finally I saw they were. I got on and got settled (behaviour). *[end of excerpt]*

14 May: I went to the Vista Rd [social] group. After a while Brett came in. A few people including me said hello to him and he answered theirs but not mine. Later on during the game he looked at me and smiled and spoke a little. I felt in love with him. I fantasized about us kissing.

21 May: *[Scrawled across the page and followed by very poor, irregular handwriting]*

AAAAGH

My parents love me so much but I don't love them as much as they love me. I feel so guilty and sometimes I feel hardly any love for them which is awful and I don't want to feel like that. I want to love them as much as they love me but I'm always guilty and then I'm in debt to them. I feel guilty for writing this. I should feel happy that they love me so much occasionaly I do. I am ashamed but I'm also frustrated and sad. AAAA

23 May [a few days after her birthday party]: Now I feel like crying. Brett probably won't even want to be friends or be the slightest bit intrested in me. One, 'cause I singled him out from the group at Martello, 2 'cause the party was a bit of a flop, 3 because Ken asked him if he was my boyfriend and I gave a horrible laugh out of embarassment so he might take that as an insult 4 Ken said "I thought Sybil had a boyfriend" and I covered my face and kept saying 'no I haven't' over and over again, all of which might have made Brett think that I told them that he was my boyfriend, which I didn't.

27 May: Ever since Myra Hindley was on the news I've kept getting thoughts coming into my head, of her name, of [her] imagined face and her evil and I feel really scared and I have to stop and think what I have done, what was doing and what I am going to do because I get this terrible powerful fear and feeling that I have or I'm going to hurt someone.

30 May [home]: I feel like I'm having to be careful and maybe tip-toe a bit [about] what I say to Molly these days, a lot because of her arguments about mum and dad. I sometimes try to make things better but then I make a mess of it. I also worry about her being angry at me and us falling out. I feel its my responsibility to keep her on the right path. I feel something like if the link between us broke down, the way her relationship is with Mum and Dad these days, she might go wayward and do foolish things and get herself further and further into a [k]not and maybe become a bad person. I don't think I'm a good person, in fact I think I'm a bad person. I feel like a lot of pressure is on me. And mum is under a lot of stress and so is dad these days. I feel like

the weekends are more about me helping and supporting them. Now I'm wondering if that is ungrateful, I feel like crying. I feel like I can't relax in this house. I'm always worrying about how things I do will affect my family even the cat, even things like watching T.V. And I can't be myself and "pour out my troubles" to them.

12 June: I got a letter from Allen [the behavioural therapist] today. Reading part of it again now before bed, I feel like I want to cry, I'm not sure why I am crying. I just now thought about Lucy [her budgie] and how she is confined to a cage and she can hear the birds outside but she is confined in a small space inside all the time and how unhappy and frustrated this must make her.

21 June: I feel a bit like crying. Molly is in a difficult, angry mood again and there is friction between her and mum and dad. I always find that very difficult. I think this is partly because I don't know how to act. I feel for both sides and I don't want to appear to be taking sides, to either of them. I often feel that I have to do or say something otherwise Molly will think that I'm automatically taking my parents' side. I also worry about Molly being angry with me. I worry about how Molly is feeling and whether she is going to do something silly. I also worry that the argument might get physical. It also reminds me of the bad days.

26 June: Jane was asking me some hard questions. Then she started talking to me like she hasn't done before I think, really plainly, I got really upset. The session was mainly about going back into my role in the family I had took on which made me ill. I feel like its my fault. I've got to do something or I'll end up ill again. I think I will reduce my weekends and I'll stop getting involved in arguments and trying to make things right. I don't know what I'm going here for. Part of the reason at least is to help my family. And its good to see them and get a change.

"THE THING INSIDE MY HEAD"

30 June: [Molly] and mum had a little argument which upset me but I told myself that it wasn't my responsibility and I felt a bit relieved.

3 July: I had been feeling really down and tearful all day. I went to the Achievements meeting at Green Lodge [Tendring Adult Community College]. When I got there I felt so nervous and panicky and still low, I wished I hadn't come and I didn't know how I was going to get through the evening. But I stayed and whats more, I decided to read my piece instead of having Sue (my teacher) do it. At the interval, a lady said she liked it. There was a really lovely atmosphere there and near the end, a wonderful feeling ebbed in, over and through me. I felt peaceful, accepted and a sort of piece [peace]. It was great. I feel more positive now, even though the great feeling has gone.

10 July: I felt more at peace with God and myself when I was ill. Well maybe not but better than now. I was a better person when I was ill. I'm a cold, heartless, tainted, selfish evil person now. I can see just a bleak picture of my future. I became ill out of faith and goodness and it has broken my faith and goodness.

11 July: Later I was also thinking about my separation from God and I realized that its gone on for a long time and that when I was ill there were times where I felt so close to him and I was sure I felt the Holy Spirit and complete forgiveness and spiritual ecstasy, really! and I wondered whether the voices were true after all and I felt lost. I feel lost now without a purpose or meaning to life.

25 July: I feel I don't want to be good all the time. I feel scared and trapped sometimes when I try and do that. I have a feeling urging me that this is important and the day of judgement is coming soon. Maybe it is from God though because they [her thoughts] seem like it sometimes. And one other worry, sensible thoughts from God or from my conscience or me or are they obsessive thoughts?

Lois Chaber

IM FED UP OF SOMETHING. I'M FED UP OF BEING CONTROLLED

Why God did you let this happen to me. I was a good Christian.

26 July: I don't know whether to start eating or not. At first I was in control but now it feels more like I *have* to stop eating and I'm getting messages telling me that I must if I want to get back to God. But I feel confused and down and bored What is life worth and all the things I'm doing worth without God?

I want help.

I don't feel my usual self. I want to eat but I can't

HELP

I feel alone and scared.

I looked up in my diary to see if it was the time of the month. It is near so then I thought it could just be P.M.T. [pre-menstrual tension]. I ate some toast and marmalade and jam and drank some milk.

27 July: I feel quite positive at the moment (now as I write). Reza [mental health client] came and it was quite good. We went for a nice walk. I just hope he doesn't think I fancy him because I don't. I think he fancies me though.

31 July [at the Crescent Cat Shelter]: Caroline [the owner] told me what she wanted me to do because she had to go to the sanctuary. This means she trusts me. I did well with my usual cats. I've got a sort of routine now. I didn't manage to brush all the cats though. One was out of reach

"THE THING INSIDE MY HEAD"

and the other, I just ran out of time and maybe because I was giving some of them so much T.L.C. [tender loving care].

When mum and dad phoned me up, mum told me she got a job. I feel pleased for her. I was always hoping she would get a job, she had been working so hard to find one. She said that she is really nervous and she starts on Tuesday, so she has a lot of work to do this weekend. She said we are all going to have to rally round her, which is perfectly normal and reasonable, but I feel really quite anxious about it as I'll have to be worrying whether I should be doing something all the time.

5 August: We were doing 'Talking to the opposite sex' in the Youth group. It was very good. I learnt a few things. I feel embarrassed because I went to shake hands in one role play and it was very inappropriate and Delia [occupational therapist] said it was a bit posh. I know she was only joking but I hope none of them think I'm posh. At least I won't do it in the real thing.

21 August: [home; when Molly changed the date on her bus pass and got into trouble with the authorities] Oh I'm so worried Dad might get violent Molly might get upset and do something stupid Oh please don't let that happen Jane would say that I'm not responsible for what they do but someone has to take responsibility. I have to. I have to make sure my sister is safe.

27 August: I wish I was a little child again and had hardly any responsibilities and I was warm and looked after. Last night I really wanted someone to mother me. I think that that is a big problem with me. I think that even at the Bethlem [Adolescent Unit], I wanted to be mothered. Maybe that was just because I felt so distressed then or maybe I have a real problem about it. Maybe its because I didn't get all the mothering I should or would normally have got or maybe its because of my mental state, and mental health

Lois Chaber

problems (which I've had for most of my life) that I feel
insecure and want to be made to feel safe and secure.
Maybe it's a bit of both.

28 August: At the Youth Group today, at first I felt
quite p---ed off because we were going to miss out on the
socialization session. But the session we did do, on work
and education, turned out to be very good. I found out quite
a bit of useful stuff and my head was buzzing with ideas,
hopes and plans at the end. But they cant be put into action,
a lot of them. Well, maybe that's not true, some of them but
I really felt eager to get a job or education and be well on the
road. But I know that I would almost certainly get ill again if I
tried to do that now, cause I'm not ready for it yet.

1 September: I can't ask anyone for a hug here [at
Granta] I always seem to want to be parented, hugged
more, or I feel more secure in a hug or being parented, by
someone other than my family. But they cant ever give me
love. I wish Roberta [her former associate worker at
Eaglehurst] loved me. My relationship with my parents is
sort of bittersweet. They are the ones, I know, who love and
care about me most and they are so good to me but I feel a
bit sort of insecure with them and always worrying that I
might hurt them and feeling/thinking they are delicate. And
so I want comfort from other adults in my life but it still
doesn't feel that good because I know they don't love me.
But if they did love me, I think that maybe I'd feel less secure
and more of a bittersweet feeling like I have with my parents.
I think that this issue is part of why I want a boyfriend. I
imagine myself secure and safe in his arms.

10 September [first day of autumn term at her
college]: I was really nervous. I kept thinking up scenarios
where I wasn't allowed in the class because I hadn't
enrolled. To my relief there was room for me and it *was*
alright to enrol on the day. The class went okay, sort of. I
started at the very beginning but everyone else, even when
they had started at the beginning, seemed to be ahead of

me. I've always been very competitive when it comes to schoolwork. I could hardly concentrate on my work because I was thinking so much about how they were ahead of me and how I wanted to catch up.

17 September: I feel a mess inside. I still have this obsession about child abuse and sexual abuse and rape. I keep wanting or wishing in a strange sort of way, that I had been abused. And what may be worse, or maybe not come to think about it, I feel attracted like a regret to anything about that subject and I take delight in and get some sort of kick from knowing, hearing or reading about other people/children, having been abused. In a terrible way I want them to have been abused and to hear about and fulfil my obsession. I cant even help people. I cant care. I've lost the ability to care or empathise. I feel like taking an overdose right now. I feel no real care inside me for people in suffering. I feel so indifferent even very slightly sadistic about it. And I feel spite for other people and want to put them down. I don't want to be like this.

18 September: I want help. For the past few weeks I've been doubting what the vicar told me; I've been wondering and seeing a good argument for all the stuff I believed in to be true. This is partly because of my lost faith. Even after the Minister told me that it wasn't God punishing me and that God wants me to be happy. You see, when I re[mem]ber the Christmas of 1992 when I really believed in God and obeyed him and threw myself into what he wanted me to do and I loved him and it was the same when I was first at the Bethlem. You see, I felt more at peace than I do now, or maybe not, but I felt a certain kind of peace that I don't feel now. This is a nightmare, what is going on since I did that sin, but it started before that, God's voice and that was before the really bad tensions at home, so that cant be why but dad had been unemployed for a year and I was at a new school and I've got no-one to hold me and make things alright, even for a short time. With or without believing in the

voice, Im lost. I really feel like I might go back to the voice and thoughts and obeying them.

24 September: I feel lonely. I don't like Marjory or Patty that much and we don't really 'click'. The last time I had really good friends was in the Bethlem.

7 October: Hazel [new Community Psychiatric Nurse] came round. We talked about making new friends with people my own age outside the Mental Health services.

19 October: On the way back on the train, near Clacton, I was listening to a family talking, and the young boy was singing really well and I heard the parents say that he goes to Tiffany Stage School and does dance as well. I felt the envy and anger, but mostly envy, I think, bubbling up inside of me until I was boiling. It felt so strong I felt a bit frightened of myself. I[t] reminded me of dancing, something I was good at and enjoyed and that was taken away from me, and is lost to me now.

I almost went to Tiffany's when I was at Jacques Hall but I didn't because on the day of the first lesson that term, Mum and dad asked me if I wanted to come home for the day or evening while Aunt Judy and Uncle Ian [actually Uncle Neville—here from New Zealand] came to dinner. I said yes because I didn't want to miss my chance of seeing them and also because I knew their coming would help me go to and be at home. So I chose to do that and next week I felt I couldn't go to the dance class because I'd missed out on the first lesson and I was already very nervous about it. So on the train I started thinking, like I had at times before what it would have been like if I hadn't gone home. Would I have got my dancing back? But I know that if I hadn't said yes to going home that time, I might still not be going home now and I might never have forgiven my parents and I might never have been part of the family again, like I am now and I might never have 'got my family back'. What is more

"THE THING INSIDE MY HEAD"

important. I think my family is [written a few months before she actually does try going to Tiffany's].

22 October: Also Diane keeps saying that I'm well. I wish that I didn't have this OCD but I still do only it is with different symptoms now, more in my head than things I do, but things I do as well.

29 October: In some ways I don't like being "well" because I'm the one who is responsible for me and my life. Maybe not absolutely and completely, I've still got a support system but it's up to me and its scary and painful. I don't want to be an adult I don't want to be a teenager, I want to be a child, I want to be a child again without OCD No I want to be dead.

I want a hug. I want Mary, Maybe Pat [nurses from the Adolescent Unit], Erica [Peter Bruff nurse] to love me and be around me. They are where I put my faith, I don't put it in me, maybe I don't put it in them but I depend on their approval and I want their love. Am I being ungrateful? I've got such loving parents. I couldn't ask for more loving parents. But I don't feel secure with them exactly because they are my parents and I worry about them and see them as vulnerable (even though they are such strong people).

4 November: I can't talk to Diane. She just thinks my unhappiness is normal, just my age. That makes me feel really horrible, It also makes me feel desperate, angry, guilty, awkward, angry alone, stubborn, afraid, frustrated, and I still feel confused.

I think Diane might have guessed about the cutting [herself]. No-one thinks I'm serious. But I am.

Part of my problem is that responsibility really really scares me. Not just for other people but for myself as well. I don't know if its got anything to do with OCD... [Sybil's ellipses]

Lois Chaber

6 November: Yesterday Hazel said that the incident I told her about *was* abuse and I didn't exaggerate it at all. I feel really mixed up about that. If it was abuse then it changes a lot of what I've been thinking and reasoning ~~and it excites excites excites excites~~

And I know this is going to sound bad, but it excites me because I've waited and waited for so long, years, to be told by someone who would know, that the incidents were abuse. I now know that one of them was and if that was then others might be. I've wanted to be acknowledged as me or my sister having been 'abused'. I know that might sound sick and awful but it isn't.

8 November: I've just been to this really awful, horrible art show—the Saatchi 'Sensations', with Molly. Now I feel horrible and its given me horrible thoughts and made my OCD worse or maybe I've 'reacted obsessively to it' but I can't help it. I wish I hadn't gone. But if I hadnt, it would have made mum, dad and Molly upset/guilty and I would have been in the house on my own.

Its because of my OCD that things like the art show really upset me and [unreadable word] I'm so afraid of myself. Am I perverted? Help Its awful I hate these thoughts and feelings.

9 November: I'm less confident and I have less self esteem than a few months ago. I think its because well I don't know. I felt proud of the achievements I had made and was making then. But now I just think 'Well, that's nothing, anyone my age could do that and a lot more, which I should be doing' It seems like the more involved and the more I become part of the 'normal', 'real' world, the more I realize how inadequate I am.

17 December [the Granta Christmas dinner]: I went to the shop I came back and when I showed Kim the little

"THE THING INSIDE MY HEAD"

black dress she loved it so I wore it and did my makeup and I thought I looked good and Kim said I did. We set off for Jackel's [restaurant]. The problem is, when I know or think I look really nice I have a funny 'look at me aren't I nice' grin on my face which is totally a bad move. I must try and stop it. I don't know if I can.

The dinner was lovely and very filling. At one point it seemed so lovely—all of us sitting down and having this Christmas meal together. And people were in the Xmas spirit. I think that Michael [Granta staff member] is beautiful, not in his looks but definitely in his personality, character and soul.

20 December: AAAAGH!

Molly and I went to Winchmore Hill (by bus) to try and get a plant for Mum. While we were sitting by the bus stop, Molly mentioned something about Nancy [Molly's friend] fancying Martha White [another Latymer student].

I started thinking about my own confusion about my sexuality and I thought about telling Molly. Something showed in my face because Molly said 'Why are you looking so worried' and I said that I couldn't tell her. She said 'Why!' I said 'Its too embarrassing' and I said that she might tell someone and she said that she wouldn't and the she had some of the world's secrets on her shoulders and that she was very trustworthy. So I said it. "Sometimes I think I might be a lesbian." I said "I have strong feelings for women but I also fancy boys and lesbians on the T.V. fascinate me and I get almost obsessed with them and I think 'I wish I was like her' and then I think 'am I a lesbian'? No I can't be because I like boys" But then I think 'I wish I was'. She said that there isn't such a thing as completely 'straight' or completely 'gay'. She also [sentence unfinished] I said 'You won't tell Nancy will you?!' She said no. I felt really weird and embarrassed. She said that she was very glad I told her. In the bus she said that if she told Nancy, she [Nancy] would think I'm really cool and 'Well done Sybil!' but I asked her not to. She also said that if I decided to tell anyone else other than her, one day, that I would probably find that most girls have had feelings like that about one person or at one time. She also said that girls even had 'crushes' on women but it doesn't mean they are gay.

I feel dirty for saying it.

23 December: She [Molly] is superior. There is a gap between us. Our relationship has gone all wrong. When I first started coming home it was really good but maybe because it was new and novel to both of us and we had a great chance then to be sisters again and get to know each other and be part of each others lives. But now as time has passed I didn't get more mature but now she has got to know me, I'm a baby, stupid, naïve and weak and I'm boring and I cling to her like an eager puppy and I hate myself for being like that but I don't know how to be anything else.

31 December: Last night when I said goodnight to Molly she said something which stays with me and casts away the shadows and brings more light and hope to our relationship She said 'It's been really good/nice (I can't remember which) having you here (!!!)' [for the Christmas holidays] That makes me feel good and it reassures me. But its not just a reassurance. Oh its great. We're sisters.

2 January 1998: Why do I have to feel so much pain in my love for Molly. Why is it so hard. I want to love but why is love so hard?

5 January: I feel a lot better now; I'm just carrying on living and doing things for now. I finished cleaning my room and airing it which was quite satisfying. Tracey asked if I'd liked to go and see her cats right now. The kittens were just lovely. It was nice to do something different and get out of the house. But some of the issues came with us. This Ken [the drug addict] thing is really getting to me. I'm torn

374

between different opinions, thoughts and feelings. I hope he does go but not in a bad way. I wish him the best and hope he gets himself sorted out but its too tense with him here.

13 January: I'm so worried about Dad. He is tired (he sounded it and said he was) and I know he is under a lot of stress and he is depressed. *Oh Oh* How can I talk about things he has done. But I need to. Oh I feel so sad for him. What am I to do?.

15 January: Molly was *so great* on the phone. She is the best sister to me. She is *so* understanding and wise and helpful. I'm worried about her. She might leave home. Mum & Dad treat me differently to her and always put her down and Molly is exasperated.

19 January: I've just talked with Hazel about a lot of 'the bad times' [in the family]. I feel all hot, a bit like I've done something naughty but a bit like I've freed something. I almost sort of feel a bit excited.

20 January: I feel so mixed up and upset. I've been talking to Molly about what I've been talking to Hazel about. I feel confused and angry. If I really take what Molly said seriously I'm weak and selfish and perverted.

25 January: I watched a Christian Programme. I broke down in tears. I think at the moment that losing your faith or love for God is the worse thing that can happen to you. I feel like it was stolen from me but part of me says I had a part in it but is that true or an overzealous conscience?

After I cried, I came to a point of, not reconciliation, and it isn't resolved, but to a resting shelf in the cliff that [is] towering above me. And while I was listening to the service I couldn't comprehend or understand it, all about God giving Jesus because he loved us so much. I feel trapped in a cage, partly a self built vacuum, angry and shaking my fist and blind to the outside, the truth.

9 February: I'm scared also about being discharged from Mayfield. I want to be discharged but I'm worried because I'll have to get my medication from the G.P. and he might cut it down. Also I might need letters from my G.P to get income support. He might say I'm well enough to work. Then what will I do. How will I do my studying, Mum and Dad will get so upset and worried and in a state. They might suggest I live with them, but I can't.

I feel under pressure. I never feel satisfied or proud of myself. Last year I thought starting english & maths would make me feel more proud of myself and less pathetic and the same with cat rescue. But by the end of the summer, I felt pathetic again and I thought a full days voluntary job added on would help make it right, but soon that felt small and worthless and I thought 'Oh when I start my GCSE's next September then I'll feel less pathetic.' But already now I feel like that isn't enough and when we go to New Zealand I'll still look pathetic. And I still haven't moved into a flat of my own. In 4 or 5 months it will be a year from when I thought I 'might move out into a place of my own in a year' and I wont be doing it.

24 February: Dial-A-Ride was good. However I heard John [the driver] and Mrs. Miles and Mrs. Mosely talking about me. I didn't really catch what they said but I think they just think I'm 'sweet' and don't take me seriously. That could mean I'm not doing it well .

3 March: I'm feeling optimistic today. I want to live life!

At one point I felt really unhappy and suicidal. It was a bit like the feeling I had at dancing about the past being irreversible and how I couldn't get back what I had then, dancing, friendship, normality, education. I still feel like that but I'm thinking positively.

25 March: I'm getting fed up with these OCD thoughts I've been getting. They are increasing and becoming more scary. It's like I'm doing something and I suddenly get a mental block and a really strong feeling that I've done something bad or something that might hurt someone or cause someone to be hurt. And the thought just stays in my mind & blocks off logic and reason & I'm not allowed to reason because someone might get hurt if I didn't check and remedy what I've done immediately. They are coming more often now and I feel like I want to challenge them and even throw caution to the wind especially now that I've decided with Hazel to work on my OCD but I think I feel that I have to wait and do it properly on a programme.

I feel like crying. I'm scared of meeting new people outside the M.H. [Mental Health] Services and making friends with them. I've always found it difficult to make friends and I always felt insecure in a group of friends without a 'best-friend'.

The insecurity will be from when I was born and a baby. But I don't want to feel angry at my parents or blame them although I do feel a bit angry now But I can't carry on blaming them.

29 March: I don't really know what I want for a career. I feel that I want to give something to people, Something important. Somehow I'm not sure I can give what an O.T. [occupational therapist] needs to give and equally, I'm not sure if being an O.T. would give me the chance to really give what I can and want to give.

I'm not sure if I could be a good psychiatric nurse after being in the system so much and so long. Plus I don't know if I could do such a hard job as that. I don't know if I could be a social worker with the unresolved feelings I have about my past, Jacques Hall kids & abuse in general. I might be using that job to resolve or as an outlet for some of my difficult and unresolved feelings, which could be very serious and wrong and bad for whoever I'm working with.

I can't see what could change to make me stop feeling bitter and feeling & thinking bad thoughts about God. Maybe if I concentrated really hard on the future & getting to where I really want to, where I could have got if I hadn't been ill & moved out etc, and if I worked really hard I could be able to see good things that have come out of it and be reconciled and have peace. I don't want to feel like this but I feel its partly defensive because I have a deeprooted fear of really believing in God and being humble & doing only what he wants, 1, because I would slow down, maybe not & 2, because I associate that with my times in hospital & the voices & fear and punishment and trapped & being controlled.

7 April: I'm tired & I'm screaming inside my head, what with the Patty dilema, the conversation about voices, talking on the phone to Mum & Dad, missing Molly's call. can't talk to Hazel for over a week Oh Help!

[On the facing page there is a cartoonish imitation of Edvard Munch's 'The Scream', with a big weight on the figure's head and prominent rings under its eyes and the following written at the top: "'The scream' (only a tired and heavy pressure from a heavy weight)"]

8 April: I know I sound like a wimp and especially because I always seem to be moaning or feeling sorry for myself or ultra sensitive but you see the bad bits more than the good because when I have good days and everything is fine I don't feel that I need to write in the diary so much. I use the diary mainly to vent my problems & negative and difficult feelings.

"THE THING INSIDE MY HEAD"

13 April: I know that Jane said I'm not responsible for my familys well being and that I would probably get ill again if I tried to be But its really hard coz I feel so responsible for Molly. She won't or can't (I don't know which) turn to her parents and I believe that her new friends are leading her astray in some ways. And she is obviously (so much to me) a hurt little girl, or a big girl who is hurting badly inside. She has obviously got serious problems from the way she is coping with school and the relationship between her & Mum & Dad. I want to, & feel I have to help her. However, it is really hard as she rarely shows her real and important and strong feelings to me & she doesn't take me into her confidence. I don't understand a lot of what's going on for her and why she behaves as she does, for instance, leaving her plates up here for so long, leaving her mess around for so long and 'going into one' when someone mentions it or asks her to clean it up. There is obviously a reason why she does it, not just pure laziness.

Last night on our way to the Indian restaurant Mum got angry & said 'Stop pushing me' 'you're always pushing me about jobs' and Dad said 'I'm not pushing you'. Then Mum shouted in a stressed and strong way "Stop pushing me. Do you want me to die of a nervous breakdown" What she said and the way she said it sounded like the old mummy before she went to psychotherapy and it reminded me of that year: 91-92. She is going backwards ever since the psychotherapy stopped. I also think that she went backwards when her first therapist left. She had changed so much and was so strong and I really admired her when I was at the Bethlem & she was seeing her first psychotherapist. She never did feel the same with the second. I think talking to her now would be a mistake and that maybe she will need to get a bit worse before she or anyone else says or does something about it. I know Jane said that I'm not responsible but she is my mother & I care and, Oh I don't know.

Lois Chaber

25 April [home]: Ive had a really good day today. The highlights were going out with June [her long-term pen pal, Molly's friend's mother] & talking about more personal things including her breakdown. Dad showing me round the garden. I liked going for a walk with Mum & having lunch with her & stroking Ali without him snapping at me.

I still feel like I'm treading on egg shells a bit with Molly & being caught in the Middle. I think of what Tracey said about 'being myself' but I don't know how I would act even then. It seems to me, that in a way, the role of being in the middle is me being myself.

27 April: I've had my review and session afterwards with Hazel. She is just GREAT! From what she said, I feel very positive about the review & things. She said that Dr. Smith mentioned (just before I was called in) that I get very anxious about seeing him, which I think is really nice & kind and even better, Hazel said its because I think he is cross with me especially [about] the Bethlem & he said he wasn't. Plus Hazel told me that he didn't really think that going to the Bethlem [Maudsley Behavioral Unit] was right for me. Plus Hazel said that when she mentioned my wanting more OCD help/work but *not Allen Brown* they laughed and that Louisa [nurse from Mayfield] said something that shows she feels similar to Hazel & me about him & they way he got stroppy & dropped me! and also Louisa said to Hazel & me afterwards, 'You know Allen!' or something like that Plus Hazel said that Dr. Smith thinks it's a good idea for me to go home less which I am pleased about. Plus he said that my family are not 'to blame' but that they are definately part of why I got ill & that they are a big stress in my life and I haven't 'just got OCD there is more to it than that'.

I feel guilty now for writing or badmouthing my family but its true & I still love & like them & want to be in good contact with them.

"THE THING INSIDE MY HEAD"

2 May: Then [Tracey] gave me a big talking to about Ken and... [Sybil's ellipses] Oh... [Sybil's ellipses] I forgot I told her that I didn't agree with her behaviour to him [Ken] yesterday. [Tracey] went on & on about how staff had tried to help him, how he refused it & all the bad things he did & how they had to be firm with him etc. etc. I felt quite worried and annoyed because of this.

But I feel worried and confused because Diane is so different about Ken & I've never trusted Reginald recently & my gut feeling is that he & Tracey are being very bad & not telling me the truth & I shouldn't believe them. This feeling reminds me of the things I used to get about people being devils. Then there is Alex [a resident] who is 2 faced and complains about Ken in front of staff but is all buddy buddy with him in the evenings & lending and borrowing money off each other.

7 May: It's not the same at Granta as it used to be. I feel paranoid & uptight or uncomfortable about & with the other residents, especially Alex.

13 May: I'm angry at Diane.

I've just had a brill talk with Diane. I feel a lot better now & not angry at her. She explained & we have come to an understanding. We also talked about Alex & she said not to take his behaviour personally & she agreed with me on all or many points about Alex & Ken & she thinks Alex is taking drugs as well. HA HA to Alex

HA

I'm sorry if that sounds immature but I'm not going to take it back!

Maths was good really good today in that we were all chatting & laughing together & I felt nervous &

selfconscious & tense but I felt like an equal part of the group.

15 May: I met up with Sue [from Jacques Hall] but it was strange and lonely and as if we didn't know each other. I miss the Old Sue. Maybe I'm finding it hard because we don't have the same relationship we had of me being a little girl, a student, and a sort of patient & she was my keyworker & my carer & my friend my guardian angel. Now we're both adults, with a lot of distance between us. I think I always wanted her to be more to me than she could. I sort of wanted her to be a mum to me.

16 May: I resent Patty for taking my time but she didn't take it, I gave it & for ordering cream cakes but that was sweet of her in a way & I felt so embarrassed when she ordered a toasted tea-cake after our cream cake & apple pie with whipped cream which we shared.

But she is not well. You can see it in her eyes. They are desperate & struggling. I feel guilty for thinking & writing these things about her but I have to get my feelings out. Now I resent her because I feel guilty. I'm a bit worried about her—I feel sorry for her. I do like her but she is difficult & I find that look in her eyes difficult to handle.

18 May: I've had a really good & busy Birthday.

30 May: It was quite a disappointment and I feel worse, and felt worse when we came back last night than I felt before we left [for the pub]. I was feeling quite good earlier on. But Kim wasn't nurturing and caring. And I suppose, to try and be positive it was good experience in getting ready dressing up, make-up, walking there, what to drink and how to drink it, how to sit how to go to the toilet and I didn't feel too dizzy, drunk etc. Am I imagining the bad things like what Kim thinks about me.

"THE THING INSIDE MY HEAD"

Later: when Kim & I went to see Tracey Kim mentioned that she hadn't really been in a sociable mood last night because she was tired.

Later—9:00: I feel empty & stupid & bored. I want to feel, to be inspired. I must fight like I did at Peter Bruff and Eaglehurst. I feel a little like crying.

Lois Chaber

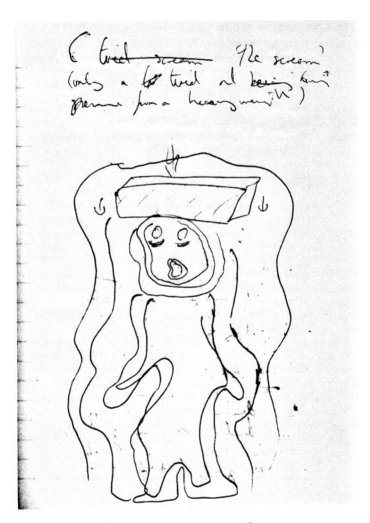

From Sybil's diary (see April 7th)

"THE THING INSIDE MY HEAD"

PART III

Lois Chaber

"THE THING INSIDE MY HEAD"

Chapter 1: Going Down

> We keep our expectations for ourselves and for our mentally ill loved ones at realistic levels.
>
> (An 'article' of the ten-point "Journey of Hope" developed in 1991 by the Louisiana Alliance for the Mentally Ill and recommended by Gravitz, *OCD: New Help for the Family*, p. 136.)

> Think positive. Don't go down!
>
> (From Sybil's diary)

By June 1998 I have come to take for granted the short shrill ring of the doorbell around 4:00 every other Friday, which announces Sybil's arrival home for the weekend. All of us by now consider the former Sybil, the bizarre Sybil, a creature exiled to the past. But Neil is under a lot of pressure at work now with The Terminal 5 project going through a reorganisation, and he is often tired, tense and grouchy around the house. And I am still teaching both my composition course at the American College and my literature course for the WEA and finding it difficult to make time on the weekends for Sybil.

Neil and I are, as my mother used to say, 'tickled pink' when Sybil organises tickets for a coach trip around the Peak District in July with her friend Ellen (another recovering patient). We regard this little holiday on her own as a high point in Sybil's ongoing quest for a 'life' and beam with satisfaction, afterwards, when she tells us how much she has enjoyed Chatsworth and the other sights, despite some difficulties getting along with Ellen ("My friend and I got a bit fed up with each other at times but we made up," she writes to her pen pal June Keyte). Straight away I shoot off several mini-newsletters by

Lois Chaber

e-mail and snail-mail to friends, boasting about this
new milestone in Sybil's progress.

As July continues, Sybil spends a good part of her
Saturdays during "home weekends" helping Neil in the
garden, as she has done all spring, particularly by mowing
and trimming the lawn—not an easy task as it is on two
levels. Neil, always overworked, even on weekends, has
begun to count on her help and is also delighted to have
Sybil's company in the garden, the two of them working side
by side. "Isn't it wonderful," we tell each other, "that she is
well enough to do this sort of demanding work considering
that three years earlier most of the time she couldn't even
dress herself." Meanwhile, however, Molly does not help in
the garden, nor do we dare to ask her. We have always
expected a lot more altruism from Sybil.

She also continues to be my companion and helper
in the kitchen on these weekends. One day, while helping
me to cut up vegetables for a stir fry, she hesitantly mentions
that some of her OCD symptoms are returning. I respond
with some soothing words, brushing it off lightly. I continue
to expect her assistance, even while noting in the back of my
mind that perhaps she is washing her hands a bit more than
usual.

We have been promising Sybil all this summer that
we will visit her in Clacton some weekend—on *her* territory—
hoping to reinforce her independence. When we finally visit
in early August, Sybil, often unkempt and usually not very
stylish, astounds us by being beautifully kitted out in a chic,
summery grey outfit with a mini-skirt, her short auburn hair
tidy and well-styled. She at once points to her white sandals
and says, apologetically, "Mum, I hope you won't be upset; I
bought these sandals with a little high heel because I
couldn't find any others I liked." A sudden, disarming picture
of myself holding forth down through the years on the
importance of 'sensible shoes' flashes through my mind, but,
aloud, I reassure her, chuckling benevolently at her timid
anxieties.

"THE THING INSIDE MY HEAD"

Sybil, with our encouragement, leads us to some attractively landscaped public gardens not far from her Granta residence, Woodland Lodge, which have only recently come to her attention. While we sit in the gardens, exclaiming over her pleasant discovery, she complains mildly, again, about the encroaching OCD; Dr. Roberts (a junior doctor on Sybil's Community Mental Health Centre team) has been making minor adjustments in her medication, including an additional dose at lunchtime, but "So far, nothing seems to be working", she says. Of course we are aware that the SSRI medications are not guaranteed to work indefinitely, but we are dismayed to learn that her Prozac, which she has been taking for two years, may now be letting her down.

We do notice, in fact, that today she has been engaging in her old habit of stopping when we walk, getting 'stuck', and then catching up. We feel worried, but still not greatly so, since she looks so well, is behaving in the main so calmly and graciously, and the sunny summer day in this seaside town is so reassuringly glorious. And the pleasant activities of the day on the beach and the pier, capped by watching a colourful town parade, lull us into complacency. The painful thought that these family outings, however companionable, are no real substitute for the fulfilling social life with her peers that Sybil so craves, lurks in the backs of our minds, but is kept at bay. We return to Southgate late that evening, buzzing with positive vibes, despite what Sybil has told us about her mental deterioration.

The next weekend, it is Molly who travels to Clacton, a visit Sybil has long desired:

At Woodland Lodge Sybil was quite shy but I think she was also obviously very happy that I was there—happy to be able to introduce me to all the clients and staff she lived with.

Lois Chaber

She showed me around her room, very proud to show me all her things.

We were to go out to meet Hazel. It was obviously a big thing because Sybil felt so much for her. We talked about Hazel beforehand, and she told me about how she'd had problems lately with her—not problems exactly—but it took a long, long time to get it out of her. Apparently, in some recent conversations with Hazel, she had kept bringing up the fact that she liked her so much, and the latter had had to keep on telling Sybil that they were not allowed to be friends—they had to keep it as a professional relationship. This had upset Sybil very much, and she was very sad about it.

I remember us just getting ready to go out, painting each other's nails. Sybil was so happy to have me there, but still intermittently anxious; she had to stop and do certain things—like pausing and retracing her steps—and she couldn't do certain other things—like play her keyboard for me. We walked up to Clacton Pier and we met Hazel in a pub. Hazel seemed very nice, very chatty. Sybil was very happy.

The next day, we sat on the beach and just talked about old times and things. I kept on offering to take her to the cinema, but she kept on saying, "No"; she wasn't ready, she didn't want to go. All in all, we did spend a lot of time just alone with each other.

Despite these two apparently successful family visits, the shadows are lengthening. One day in August, when I am returning home by tube after a day's teaching in the American College summer session, lost in a book as

"THE THING INSIDE MY HEAD"

usual, I feel someone tapping on my knee. It turns out to be the father of Purnimi, Sybil's old friend who has been out of touch for at least three years. He enquires after Sybil, and when I boast of her great progress and her regular home visits, he starts crowing about Purnimi's longstanding admiration of Sybil; she will be eager to call her at home in Southgate when she hears the news. Suppressing unpleasant memories of their awkward meeting in the Bethlem Adolescent Unit, fantasising about a reunion of the two girls that will be one more sturdy prop for the recovering Sybil, and, as ever, assuming I can transform Sybil's social life, I am totally taken in by Mr. Shah's enthusiasm, and I impart my hopes to Sybil.

Over the next two weeks this situation turns into a distressing fiasco. Twice again I fortuitously bump into Mr. Shah in Southgate, and each time I am gulled by the Eastern proclivity for saving face when he makes slavish excuses for Purnimi's silence. I even persuade a dubious but hopeful Sybil into herself phoning Purnimi's home three times, but she is met only by a barrage of excuses as to why the her old friend is temporarily unable to come to the phone. In the end, the two girls never speak; Sybil is deeply humiliated, saying little but silently absorbing the crushing pain of the snub.

All too soon, Sybil is buffeted by another rejection— one that is understandable but similarly hurtful. Marjory, the thirty-something year old whom Sybil met originally in the Peter Bruff Ward back in 1996, has played an active role in Sybil's very small circle of friends up to this point. After a few spells in hospital and some time in Eaglehurst, Marjory, like Sybil, is trying to create a 'life' for herself, in this case by moving out of her parents' home into a flat, unbeknown to Sybil. For some weeks, Sybil phones her at her old home but repeatedly gets the run-around from her parents and no calls-back from Marjory. Finally, Sybil receives a polite but admonitory letter from her advising Sybil to socialise with Ellen and Patty, young clients her own age, while she,

Lois Chaber

Marjory is moving in a different direction and hoping to make friends closer to *her* age.

One weekend in August after these two distressing episodes, she is unable to help me in the kitchen at all, and, at the next, she phones to tell us she no longer feels capable of travelling by herself to our home in London. She says she feels unwell and complains yet again about the accelerating OCD.

Meanwhile, on the back of our successful Warwickshire excursion last summer, we have been planning for months to take Sybil on another long weekend at the August bank holiday. The plan is to use the home of good friends in York as a base to explore some of the Yorkshire moors and dales. However, Sybil phones us near the time and timidly tells us that she no longer feels up to going on the trip: "Mum, I don't think I can handle it." Upset and disappointed, genuinely convinced that a little holiday break will cheer her up and that she is, as usual, underrating herself, we wheedle and coax, reminding her that she has improved on family trips in the past (the Scotland trip always our benchmark). Reluctantly, she agrees to go, but I write guiltily in my travel diary on August 26, "We have virtually browbeaten her into it."

Arriving at our friends' home, we are relieved to see Sybil interacting happily with our friends' fifteen year old daughter Suzi. Sybil can relate quite well to younger girls; she also has an ongoing pen pal friendship with Alice, the fourteen-year-old daughter of our old Qatar friend in Reading, though not with Alice's two older sisters. Because Sybil is generally slow in getting ready for anything, particularly when her OCD is dominating her, I comment in my diary with pleasure and surprise the next morning, "Sybil miraculously gets ready for breakfast quickly."

A day later in a B & B cottage in the small town of Hanlith, the three of us enjoy a quite relaxed walk to a pub, but an awkward incident occurs when, on our return, the

392

"THE THING INSIDE MY HEAD"

very pleasant owners stop us in the entryway for a brief conversation. They say to Sybil, after asking her age, "Oh, you must be in university now." Sybil, who hasn't even done her GCSEs yet and is taking remedial secondary school courses, blushes, and is silent, suffering intensely the stigma of not being a 'normal' twenty-year-old. I feel myself going hot and cold with anxiety for Sybil, but know that to answer for her will be even worse. The woman maddeningly persists in quizzing Sybil, so Sybil finally has to stammer out, "I'm going to special classes," and Neil and I hasten to change the subject.

We spend a very active day hiking at rocky Malham, in Gordale, with Sybil holding her own in this strenuous activity and appearing to enjoy it, except that, once again, she frequently stops and starts awkwardly. We have to periodically wait for her to catch up, though this does not deter Neil and me from feeling exhilarated by the exercise and the spectacular scenery.

Back at our Yorkshire friends' home later, Suzi eagerly informs Sybil that a very sensitive and intelligent older friend of hers is going to join the group for a barbeque the next day. Because this young woman is closer to Sybil's own age and because Suzi thinks so well of her Sybil finds this prospect extremely intimidating. The next morning, her terror of this stranger as well as the general wear and tear on her psyche from sustaining herself throughout this trip, leads to a mini-breakdown in her room: she can't get dressed or even take her medication without my assistance and coaxing. Also, her personal hygiene is ominously deteriorating; her hair is scraggly and unwashed and she refuses to change her dirty T-shirt, dank with sweat, which she has been wearing the entire duration of the trip. In the evening, despite the fact that she *almost* refuses to come down from her room, the much-dreaded get-together with the young woman eventually passes off quite well, the three girls chatting away and tinkering with our friends' piano.

Lois Chaber

Nevertheless, during the tedious four-hour journey home in the car the next day, Sybil, strung out and now quite obviously ravaged by OCD compulsions, is totally silent for long periods, refusing to answer us, her face distorted in pain, her hands on her head or covering her ears. A few times, Neil, with whom she is sitting, manages to draw her out of herself by talking about popular music, when she becomes virtually transformed into a 'normal' teenager for about ten minutes, but we travel home with a sinking feeling. Leaving her with one of her careworkers at Woodland Lodge, we emphasise Sybil's ability to manage during the larger part of the trip, proclaiming, "She was brilliant!", but the pathetic and downcast condition she arrives in causes the staff to permanently regard our Yorkshire excursion in a baleful light.

We assume we won't see Sybil again for a fortnight, but she phones to ask if she can come next weekend anyway, as there are going to be strangers, 'agency staff', on duty, which she finds threatening. We have been expecting three elderly friends from Kent, a retired professor, his wife and the professor's even more elderly aunt-in-law, for dinner that weekend, but Sybil knows them, so we are happy she wants to join us, even though it means Neil making the 160-mile round trip to fetch her on the day of the party. During dinner Sybil makes a point, ill as she is, of talking to and drawing out the eighty-five-year old aunt, a very shy and unprepossessing woman, a timid bird like Sybil herself, whom the rest of us unconsciously but effectually exclude as we babble on about ostensibly sophisticated topics. Sybil puts us all to shame. Later, privately, she lucidly expresses her anger at our inconsiderate behaviour. But once our guests depart the next day, she becomes quite distraught, lingering in her room, whimpering, 'repeating things' and having difficulty getting dressed to go back to Clacton with Neil.

This is the last time Sybil ever comes home.

"THE THING INSIDE MY HEAD"

Over the next couple of weeks, she continues to deteriorate, and soon she can barely manage to carry on a phone conversation. I get a call from Hazel. Sybil, she tells us, has stopped communicating at all with *anyone*, has not been taking care of herself, has not been eating, has needed constant assistance, and the limited staff of Grant's half-way house can no longer handle the situation. She has been re-admitted to Clacton hospital. We are shocked and upset, finding it difficult to take in the disappearance of the resurgent Sybil we've known for nearly two wonderful years. We soon learn from the Peter Bruff nurses that Sybil has fallen back into two old delusions this week: "God is punishing me" and "If I see my parents, I'll harm them." Visits and phone calls from us are proscribed. Sybil has gone full circle, back into the very hospital where she started out in Clacton.

* * *

We hear, shortly after Sybil's re-admission, that there is going to be a formal review of her current crisis, and Neil is so concerned about Sybil that he takes time off work to attend it in Essex:

> *The review was late; I let people know that I was there. Beforehand, I had asked Lois to write up her observations, from July through to this point, to let her team know what we had been seeing. I sat, first of all, in the dining area of Peter Bruff and perused the various papers that I had, just to collect my thoughts because it was all very detailed, specialist information, a lot aimed at the medical profession.*
>
> *But nobody came to get me, so I started making inquiries. It soon became apparent that the review was in process because I had seen Sybil come out just before, with a young woman from Granta [Kim]; probably her part of the review was over. She was very distressed,*

crying, not looking at me (may not even have seen me). So I then spoke to reception, telling them: "I came for the meeting; no one has let me know. You're obviously having the meeting; I need to talk to Dr. Smith." The person on reception went down the corridor to where the meeting was being held. Eventually, someone came out—I believe it was the senior nurse (male), Tony—and said that he'd ask Dr. Smith if I could join them, but I didn't wait; I just followed him and joined them in the room.

I was very polite; I went around and shook everybody's hand, and as they didn't introduce themselves I asked who they were. It was very evident that Dr. Smith was on the defensive from the very beginning, probably why he wanted to get through the review without letting me in there. I said I wanted to know what the situation was. Dr. Smith seemed, in his attitude and from what he was saying, to be working from the premise that I had come to complain that Sybil was back in hospital, whereas, in fact, I'd come to discuss the situation and to give them our notes and observations on the decline which had brought Sybil, understandably, back to hospital. He said that he wouldn't tell me their views. I tried to talk to him about the drug therapy, pointing out that best practice had shown that they should now be trying out another of the SSRI drugs, the procedure usually recommended when one SSRI- type drug becomes ineffectual. Dr. Smith would not talk to me very much, but one of the junior people did speak to me more. He assured me that though the drug they had put Sybil on was an anti-psychotic, it was not being used for that purpose. I said that yes, I understood that.

"THE THING INSIDE MY HEAD"

At some point, Dr. Smith wanted me to leave. First, he wanted to leave himself, and I blocked his way, saying, "I've come for information; are you denying me information?" Basically, he said that he was. Then he changed his tack to saying that I was to go and that he would call for a nurse. I said, "Fine". He then said he'd call the police. I said, "It's not a problem for me." In the end, he backed off, we talked a little bit more, and then I handed over our notes to him, which he just immediately passed to his junior, telling him to put them in the file and look at it later. I believe the meeting broke up then, and I returned home, very upset.

This confrontation of Neil's forms part of what our family perceived as a pattern: medical institutions intermittently trying to exclude us from Sybil's care. This is to get worse.

In the incisive and forthright series, "Why Doctors Make Mistakes", broadcast on Channel 4 in October 2000, the medical profession as a whole was accused of engaging in a "conspiracy of silence" during and after its treatment of patients. The NHS at one point has even been characterised as a culture of "institutional arrogance", by the official inquiry into the Bristol heart surgery scandal resulting from one hundred babies dead (*The Sunday Times,* 11 February, 2000). Neil's experience at the September 1998 review, we feel, can be understood in the light of such criticism.

* * *

Back in June, in Woodland Lodge, Sybil's keyworker Diane had decided to leave for work in London—despite her deep concern for Sybil—because she could no longer tolerate Clacton's claustrophobic small-town atmosphere.

Lois Chaber

She was replaced by Michael, a slim thirty-something Granta careworker, sensitive and laid-back, with a prominent shaved head; he puts me in mind of a benign otherworldly mentor from one of the recent fantasy films. Michael, who like Diane, puts people before systems, has shared with me his observations on Sybil during roughly the same period I have just described, June through September 1998. Her troubled thoughts were more in evidence to him early on:

She would often talk about her "horrible thoughts," but she wouldn't actually say exactly what they were. And she would often come and say, "I'm a horrible person, I'm a bad person, I think badly of people." One night she came in saying, "I'm having terrible thoughts. I'm really angry with my dad, I'm really angry with him!" I can't remember what it was about, but I said, "But that's not a problem, Sybil. We all get angry. It doesn't make you a bad person. When I get angry (this produced a little laugh from her)—does that make me a bad person?" (Another laugh.) "No, you're a nice person," she responded. So then I said, "Yeah, but that's what I did, that's what I felt. So, does that make me a bad person?" She said, "No, not really." So we just talked them through, these concerns, and often, she would agree, say goodnight, and walk away quite happily. But you know, I could tell by her reactions, that this was not what she wanted; I think she was looking in many ways for some sort of absolution. But she couldn't articulate this. She was slowly drifting.

Admittedly, some of her OCD thoughts would sometimes be to harm others—like you or me. One day, she was sitting there and she went like that—just kicked her leg out at me.

"THE THING INSIDE MY HEAD"

She then ran out of the room. I said, "What's wrong, Sybil?" She said, "I just wanted to kick you." "Why, because I've accidentally upset you?" " No, I just wanted to kick you." "Why?" She went, "Oh, I don't know why, because you're here." I responded, "And we can't have any physical contact, can we? I'm staff. Yes, we can't touch and the fact of the matter is you want to touch me, but you obviously can't do it". "No", she insisted, "I wanted to hurt you." And I said, "Does this often happen?" and she replied, "Well, yes it does; I sometimes just get this thought: I've got to hurt somebody." She explained how sometimes in the kitchen, there'd be some knives there, and somebody was there, and she'd have the thought that she was going to hurt them. And that's when I realised that I was obviously misinterpreting what she was telling me when I asked her why she wanted to kick me; it was for more clinical reasons. And once I began to realise that, my concerns increased.

There were a couple of times when she was a bit depressed. I remember once being on a sleep-in and hearing a knock on the door. I said, "Who's there please?" A little voice said, "Me, Michael, can I have a chat?" I said, "OK, go and sit down in the lounge. I'll get changed and dressed." She was sitting in there; she had on her dressing gown and her pink slippers that she always wore, and I said, "What's your problem?" She said, "I feel like I'm going to hurt myself." I said, "How do you mean, Sybil?" "I feel like I'm going to harm myself." We talked through why that was, and it was because she felt a couple of other female students in her evening class were against her; they wouldn't speak to her. What I saw was a young woman bravely dealing with problems that would break many people, and, in truth, it was these girls who should be humbled by her. We spoke at length about self-doubt, and how difficult it was to overcome.

Then she started speaking about seeing the chaplain and God started coming into the picture. That became even a greater concern, and she made arrangements for going to weekly or fortnightly sessions with the chaplain. I expressed to her that I thought it wasn't really a good idea; I said to her, "It's your choice." Perhaps, I suggested, she needed to take a step back, try to think of some different things, give herself some space intellectually. But it seems that was impossible for her, because she was pretty adamant to see the chaplain.

Sybil was a very bright individual; very self-aware and intellectually capable. Her understanding of life and people proved to be quite profound at times. But as soon as any discussion took on a religious dimension, things changed. Her reasoning became very confused yet rigid. She was looking for answers to profound questions without recognising the complexity of the subject. About her religious obsessions, it was really hard because she didn't actually speak much about them, except that she thought there was this dimension of 'badness' in her. We reckoned she was becoming ill.

What I have been saying suggests a long-drawn-out process; it wasn't. It happened in a matter of weeks. It did really get quite intense. As she was regressing, we tried initially to manage her environment. We tried hard to keep her out of hospital.

"THE THING INSIDE MY HEAD"

She was very ill one morning, and we had made arrangements for her to see her psychiatrist on an emergency basis. I went up to knock on the door. She answered in a small voice. I'd say, "Do you want your medication?" She said "Yes, but I'm not dressed." Later, I knocked on the door again, "Do you want to take your medication?" "In a minute, Michael." "Are you going to come to the door and take your medication now, Sybil?" She said, "OK Michael. I'll have to dress myself." I must've waited for something like five minutes. Eventually, she came to the door and took the medication, and I said, "Well, we need to go see Dr. Roberts today". She responded but closed the door.

Alas, it nearly took me an hour and a half to two hours to get her to come downstairs. I was getting to the stage where I needed to take her to the appointment immediately, but obviously I could not go in her room in case she wasn't dressed (Sybil would dress and then undress, repeatedly). So, I was really patient. I was getting nearly to the point of asking a female member of staff to come in specially and enter Sybil's room. I told Sybil, "You must really try hard for me, Sybil; really try hard Sybil to get yourself ready. You know I can't help you; you know I can't come into the room. I know it's very difficult for you; but if you'd do that little thing for me I'd be most grateful." Finally, she responded to that, and appeared. Even then it took me another half hour to get her downstairs and to get her into the car because she kept retracing her steps.

Meanwhile, at Granta, we tried a variety of things. She was seeing Dr. Roberts, who gave her diazepam [Valium] for instance, to try and control the panic attacks she was having at the time. She would sometimes get panic-stricken and just run around the house. She was also having difficulties in getting to sleep. We gave it to her 'as and when' because obviously we didn't want to create a dependency. There was concern about her reaction to haloperidol [an anti-psychotic medication], its interaction with other medication, in case the levels in her blood might become too high, so the doctor tried to give different dosages just to see what effect they had, at the same time carefully monitoring that she'd be okay.

Soon it became very clear, however, that we couldn't manage Sybil's illness at the project. Dressing was a big problem for her; plus we were often prompting her to eat, to drink, and, unfortunately, she had been neglecting herself as well, so we were prompting her in all aspects of her self care. We just could not give her the level of attention she needed, which was very upsetting for us. For one thing, they really needed to get her into a hospital environment to reassess her medication in a more comprehensive way.

Sybil had been offered, a couple of weeks prior to that, an opportunity to go to into hospital by Dr. Roberts, but had said, "No". We were just about coping with her behaviour at the time, so we thought, let's give her a chance, but it wasn't long before we had to concede defeat; and that was when she was voluntarily hospitalised.

Tracey, one of the female staff members close to Sybil, expresses frustration similar to Michael's:

"THE THING INSIDE MY HEAD"

You know, we really kept a lid on it with Sybil for a long time, sort of trying to look after her to keep her in a stable environment she was used to with the people she was used to. You know the many times that Sybil stood in the toilet and didn't want to come out. We were very anxious, and we used to follow her around, everywhere, just to keep her occupied and out of the toilet. It got to where we couldn't manage it; she needed specialised care.

Sybil's state of regression upon her return to Peter Bruff Ward in September is graphically described in the official case report. It recounts such obsessional behaviours as jumping, hopping, repetitive movements, and occasionally the hiding of her head inside her jumper or behind her hands—behaviour not seen since her worst days at the Bethlem Royal. At her admissions interview, she barely responds to questions. She does indicate that she is being battered by intrusive thoughts revolving around God, evil and the like. Dr Smith, in the report, describes them as verging on blasphemy at times. He seems to be morally shocked, but Joseph Ciarrocchi in his book *The Doubting Disease* (see Pt. II, Ch. 2) points out that 'blasphemy' is a standard clinical symptom of OCD scrupulosity.

Sybil, it seems, is aware that she has undergone a relapse, but she refuses to eat and drink, and there is evidence of self-neglect and self-harming, not to mention food deprivation, probably from extreme anxiety. According to the report, there are no visible signs of intended suicide, but there is a concession that assessment is difficult at this time.

Was this the same Sybil who a couple of weeks earlier had skilfully created conversation with our friend's elderly aunt at the dinner table? Yet, the signs had been there for some months.

* * *

The question on everyone's mind, then and now, was "why had she regressed?" Michael articulates his frustration on this point: "This is the biggest mystery. She would converse with me about anything—her family, her problems, her care, her past history—but as soon as it would become her illness and other worries that overlapped with that, she was very loathe to discuss that at all and she became very distressed."

To be sure, the literature on OCD tells us that patients do frequently relapse, particularly when there is comorbid depression, and that once-effective medication can gradually or suddenly become ineffectual; moreover, since Allen, the behavioural psychologist, had withdrawn from Sybil's programme in 1997, Sybil had been receiving no other therapy at all, and all the OCD literature explicitly declares that the long term effectiveness of medication can only be ensured when it is accompanied by some form of behavioural therapy, particularly cognitive behavioural therapy, which can change the patient's way of thinking. In Sybil's case, however, there were some specific external pressures, on top of her ongoing disappointment in her dismal social life, that were probably ratcheting up her stress. Her diary entries in the next chapter will make evident also her troubled religious thoughts during this period, a return of the 'scrupulosity' she experienced at the Bethlem Royal, but whether this latter should be regarded as a *cause* or as an *effect* of her regression is another enigma.

Granta staff had hoped Sybil was stable enough by the summer to absorb the shock of her keyworker Diane's departure, but Sybil always (like myself) had great difficulty adjusting to change—particularly change in careworkers to whom she was strongly attached. Notwithstanding Diane's own views on this subject, in her cheerful, no-nonsense,

"THE THING INSIDE MY HEAD"

confident carer Sybil seemed to have found the secure and stable surrogate mother for whom she had been yearning. Despite Diane's initial optimism, the at-least-partial link between her departure and Sybil's decline emerges from her own account:

> I remember when I decided to leave Granta, the first person I told was Sybil. At first, she started to get very upset with me. And I sat her down and said, "Gee, we're not doing either of us any favours." I said, if it was her moving on, what would she expect from me? She said, "I'd expect you to be happy for me and I'd expect you to support me." So, I said, "What do you think I expect from you then now?" She answered, "Oh, the same thing". I said, "Fine. I know you're going to be upset; however, friends don't just disappear. Friends will stay in touch." She thought it through, and then she came back and said: "You're right. I would expect you to treat me with respect if I were moving on; I have to do the same." And after that, she was fine.

> We'd sit and read through my application forms, and I'd tell her about the interviews. And when I applied for a particular job, and said how much I wanted it, and finally got it, we went out and had a cream cake—to celebrate. And I reassured her that London is not far and she's always coming up to London, and I go down to Clacton-on-Sea.

> I left in the June, and for a few weeks after I left, she was phoning me from the office, and I was phoning her; she wrote me a couple of letters, and I wrote back. But instead of being long letters, they started being little short things,

*and Mike said that she was not very well.
Before she went on holiday [with Ellen], she
was very stressed up, and we thought it was
because it was the first holiday on her own, but
that must've been the beginnings of everything
escalating. We planned that when she got back
she was to phone me and we would meet up in
London for coffee and cake and she could show
me the photographs.*

*But she never did that. Things went
wrong, badly wrong. When she came back she
got worse and went downhill and then she
started saying to Mike: "Oh Diane wouldn't
want me to write to her—Oh no, I better not
phone Diane." And Mike would make her
phone me, or he would make her come to the
phone when I phoned up, but all I got out of her
then was "yes".*

*And when she was in the hospital, I
phoned there a couple of times, and I even said
that I would come down, just for the day, and
take her out. And they said that there was no
point me coming down; she wasn't well enough
to see me. Unfortunately, I believed them.*

In a letter to her pen pal June Keyte, Sybil,
struggling to appear 'with it' and mature; describes her new
keyworker Michael: "He's a nice bloke," but 'bloke' is
crossed out and written again. For not only did Sybil have to
resign herself to the bowing out of yet another maternal
surrogate, but she also had to adjust to having a male
keyworker—and to the loss of certain intimacies. Michael
himself was particularly sensitive to the situation:

"THE THING INSIDE MY HEAD"

Granta staff felt that because Sybil had been in the care of professionals in the system for such a long time, she hadn't really had any chance to build relationships with males, to communicate with males, in a normal setting, in a normal way, and they felt that having a male keyworker would be give her an excuse to relate to men. I'm also a very easy-going individual. That would be beneficial to her, to get away from the sort of psychiatrist, CPN [Community Psychiatric Nurse] relationships and get her to engage on a more social level, so that a male could be just another human being. I think we did have a good relationship, a working relationship that came about naturally; any things that were really of a personal nature, she would always refer to female staff anyway. I think that because I was only her keyworker for such a short time, however, the impact on any change was very, very small.

And even the laid-back Michael cannot quell Sybil's by-now-cumulative sense of loss, deepened by Diane's departure:

Once, when she was feeling quite well, I took her for a walk around the seafront, and was just chatting through her concern about the past, and she said to me, "All the people that I've got close to in life, Michael, have always left me." She was talking about the people in the care profession. I said, 'Well, unfortunately, that's the case." She was concerned that staff leaving here was always a thing that she would find quite stressful. She said, "And you'll go as well." "It's possible, Sybil, it's possible. You know, Di's left. It's possible that sometime I will

407

leave. That's why you mustn't get dependent on us, you know, emotionally, or anything. Yes, we're there to support you, we're there to help you, and we always do, but maybe another Michael will come along, there'll be another Diane, another Kim; but really, for you, you must build a life for yourself, have friends and companions outside the project and the mental health field."

Sybil recognised this and had talked earlier about going on an 'outward bound' holiday to meet new people. We had said to her, "If you want to meet somebody nice, that's just the place you'll do it." She wanted to live independently and have her own friends, but achieving this was the problem. I pointed out that that was what the project was there for, to help her achieve such aims. We understood that it would not be easy.

In addition, in the summer of '98, things had come to a head over the drug-addict at Woodland Lodge. Ken was still refusing to leave the residence, and the Granta management had eventually taken legal measures to evict him, resulting in uncomfortable courtroom battles. Sybil's compassion and sensitivity put her in a stressfully ambivalent position: she sided with staff in rejecting Ken's anti-social behaviour and his illegal addiction but she also sympathised with him, *mistakenly* feeling that staff members were persecuting him and did not care about the possibility that he could become homeless.

She was similarly stuck in the middle in the ongoing confrontations between Neil and I on the one hand and Molly on the other, as Molly strove to forge an identity from rebelling against all authority—at home, in school, and in the culture at large. Sybil could see the dangers and detriments of Molly's intermittently anti-social behaviour and could empathise with our aggravation; however, she also sided

"THE THING INSIDE MY HEAD"

quite urgently with Molly when fierce rows arose in the house, her sympathies quickened by sisterly devotion and her belief that we had always treated Molly 'badly' and favoured herself. With ongoing conflict and disharmony in both her 'homes', it is no wonder that Sybil felt trapped, unable to cope any longer.

Meanwhile, back in June, Sybil's remedial classes at Tendring Adult Community College, "Improving English and "Improving Maths," had come to an end and she had sat an exam set by the Royal Society of Arts in Stage One of English that was to lead into GCSE classes the following autumn. Despite our encouragement and praise when she received the exam result, Sybil, feeling its relative insignificance when compared to the A-Level examinations the younger Molly was concurrently taking at the Latymer School, dismissed our compliments with characteristic self-contempt. To make matters worse, she was told that she needed further work in 'Improving Maths' before taking the exam in that subject, and Diane recounts her distress:

She was quite upset because she'd done one little test but they'd advised her not to take the other one, the Maths one, because they thought it would be too much for her. At the time I didn't think much about it, but, thinking back, it was all out of context, so distraught she was about not being able to take that exam. Although *I* was saying, maybe they're right; it was a test she could take the following year, *she* was saying that she'd let *you* down, she'd let *me* down, she'd let *the teacher* down. And it went on for days; whereas, normally, I could snap her round, to look at something not as a failure—as far as I'm concerned, the word 'failure' should be wiped out of the language— but as a setback, not one that would do her any damage, this time I couldn't seem to talk her round that one. Then, I left a couple of weeks after that.

Lois Chaber

One of Sybil's later diary entries confirms her intense anxiety over these academic matters: "I want to get qualifications and good marks & please & impress & live up to expectations of family & friends including 2 GCSEs." Neil and I, who had invested enormous value in academic achievement all through the girls' childhood, unconsciously made matters worse by gently but insistently urging Sybil to regain 'normality' in her educational programme, not realising how far she had come, how fragile she was, and how gradual the rehabilitation needed to be. When it had become apparent that she wasn't yet ready to take GCSE Maths in the autumn, we encouraged her to take another, second GCSE course (Human Biology) along with the English class.

Michael recognised this problem:

If pressed, I would put the change in Sybil down to the high expectations of her, and indeed the expectations she had for herself. It was all too much, and this was probably what brought about the relapse. I would typify this by the concerns Sybil had about her GCSEs, her fear of failure and of how people were going to react to her possible lack of achievement. Knowing what we did of Sybil's history, it was amazing how far she had progressed—but perhaps just too quickly.

Finally, there was Sybil's anxiety over the family's proposed trip to New Zealand at Christmas time 1998. We had not been there as a family for twelve years, since our exodus from Qatar, what with Neil's unemployment and Sybil's illness. With Sybil so well in 1997 and the trip to Bruges so successful, Neil enthusiastically began to plan a complicated family trip to his homeland in early '98. To visit there with a rehabilitated Sybil would fulfil his deepest yearnings. When Sybil's deterioration became evident to us

410

"THE THING INSIDE MY HEAD"

in late August, the big question was: would she be well enough to travel to New Zealand? Optimistically, Neil carried on with his preparations. Michael, knowing our wishes, even took Sybil out of hospital later on to get a photo so that Neil could renew her New Zealand passport. For Sybil, however, the trip became, increasingly, a threat; she feared meeting our friends and relatives there, many of whom she hadn't seen for so long, and who she imagined looking askance at her thanks to that long, terrible illness.

At the time, we, especially Neil, averted our thoughts from her fears, and Sybil, typically, avoided the issue, but the prospect of the trip aroused concern in Sybil's careworkers, such as Tracey: "She seemed worried about going to New Zealand. Because Sybil always liked to please, didn't she? She always cared about people's feelings, and I think that was the answer—not necessarily *because* of the holiday, but her deterioration seemed to start about then."

Dr. Smith, in his clinical report, also claimed our New Zealand plans were causing Sybil additional distress. Despite a lifting of mood after another course of ECT when she returned to hospital, she grew increasingly agitated as the weeks went by. Unfortunately, none of these professional views were communicated to us at the time, so we continued our blinkered assumptions of Sybil's assent.

It seems to me that none of these factors *alone*—the loss of her beloved keyworker, the crisis over the drug-addict, her piggy-in-the-middle position at home, the impending challenges of the GCSE courses and the New Zealand trip, or even our complacency—adequately explains why Sybil lapsed back into severe OCD behaviour and mentality. Just as no *one* event explained her total breakdown in 1992, here we may also assume a cumulative effect, in conjunction with the well-known undependable chemistry of Prozac. Whatever the causes, Sybil's diary entries during this period leave little doubt of the spiralling turmoil she was bravely enduring.

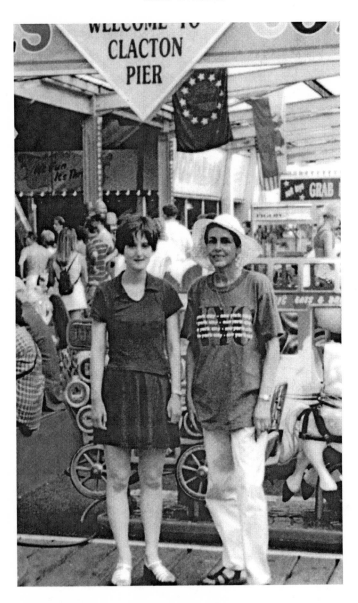

Sybil with Lois at Clacton Pier, 1998

"THE THING INSIDE MY HEAD"

Chapter 2: The Return of the Voices

Excerpts from Sybil's Diary
June '98—August '98

> O Eve, in evil hour thou didst give ear
> To that false worm. . . .

> (John Milton, *Paradise Lost,* Bk. IX, ll. 1067-68.)

1 June: Diane is great.

I feel stressed about Patty, Molly, Mum, my exams, my OCD, my spiritual problems, Diane leaving, orthodontist. But Molly sounded much happier on the phone today & I'm less worried about her & we had a good laugh & she said 'I love you' to me! On [word missing] I'm going to get a hug from her.

3 June: I had a difficult chat with Michael and Diane, but it was okay in the end, well sort of. I'm scared about Diane's leaving. I'll miss her.

I still feel very uncomfortable with Michael & still feel resentment towards him. I'm worried that our relationship is ruined for good or at least a long time & it will be horrible without Diane and with him as my keyworker.

I feel horrible and like crying. I feel like I can't go to Michael, when I feel bad, anymore.

Later: I can talk to Michael. I've just had a good chat with him.

6 June [home]: I didn't want to go through the process of getting up this morning. It's odd and worrying that I still feel that about getting up even when it's quicker

than it used to be, but I feel like it's getting worse. The intruding thoughts that I have, or will, hurt someone, when I'm putting on my clothes are really aggravating me.

I wrote most of a letter to Alice [the 14-year old daughter of old family friends], reading her latest one beforehand. It was great. I really like her letters, they make me feel that she is confiding in me, that she is my friend. I found myself wishing that I was 14 now and could be a proper friend with her, but it wouldn't have worked then. I've got a bad problem of great insecurity which hinders and harms my relationships with people. It definitely did when I was a child and teenager.

The printer has broken down and Dad spent virtually the whole day trying to fix it and not succeeding. He was really tense and kept snapping with Mum. I got quite worried and a bit upset about their snapping etc. But when Mum and I were doing the fruit salad she said that Dad was in a bad mood because he was so frustrated about the computer and she understood. She loves him a lot.

After dinner there was a scene between Molly & Mum about revising [studying for A-levels].

I feel like a hug from Diane.

7 June: [I] Did comprehension [in practice for her upcoming Royal Society of Arts English examination]. I found it very hard, much harder than I expected and I panicked. I didn't finish in time. It wasn't very good. Went swimming, felt dirty and irritated afterwards. Mum washed swimsuits which was a welcome relief and then Mum marked my RSA paper. I felt really anxious. I always do when submitting work to her. She found lots of bad mistakes. I felt embarrassed and ashamed. I felt she was disappointed in me. However, at the end, she said that I will definitely pass but it's how well I will pass. This eased my mind a little and also made me feel a bit more pressure because of her wanting and expecting me to do well.

"THE THING INSIDE MY HEAD"

9 June: I had a good day today. Dial-A-Ride went well. Ian asked me about more voluntary work. I said I'd think about it but I've decided it wouldn't be wise as I don't really have the time. However, it made me feel good that they must like me to ask for more or maybe they were desperate. I don't think so. When he started to ask me, they way he was speaking (plus my fantasies) made me think he was going to ask me out. I was quite disappointed when he didn't. I must do something about my appearance. I need a haircut and some new clothes. I had some good laughs today. I made a joke myself and then laughed and lingered on it. I ruined the joke a bit and I felt quite embarrassed.

I enjoyed today. I like doing the Dial-A-Ride. It gets me out, keeps me busy, gives me more confidence and self-esteem and it makes me realize how lucky I am.

10 June: I was watching E.R. ["Emergency Room"] I suddenly felt a panicky feeling about what working as an occupational therapist [would be like] and how stressful I would find it and how I would remember and then I had a thought that maybe I would be panicky and anxious all my life and was it worth carrying on?

11 June: I'm fed up, I'm fed up of OCD. I wish death was the end, sometimes, so I could go there and have peace, nothingness and not go to hell. I feel imprisoned by my mind.

13 June [After Diane's leave-taking party]: Now it's beginning to hit me. I'll miss her being here and being my keyworker. I feel scared without her. It's another person moving on, another change in my life of many changes and moves on. I'm glad I can be her friend now and we can see each other.

[Undated; probably 15 June]: Things to remember from Hazel's session:

415

Lois Chaber

I told her about the smear test letter [inviting her to have an NHS cervical smear]. She said that I don't need to rush making a decision. She said that I don't have to but it would be sensible. She said to weigh up the pros and cons. She said she is quite happy to talk to me about it. She said I could request a woman doctor to do it. She said that it would be done in a very detached, clinical way.

I asked her if they could tell anything about you when they do it and she said that they can tell whether you're a virgin and when your last period was. I think it would have been better with me if I hadn't asked that. I almost told her about masturbation. I wish I could but I'm going to keep my mouth shut until I know for sure I can talk about it with her.

I wish Kim and/or Hazel would volunteer that masturbation is normal and healthy and it would be better if they could admit doing it themselves or having done it so then I could admit to it and get it off my chest, in general, as well as about the smear test worries, and also not feel dirty anymore.

After Hazel's visit I felt a bit brighter.

16 June: In the song "Greatest Love" by Whitney Houston, it says about everybody looking for a hero but her not finding anyone who could fill her needs, so she learned to depend on herself. This really struck me yesterday at aerobics and today when writing this. This is because I'm always looking for a shelter, a rock, someone who I can depend on, believe, and look up to but there isn't anyone. I've felt for years that it can't be my parents for a few reasons, one of them being that I'm always conscious I worry about their vulnerability.

I used to find my 'hero' in nurses, staff, but the ones at Bethlem showed they weren't, and I found for myself they weren't. I used to feel that way about staff at Jacques Hall, but this couldn't fulfil my needs. At Peter Bruff I took Erica and Jenny & Valerie. Valerie wasn't, after she got fed up of me Jennie didn't want to stay in touch & tonight I saw at aerobics that the Erica I remembered and hoped for (a motherlike, guardian angel-like figure) was gone and maybe wasn't ever there.

Anyway, there is no-one on earth who can give me what I want and fulfill my needs. In the song the writer decides to depend on herself but 'me' is the person I trust least. I feel so insecure and lost. I know God wants me to come back to him but I feel I can't yet. Can he fulfill my needs or do I need to depend on myself as well?

I think I do. I hate my OCD & distrust myself.

AAAAA

18 June: My clock was wrong this morning. Kim gave me a lift. I think that I manipulated her. Maybe Terry Lee [from Jacques Hall] and Maggie from the Bethlem were right; maybe I do, and am good at manipulating people.

20 June [home]: Molly & I had a really good chat. We talked about memories and she said it's normal for the memory to block things out and we talked about staying and losing touch with people and old friends. We talked about music bringing back memories & I told her about Queen & my reacting to certain music which brings back memories.

She offered to help me with dinner. Then she said that I look good at cooking which really surprised me but was lovely. Oh she is a great sister. She does love and like me.

26 June [home]: The day started off well.

[*Scrawled across several pages in messy handwriting*]:

anxiety—I hate OCD depression I hate my feelings AAA

I was feeling good but now after talking to Mum & Dad I feel awful— like screaming & crying. It's not their fault. I feel guilty for having such a good time and life when they don't. I feel upset and worried about Dad. Poor Dad he needs all the relaxation he can get & then he has an accident because he is so tired. His boss is giving him too much work. He is overworked. He has no choice. It's wearing him down, physically & mentally. There is nothing I can do except be good on weekends.

27 June [after a birthday party for the nurse Erica's daughter]: I'm not really in the mood for writing my diary but I've got to say something because my time at the party, overall went really well. I got all dressed up and looked nice.

"THE THING INSIDE MY HEAD"

I feel weird. I still feel in party mode but I feel like getting emotional and crying. That was the first proper party I'd ever been to. I feel more confident and better about myself. I think I've been getting misconceptions from trying to model myself on Kim.

[Parallel to her diary for June 1998, Sybil intermittently kept a sort of spiritual diary on sheets of loose-leaf paper]

1 June: I have been thinking again [of] talking to a minister or chaplain about my spiritual problems and my illness, but now I am feeling like I mustn't refer to the voices as 'illness' because they might really have been real after all. Then I contemplated the idea that it was real and it seemed to make more sense and be more congruous than when I don't believe in them, but now after writing it I feel less so and that they were *in*congruous, but I still feel as though I can't, mustn't refer to the voices or that side of my illness.

I don't know what's the truth anymore. I don't know what to do.

2 June: I still had the thoughts today. I kept being stupid or foolish but then if I am being foolish then maybe God hasn't answered that prayer. Just before [Hazel] came I was worried and felt guilty and the thoughts said to go to the toilet downstairs (because I needed the toilet) only a couple of minutes before she came & I didn't want to be rude and embarrassed by going to the toilet just before she came and being in there when she arrive[d] like, I think, the last time. So I didn't. I was confused about what to do to make the [Hazel] meeting and the chaplain meeting alright [the Rev. Richard Smith, chaplain to Clacton Hospital].

How do you know when it's God talking to you and not just yourself thinking or your illness?

Ask about that passage in the Bible [*probably referring to Mark 3. 28-29*]

Lois Chaber

Ask about forgiveness.

But what will a minister know? What if he has been swapped with the devil because of my mistakes today?

Will I ever know I mean I've always had thoughts telling me to do things and making me scared and unhappy since I was about 6 which is around the same time as my interest in Christianity started & my OCD started, but maybe it wasn't OCD but God's voice in the early days, like that sacrifice. That was quite similar to times since I was 13 when I was 'ill' & God telling me to do things and me panicky & faithful & distressed.

Oh dear I feel like crying.

But if the voices/thoughts aren't true then why did God let this happen & why do I feel like there's a big wall between me and him and I feel estranged.

I've just thought about asking Roberta about them but the thoughts have been warning me not to.

The thoughts are telling me not to get a hug off Diane & I shouldn't & God will help me if I don't

28 June: I'm getting more thoughts the last couple of days when & since I've been thinking about talking to the chaplain. It's frustrating and frightening & sometimes when I do what the thoughts want me to do I end up feeling more peaceful and happy & more at peace with God & happier. I'm scared. I don't want to be frightened anymore.

[undated—a torn slip of paper]: I'm still being punished—but then again I am still thinking bad things. However sometimes I don't know or am, at least, not sure why I am being punished & sometimes I wonder if I'm being punished for nothing. I'm still getting threatened, & apparently some of these threats have been carried out, and the people who I need or care about me or are around me

"THE THING INSIDE MY HEAD"

will be replaced with devils to punish [the paper is torn off here].

[Main diary continued]

1 July: During the session [with Hazel]:

Stress with Ken:

Same as before. Keep a clear conscience but remember it is up to him in the end & he [broken off]

Stress with Dad:

Show him I'm there and show support & care but (*is important) don't push support on him. It's his responsibility in the end He's an adult. He's my dad.

Friendship with Theresa [classmate from Green Lodge College]:

Ask for her number to arrange to meet up in summer hols. Tell her only what I want to tell her. Tell her only a little at a time and see how she responds to it before telling more.

She (Theresa) has shown me that I look like a normal person; I don't look like a mental patient.

3 July [home]: I feel so angry and agitated and upset & frightened & alone. I feel sort of like I did the summer 91. I feel scared. If it isn't God talking to me, God didn't answer those stupid prayers of mine. Where is God, who is God, where & who am I & where do I stand & where does God stand & I feel without God. I'M SCARED AND CONFUSED. WHAT IS THE TRUTH?

I feel like I did at those times in the Bethlem when I had told about or challenged the voices. I feel restless and confused. I want to be in Peter Bruff, I want Hazel. I can't phone Kim up. She would be completely the wrong person to talk to. I feel calm now. I don't rave. I feel suicidal

HELP HELP HELP HELP

I wish I had let myself cry I wish I had cried naturally then the chaplain would know I want seeing about. But I think he knows that anyway cause 1) he wants to see me regularly for 1 hr. 2) he said I was very frightened.

I just weighed myself. I'm 8 st. but I feel so fat. Do I have anorexia? Part of me wishes 'Yes'.

I want to kill myself. Life is too hard & pressured & painful. I feel angry with God for making life like this. It is the devil who did really but why did God let him.

[Scrawled across the page]

I WANT TO TAKE AN OVERDOSE AND END UP IN HOSPITAL & PETER BRUFF. I CAN'T DO IT HERE. WHAT WILL BE THE BAD THING IF I DO [word illegible, probably DIE] *NO-ONE AT LEAST WILL UNDERSTAND.*

I feel very unwell. My mind is in tumult.

I WANT TO DIE

5 July: I don't know if I'm taking on the role of protector, responsible with my family again. Some part of me enjoys being in this role. It gives me a warm feeling, a feeling of usefulness, self esteem, and power and something else. Is that sick? Am I being bad? Will I be affecting my mental health?

"THE THING INSIDE MY HEAD"

6 July: I'm angry. I'm angry that I have to be in this situation with Ken etc. AAAAAGH. Think positive. Don't go down!

Good things about today:

I got my own laundry done. I got 2 belts & feel I can get more. I got my smear test over & done with. Hazel isn't angry at me. I had a nice, if still stressed talk with Shirley [Granta resident]. We talked about how terrible it was with all this business with Ken going on. She thinks I'm a good cook. Dinner was nice.

8 July: I got a letter from DLA [Disability Living Allowance] saying that I wasn't entitled to Mobility Allowance, starting from the 11.5.98. I was surprised how disappointed, & even surprised, I was as I knew this was likely. I'm worried about paying the back dated money from 11.5.98 till now. Michael & I are going to ring up social security tomorrow to find out. I'll also be short in income now which feels horrible.

11 July: [home] I feel like I have to do, or not do, things, in order to reduce Mum & Dad's stress. I'm so scared when I see how haggard, tired, worn & unhappy Dad is. He is old before his age. I don't want to mow the lawns tomorrow but I feel & think I have to otherwise Dad will get more stressed. He asked me if I would but they (Mum & Dad) always expect me to do things when I'm home & I don't like it. Sometimes it's okay but others, I really don't feel in the mood & I hate mowing the bottom lawn. It seems I can't even sleep in or relax tomorrow morning even though I'm ill. Dad is ill too though. But I'm fed up with it. He has to do something to change his lifestyle & his stress. I can't take the burden anymore. But how can I stand back when he is like this? I don't want to come home again for a long time. I want to be at Granta this weekend.

Lois Chaber

13 July: Ken is meant to leave tomorrow—a whole baggage of emotions. I feel torn. I want him to leave but I don't want him to be homeless.-

15 July 98: *Gwendolyn* [former teacher from the Adolescent Unit] *just phoned I'm so excited I was so pleased now I feel nervous but I'm feeling good about it as well. Oh what a surprise. I found it hard to believe. OH YEAH I feel hopelessly nervous & pent-up after Gwendolyn's phone call now* It's like how I felt when I agreed to meet up with Michelle & decided to ask Brett to my party & had a crush on him. It's very important to me and I want it to go well & I'm excited but I get tired of being excited. Oh, it's hard to explain.

16 July: I went to the cat rescue. I was making a fuss of Lucky. She put her front paws on me and leaned up to be picked up which was lovely but then I smelt poo and saw her bum was near my face. I couldn't move it. She climbed around me and onto my back and shoulders. When she got off I saw poo on my arm. I was disgusted. I disinfected it off but I still smelt it & I thought it had gone on my jumper & hair as well. I felt disgusting & quite uncomfortable. I tried putting that anti-bacterial soap all on my hair & right shoulder while I was alone washing my hands and the clothes. Didn't help. When I got back I had enough time to have a shower which I did.

19 July: I had a lovely lunch but I ate it all even though I began to feel sick because I was too full. Reginald obviously went to a bit of trouble especially for me. Sometimes, like at one point this morning, I think he is the devil. Right now I don't.

Mum [*on the phone*] said that Molly's boyfriend slept in her room last night & they didn't emerge until about 4:00 PM & they were quite quiet. Mum & Dad thought it strange & had ideas about what they could be doing but didn't interfere. I feel angry, frustrated, disappointed, disgusted & worried with & about Molly. I hope they didn't do it. I feel angry because she hadn't even told me she's got a boyfriend. We can't be that close then, not as close as I thought, hoped we were.

I hope the [coach] holiday goes well. Mum gave me some good advice to not let the hiccups & changes & things going wrong upset me as they are bound to happen. I feel excited. I feel ~~horrible~~

25 July: Alex [Granta resident] came out. I didn't want him to be there. He asked about my holiday. I felt threatened by & sort of jealous of, him. I think it's because I'm competing with him to be the most active, independent, forward moving, well resident here, now that he is getting himself together & passed his Access course [an accelerated alternative to A-levels for mature students] & has been accepted to be a 'Mind' Advocate. I think it's also because I can't nag him & put him down, in what I do, say & think, so much anymore. I think I enjoyed the sense of power I had. In a sense I was, & still am, a bully, for instance I often realized when thinking that I didn't want Ken to change & behave better & pull his weight because then I wouldn't be able to put him down in what I do, say & think or brush him aside or treat him how I used to. I think it is because I feel so insecure about myself and my relationships with people.

28 July: I want the care and comfort of Peter Bruff [Ward], although I won't have it and never have had it to the extent I hoped for, wanted.

No-one can help me but myself.

[*The following description of her meeting with the Reverend Richard Smith, written under the same day's entry, is systematically scribbled over. Did she want to entirely repudiate this experience?*]

~~I went to see the chaplain at the hospital. Now my head is buzzing & confused & going around in circles. I feel~~

scared and like I've been brought up in a cage and suddenly the door has been opened. The chaplain was very nice. I struggled down there but God had mercy & with work I got there and waited for him [the chaplain]. We went up to the chaplaincy. I thought I'd never get there alright. Then I had to tell him why I was there. I said I didn't know how to start. He said, 'Just start anywhere'. I kept stopping and he kept urging me on nicely. I found it very hard. I started by saying I wanted to be at peace with God and that I used to be at peace with God and that I used to be a happy Christian. I said that I started to become interested in God when I was 6 or 7 and at that same time I got OCD, although I didn't know it at the time. I said that I felt angry at God and guilty. He said that it was alright to feel angry at God, and that I didn't need to feel guilty about it. He said that if I felt angry at God at least I believed in him and some sort of relationship with him. He said that usually when we were angry at God we are really angry at someone else and somehow it gets put on God, and we think he should be doing something to stop it or something. Then he said that I might be angry at a father or a uncle, then he paused. I didn't say anything. He was referring to sexual abuse and I think he thought I had been. I didn't. I told him about my OCD bad kind of thoughts until I was confirmed [in the Methodist Church]. Then how I shed them & then got dirty thoughts when I prayed etc. & then said about the passage in the Bible about the Holy Spirit [Mark 3: 28-9] & my OCD thoughts (though I didn't know it was OCD then), my half asleep saying mistakes & then what I said out loud. I also told a bit about the thoughts which said they were from God. After a while he said they weren't from God. He said it was all an illness. He said that God wouldn't punish me for thoughts that were an illness, not premeditated. Then I said some of my thoughts are premeditated. He didn't answer.

He said I should stop reading the Bible for now after I told him about Jesus being strict in the Bible. He said it was a very hard book to understand; we need guidance when reading it. He said God loves me & I said if he loves me why does he send people to hell. He said he doesn't

"THE THING INSIDE MY HEAD"

~~believe God sends people to hell. I don't know…[broken off]~~
~~I felt like crying. I don't know what he meant by that. He~~
~~said that God wasn't punishing~~.

28 July: I'm angry because I am weak as a human being & keep sinning & then I'm guilty, then I'm dependent on God's forgiveness & mercy & I am scared & have reason to feel bad about myself & continue to sin.

In the Bible it says that it is Adam & Eve's fault that we know the difference between good & evil now & can sin now, but why should we, countless generations, have to suffer because of them? Why did God let the devil tempt Adam & Eve? Why did God plant the tree of knowledge within human grasp where we could fall? Why did he let us lose our innocence? Why did he let the devil fall? If God is good how can anything he creates (and he created everything that is) be evil? Why did he let the devil get to us as well & continue to? I feel angry at God for letting all this happen. I also feel angry at God that a woman sinned before men & we have to feel guilty & bad about our sex now.

29 July: I feel like I want to be in Peter Bruff & cared for, mothered. It isn't like that though. I want people like Hazel to know how much I'm hurting.

I feel like I'm not coping, part of it is anti-climax after the [coach] holiday. If this is what holidays do to you I feel worried about going on one again. Even the N.Z. holiday. I'm worried about that, very worried. I wish we weren't going. I used to look forward to it so much. Now I'm dreading it & really worrying about it. Will I be alright without Hazel or staff to talk to, I won't have my room & privacy & T.V. & radio to fall back on.

Mum phoned & I spoke to her & Molly, which has really helped lift my mood.

Lois Chaber

I keep thinking, feeling & being told I might probably murder someone.

Will I?

Evidence for:

I tried it [in the] Bethlem.
I let myself do evil things.
I do evil things.
I think evil things.
I feel evil things
I feel like the devil or evil is in me or I'm letting it take me over.
I feel a bit like hurting people sometimes.

Evidence against:

My prayer to God.
I don't want to, when I'm thinking rationally & search inside.
Sometimes I feel I can't when I'm told to or given a sort of opportunity to
I haven't hurt anyone physically for a long time. I don't remember feeling like I'll hurt them through the devil, so much as recently.
I don't want to & I am in control.

Sometimes I think bad thoughts when I think that God can't punish me or he isn't real & I want to be adventurous or live dangerously.

Sometimes I do it to rebel against the voices or thoughts or my conscience or OCD or anything & sometimes I think they are God.

I feel scared & like I am going downhill but Hazel can't [broken off]

"THE THING INSIDE MY HEAD"

4 August: I keep getting messages from God. I'm obeying most of them or having a go. I wish they weren't from God & I knew they weren't but at the moment I think they are & my brain feels funny & overloaded & like it did when I was ill. That could be partly because I don't drink enough which I also did when I was ill.

Or I could be getting ill.

Or it could be real.

I feel like I'm in the bad way again

[Most of the rest of this diary is scrawled in a nearly illegible handwriting]

I feel so angry I feel like exploding.

I FEEL SOO ANGRY

And like I will blow my lid. I feel so angry & hurt by God.

I FEEL SO ANGRY FOR GOD MAKING OR EVEN LETTING MY LIFE BE TURNED UPSIDE-DOWN.

I FEEL SCARED AND LIKE I HAVE TAKEN ON TOO MUCH.

7 August: I feel so FED UP

I couldn't see Richard the chaplain because of his having to go to an emergency.

Lois Chaber

I feel so alone with only the devil's company which I *don't* want! Tracey is there though she said I can chat to her.

I feel so angry at, & so distanced & estranged from, God. Why did He do this? He probably called Richard [the chaplain] away either to punish me or maybe the voices & thoughts use him. Maybe He knew I'd make a mess of it but that's not fair because he is the one who is threatening to replace the chaplain with the devil when I see him. I feel a strange sense of calm while I don't know if it's the devil or God. I was going to ignore the voices if I couldn't see him [the chaplain] but now I'm not so sure. Yet there are still so many thoughts & feelings of anger that I feel like I'm being pulled here there & everywhere.

I've got my conscience,
I've got my sinful flesh wants
I've got my intellectual thinking about the voice/thought
I've got my ANGER at God
I've got my ANGER & frustration in general.
I've got my OCD thoughts and feelings
I've got the 'child/baby' in me.
I've got the confusion, anger fear anxiety & hurt & bewilderment because of the voices/thoughts, punishments & things from the Bethlem & at home in 91/92 & Hill End etc.
I've got the 'grown up' sensible good side of me

> Molly's phoning me back later

There's the devil tempting me.
There's my adrenalin making me high & nervous & maybe relaxed
There's my tablets making me I don't know—relaxed & stimulated I think
There's the thoughts which threaten to replace people with the devil

"THE THING INSIDE MY HEAD"

There are the thoughts saying they are from God.
I get compulsions to do bad things.
~~good feelings~~ ~~good feelings~~ ~~good feelings~~ good feelings

calm

Later: 7:00 PM

I feel so much frustration, anger, agitation that sometimes I feel I might kill someone or do something terrible. I feel like I want to <u>really really really</u> rebel.

I DON'T WANT TO THINK BAD THOUGHTS. I WANT TO BE AT PEACE & PURE & STRONG.

I CAN BE STRONG but I'm afraid of all the pain & loneliness & fear that goes with it.

~~Tracey help~~

I feel like screaming. I just did!

Hazel phoned. She had spoken to Dr. Smith & he had said (& she agreed) to increase some of my medicine, my haloperidol [anti-psychotic drug]. I was really pleased. She sounded very caring. She came and gave the meds to me & said she couldn't chat much as wished to because she was swamped on urgent duty. She said she'd see me on Monday & then arrange a time to take me to see [Dr.] Roberts in the week. I wish she would adopt me as a big sister or Auntie or something. She is *so lovely.*

I was really pleased about the medication but I wish he had upped the Prozac as well. Still, I musn't grumble as the haloperidol was upped & procyclidine to counter side effects & more diazepam [valium] if I need it. I don't want to

431

get addicted & also don't want it to mask the effect of the haloperidol.

Molly called. It was a really great conversation & she was lovely & she really cared a lot.

We joked & chatted & helped each other.

Mum & Dad are coming tomorrow.

I'm fed up of restrictions.

AAAAAGH

8 August [day of our visit to Clacton; All Sybil has written is "~~Mum and Dad's~~"]

9 August: I think when I have a relationship with someone I don't want it to be like in movies, or like when couples pinch or pat each others bottoms or make what I think are degrading jokes. I want sensitivity, gentleness, shyness, respect, honour, regard & a humble, faithful love.

11 August. I don't live my life. I thought of 'The Greatest Love of All' again & realized again (to be continued)—

~~I WANT TO BANG MY HEAD~~

—that I needed to do that—love myself. I need to like myself, feel confident, not be afraid of myself, I need to believe in myself.

12 August: I just had a great/wonderful conversation on the phone. Patty phoned earlier to say she couldn't come and I could tell by her voice that she wasn't feeling good. I phoned back just now because I felt worried & guilty that I'd

been a bit harsh or nasty to her on the phone. She said I hadn't been & it was her. Then she said her Mum wanted to speak to me. Her Mum said that they thought I was A VERY NICE GIRL

Sorry, but I am feeling agitated & getting bad thoughts.

And it wasn't my fault & they looked forward to seeing me & Patty's lucky to have a friend like me. I felt a bit guilty about this knowing that I have been not so nice & my feelings about Patty But then I felt really happy & cheerful.

But now I'm worried that Patty would feel hurt because her Mum kept saying that it wasn't my fault but Patty's.

15 August [after Molly's visit]: Molly saw me doing stuff & even on my own I'm doing stuff that I thought I'd left behind ages ago like walking back, walking backwards, stopping.

I'm having troubles speaking without checking or being 'ready' (rituals) first & without stopping in the middle or not saying it at all.

I FEEL SO FED UP. AAAAAA. I HATE OCD.

The weekend with Molly went *really* well. I feel touched & emotional. It was hard but it paid off. I'll write more later.

[Scrawled across the next few pages]

I HATE THE DEVIL

Lois Chaber

I HATE THE DEVIL

I HATE EVIL

I HATE MY BEHAVIOUR I
KEEP GETTING COMPULSIONS TO
BE [word unreadable] OR ~~DEVIL~~

I feel I haven't even been able to write my diary properly because of the OCD I want help—I'm getting help already AAAAAAAGH

~~Hazel stayed with Molly & I all last night. She is great~~.

16 August: The OCD is getting worse

But at least I can now tell Hazel everything or the priest everything

Oh no! Maybe I can't tell Hazel everything because I'm still getting thoughts telling me to do things which might be from God.

I WANT TO TELL HAZEL
EVERYTHING I WANT TO BE ABLE TO

My writing is being affected badly now.

& my praying I can't pray or at least it feels that way I can't speak into it I can't speak into a telephone I maybe can't speak. I'm angry & frustrated & scared.

I wish I saw the chaplain sooner but it will be good seeing him (or maybe not while I'm like this). I went to see the vicar this Friday [I have not been able to identify a 'vicar'

434

in Clacton who saw Sybil; it is probable that she means 'the chaplain' here]. AAAAAAA

The vicar gave me lots of things to think about. He said that the voices about punishment about turning people into devils wasn't God. HOORAY! He said it was fine to be arguing at God. (good) He said that I think bad thoughts on purpose because I'm angry at God. He suggested that I deal with my anger in better ways, which I agreed to.

He said that one way would be to talk to him about my feelings & thoughts about God.

That sounded ~~good to me~~
~~goo~~
~~good to me~~ me
good to
I hate O.C.D.
me

I'm worried that now he thinks all my bad thoughts are on purpose which they aren't. He understands about OCD thoughts. Most of my bad thoughts are OCD related. Some aren't; of the ones that are, some I can't help & some I can to a certain extent.

I told the chaplain that I was angry at God because my life had been turned upside down since I became ill when I was 13.

He said, 'That's a difficult age for girls and boys.'

I told him about my dancing & flute, I didn't get to tell about school. I told about my faith till then. I mentioned family problems that year. I told him about Dad's unemployment, Mums saying she was going to kill herself, Molly's worrying behaviour & my problems moving to a new school all at the same time. I hope he didn't think I was boasting about the 'grammar school' or thinking that the 'family problems' were small. I can't remember what he said about all that.

He asked why I wanted to see him. I said to sort out my thoughts & feelings about God. He said I'd be welcome at the church services & everyone is really supportive to each other. I can't go to church at the moment 1: I'm too bad 2: I'm too angry.

I told him about when I was 7—the OCD, Christianity & the voices/thoughts. He asked me what was going on at that age. I told him. I'm worried he will think it's nothing.

He said that God is a loving God & not a punishing God & that we punish ~~ourselves ourselves ourselves ourselves ourselves~~ ourselves.

I HATE THE DEVIL, OCD & MYSELF. I'M ANGRY AT GOD, BUT HE IS GOOD, BUT WHY IS HE LETTING ME SUFFER.

[Scrawled over two pages]

I   HATE   ME.

17 August: I feel calm but there is a tight ball at the bottom of me—somewhere. I can't even phone the chaplain.

Last night I asked Michael to help clean the kitchen out, like I had done with Kim in the morning. I decided to talk to him instead as I felt crap. Much of what he said wasn't helpful at all but there were a few good bits and he ~~made me laugh &~~ rambled on until we both didn't know why we were talking about that & I felt relaxed & sleepy. Then we cleaned.

"THE THING INSIDE MY HEAD"

Then I phoned home. Mum kept saying 'remember I love you so much' & she sounded sad. I had been thinking of suicide seriously yesterday or at least attempted suicide for help, & then I thought I can't do it because of Mum it would devastate her. But I'm still thinking about it today. I don't feel that Hazel is taking me seriously enough. However, she is brilliant, kind, intelligent, knowledgeable, experienced & lovely. I still can't get over her spending Fri night out with Moll & I.

In some ways part of me wants to be in hospital—where I don't have to worry about cooking, cleaning, voluntary work, going home etc. & I could just work on my problems & feel sort of protected, like in a mother's womb, but I partly know that part of that is a fantasy. I would be bored, upset by the people, lonely, & probably get less 1 to 1 time there than here & it wouldn't work. I just wish I knew a better solution because I'm really struggling & it feels like I'm losing a bit, gradually.

I really want to do something silly for a cry for help. But I might anger them & get less help & sympathy. Am I being ungrateful for all the help I'm getting? YES. But I feel so distressed & I'm not used to it anymore & don't want to cope with it & live with it now.

AAAAAA

HAZEL

MICHAEL

don't realize how serious this is

AAAAAA

[Sybil's diary for August ends here. There does not appear to be a September diary.]

Lois Chaber

Chapter 3: "The Worst"

There is one grief worse than any other.

(Ellen Bryant Voigt, "Daughter", in *The Forces of Plenty*, WW Norton & Co., 1983.)

It's a Sunday in early October, 1998, and Molly, Neil and I are on our way—at last—to see Sybil in Clacton Hospital. We have had to wait some weeks since her re-admittance for her to voluntarily contact us, and then after a couple of these brief, timid calls, for her to give us 'permission' to visit. Outside the car, the autumn rain is beating down relentlessly, making the old familiar journey to North East Essex even drearier. My classes have resumed after the summer, and I'm using the journey, despite my increasingly queasy stomach, to red-pencil student essays, leaning awkwardly on a large book in the back of the car. I am greatly worried about Sybil and eager to see her after a month's gap. But I am also slightly resentful that, with so many tasks piling up at home, once again we have to make this time-consuming and tedious journey; I wistfully recall the days of Sybil's independent travel down to Southgate. A recent phone call from Hazel, warning us that Sybil's stay in hospital may be longer than expected since she is not making good progress, has not lightened my spirits any, either.

With great trepidation, we eventually enter the familiar doorway of the single-storey Peter Bruff Ward. Sybil will see us only in the glass-enclosed visitors' room, a goldfish bowl sealed off from the rest of the ward. She is extremely anxious and extremely reticent. We do most of the talking, purveying all the titbits of 'news' we can summon up but studiously avoiding any direct references to her relapse or her present dreadful condition, which we know Sybil won't countenance. She cannot take too much of us, and before long we are leaving her behind, a small, haggard figure hesitantly waving goodbye from the hospital foyer.

There are several of these dismal weekend visits; Molly's participation is erratic, I decide to go every other time due to my busy schedule of household chores and teaching prep on weekends, and Neil makes the journey every week. I tell myself: "After all, Sybil gives us a lukewarm reception, and surely her deplorable state is only temporary. Neil's soothing presence will be enough to sustain her."

Members of the staff from Woodland Lodge also visit Sybil regularly this autumn, willing her, as we do, a speedy recovery; Michael explains: "We felt it was important to stay in contact with Sybil when she went into hospital in the autumn because we obviously hoped for her (potentially) to come back home." But Tracey, one of her most frequent visitors, comments revealingly on Sybil's attitude towards being in hospital again:

She said she felt happy at the hospital because there were no pressures; if she couldn't do something, it didn't matter. I guess when you're unwell, that's fine. When she was well here at Granta, she was doing everything that she wanted to do and being independent and doing everything that was expected of her, same as if she lived at your house—cooking, a bit of cleaning and shopping. In Peter Bruff she didn't have to work hard at all. I think in some ways it was easier for Sybil to cope when she was in there, because they didn't have so many expectations of her.

* * *

Meanwhile, Sybil's support team is trying new measures. They switch her main OCD medication from

Lois Chaber

Prozac to a new drug, Venlafaxine, with a different chemical structure that acts not only upon serotonin (like the other SSRI drugs) but also on the brain chemical norepinephrine. Worryingly, we find from the Internet (now at our disposal) that, at this time, Venlafaxine has only been studied for periods of administration up to six weeks and has been restricted to patients diagnosed with Major Depressive Disorder. *OCD: A Guide*, published the same year as Sybil's treatment with the new drug, comments: "The only small controlled trial reported to date had mixed results, and more careful work is needed to establish the proper role of Venlafaxine in OCD." A contribution by Dr. Greg Wilkins to a "Psychiatry On-Line Forum" in early 1999 also indicates that the effects of Venlafaxine have not yet been thoroughly explored. Wilkin cites the case of a 37-year-old female patient who twice reacts to a new packet of the drug with "a marked recurrence of depressive symptoms (old) and anxiety symptoms (new)." Although changing the batch each time has reversed the symptoms, Dr. Wilkins ends with an appeal for help regarding this really quite experimental drug: "Has anyone else witnessed a similar phenomenon?"

It is not only that we are concerned about the choice of a relatively untested drug on Sybil, but also that, by now, we are reasonably well-read in the literature on OCD and know that the recommended line of action when one SSRI drug (like Prozac-fluoxetine) is or becomes ineffectual for a patient, is to try switching to another of the same family (fluvoxamene, paroxetene or sertralene) because they each have a slightly different molecular structure. With difficulty, I manage to obtain access to Dr. Smith by phone to discuss this issue, but, in a tone that seems to me by turns patronising and tetchy, he insists that Venlafaxine is the best choice because Sybil's OCD is complex, combined with other factors. We are not convinced, but there is little we can do except wait and watch the results of his choice, marking time until we can say "Look, you've tried it and it doesn't work; now please follow the conventional recommendation of switching SSRI's." We cling hopefully to this plan.

"THE THING INSIDE MY HEAD"

Around this time, also, her team arranges for Sybil to receive cognitive behaviour therapy (CBT) from a young specialist living outside Clacton, a long overdue step that we've been pressing for, Sybil not having had formal therapy of any kind since she refused the Maudsley programme and Allen Brown resigned from her team, and since Jane Clark, her former CPN who had given Sybil cognitive behavioural therapy, left her position due to illness. By now we have learned that CBT, ideally accompanied by exposure and response prevention, is the treatment of choice for OCD sufferers because it aims to change the patient's thinking— particularly the catastrophic type of thinking behind the rituals (the Maudsley CD-ROM's example: "Because I didn't remind my mother to wear her seat belt, she's going to die in a crash"). It is possible that Sybil's relapse might not have occurred had she been receiving such therapy in late 1997 and 1998. Although this new CBT treatment is now scheduled weekly, due to administrative errors and contingencies that arise, Sybil only gets to have about three sessions from mid-autumn through the end of the year. It is too little, too late.

She is also given a course of ECT (electro-convulsive therapy) once again during this autumn period, but unlike the dramatic improvement we saw in 1996, it now has only a very modest impact.

* * *

Throughout November, we continue to visit Sybil in hospital, and there is even a successful family outing to a low key Clacton restaurant to celebrate Neil's and my birthdays, which fills us with fresh hope. The countdown towards the New Zealand holiday begins, with us getting increasingly anxious as to whether Sybil is going to accompany us or not. Neil delays buying the tickets (for three or for four?) as long as possible; then he buys four anyway, hoping he won't have to cancel Sybil's at the last minute. Sybil remains non-committal.

Lois Chaber

Near the end of November, although not vastly improved, Sybil seems well enough to be discharged from the hospital into Eagleton Assessment Unit once again, to undergo a programme of gradually increasing visits to Granta Housing, in the hope she will be able to return there eventually. Are the hospital and Sybil's team nudging her along willy nilly towards a specious 'recovery' simply to get her off the ward's hands? We wonder. We hear that her behaviour during these visits to Granta is erratic, at best, as Michael explains:

> Basically, when the hospital staff was talking about discharge, we were concerned about our ability to cope with Sybil. We needed her to be showing good signs of improvement and of being able to care for herself. We were advocating a staged discharge so we could assess Sybil, and also reintroduce her to the project in a way that took some of the stress out of the process. The success was variable. Sometimes her behaviour gave us optimism; other times it was obvious she was just not coping and finding things very difficult and stressful.

On one of these days we call up Granta because we've heard she's going to be there overnight. We get Reginald on the phone, and, before asking to speak to Sybil, we inquire how she's managing on this particular visit. Just as he's in the middle of saying, "She's not doing all that well," he suddenly yells out—"My God, she's just cut herself! I have to go!"

Sybil has cut herself on the wrist, we later find out, and staff members have to go through all the necessary emergency procedures, even though it's not a serious

442

wound. Michael further enlightens us about her history of self-harming at Granta:

> I recall how we would occasionally hear some banging, but did not immediately realize its significance. We thought it was doors banging etc. Then we noticed a little bit of blood on the wall of Sybil's bedroom just before she was admitted to hospital. She'd been banging her head against the wall. There were some other, isolated incidents of self-harm. Once, when she was becoming ill again, she did make some sort of attempt to cut her wrists. Staff were made aware of this very quickly and went through the usual procedures we have for those cases. I can only think of two occasions on which that happened, and the self-harm was not extensive in any way. But the attempt was genuine enough.

* * *

The precise state of Sybil's mental health is still unclear by late November, and we remain in suspense about the New Zealand visit. The plan is for Neil and Molly to leave very early in December, while I set off a few days later in order to see through my American College final examinations. And Sybil? On the final weekend before Neil's departure, the two of us travel up to Eaglehurst to wrest a final decision from her. It is the first time we are visiting her at Eaglehurst this time around, and from the minute we walk in we feel uneasy; there is a subtle atmosphere of remoteness towards us in the house, unlike anything we've sensed before. I intuit that Sybil is not really being cherished in the unit as she was in her first stay two years ago; she is here on sufferance only, we feel.

Lois Chaber

Sybil is in the long, narrow kitchen, very diffident and anxious, hovering near the work bench; *we* know that *she* knows that this is the decisive moment. She flits in and out of the room and finds it very difficult to concentrate on making Neil some tea. With great difficulty, we manage to manoeuvre her into the more private, more comfortable parlour, with its shabby genteel arm chairs and sofa. She is well into her OCD behaviour, pacing back and forth from the parlour to the kitchen, unable to sit down, barely able to talk to us. Very tense, we summon up all our patience and resolve, waiting for her to settle down, sipping tea. Finally, she stabilises enough to tell us, with a great effort, that she has made up her mind: "I'm not going to go on the trip; I don't think I'm up to it."

For the next hour or so, we make a sustained effort to persuade her to reverse this decision, pleading argumentatively, like two barristers—that is, whenever she is able to remain in the room. Perhaps it is wrong of us not to simply accept her decision and drop the subject. Perhaps that might enhance her self-respect and diminish her guilt and self-torment. But, caught up in anguished longing and convinced the trip 'will be good for her', we don't seriously consider this option. She tells us she is wary of relatives and friends in New Zealand "looking down at her" because of her illness, and no amount of reassurance from us about how they will be loving and accepting of her puts these fears at rest. We tell her we will book an earlier return to England for her and me, so that her part of the visit will be curtailed, but even this possibility does not allay her many anxieties and her self-distrust. While I grow pessimistic, and resigned, about the outcome of this discussion, Neil is becoming ever more impassioned in his pleas and, as I can see, distressed; he has really counted on being able to move her. By the time we finally give up and prepare to leave, Neil is distraught and in tears, though trying to hide it. We will have to cancel that fourth ticket after all.

Sybil's decision leaves us in a very difficult position; we are deserting her, in effect, at that time of year that has

"THE THING INSIDE MY HEAD"

always carried a huge amount of emotional baggage with it for Sybil. My conscience and my worries assault me, and I resolve to stay here and forego the New Zealand trip so that Sybil at least will have part of her family at Christmas. This resolution comes fairly readily for me because I'm not as wildly enthusiastic about the trip as Neil is, and I can see some compensation in staying here, although I am much saddened by the thought of separation from Neil and Molly. Neil assents sorrowfully to what I say, but I decide to check it out first with Hazel. To my surprise, she is quite adamant that I not stay behind for Sybil's sake: Sybil will feel terribly guilty over this, Hazel is convinced, and that will defeat the whole purpose. It's important for her to build up her independence and self-reliance; this will be a true test of Sybil's mettle and will promote her improvement and growth, she reassures me. Part relieved, part guilty, I yield to her reasoning and say nothing to Sybil.

Neil and Molly depart mid-week. I work assiduously at marking my class's exams, organising my packing, and orienting a young couple from New Zealand who are to house-sit for us to the appliances, the plants, and the cat's needs. Miraculously, I find that I have a small window of free time—about a day's worth—before my flight leaves, and this throws me into a quandary: On the one hand I am tempted to use that time to resume work on a long and complex scholarly book review, well overdue, that I am in the process of writing for the journal *Eighteenth-Century Fiction*. However, in the depths of my heart I am well aware that I should make one final visit to Sybil before my departure... and how can I doubt what is the right thing to do? Nevertheless, there is still that nagging conflict within me between my child's needs and my own vocational drive, between motherhood and career. A visit to my current junior psychiatrist at the local hospital helps me to resolve this conflict in favour of Sybil. (Later, in New Zealand, Neil is amazed that I even hesitated—but he, of course, worked at his job right up till the day of his flight!)

Lois Chaber

The first thing Sybil says to me when I enter Woodland Lodge on Sunday, is, "Do you think Dad will ever forgive me?" Her words stab me and I do my best to reassure her: "Although he's sad, he's not in the least bit angry with you!" Before I go, I make a point of talking to Rebecca, Sybil's young female keyworker at Eaglehurst, someone completely new to me and of very recent acquaintance to Sybil. I feel compelled to remind her to be especially attentive to Sybil while her family is absent, although I can't say this outright as Sybil is lingering nearby. Neil and I have given Sybil and Molly each £100 to spend on themselves for Christmas (Sybil always badly needs clothing, subsisting as she does on state benefits), and I enjoin Rebecca, "You'll be sure and take Sybil shopping to spend her Christmas money, won't you?" as if my words can will her to act kindly to Sybil if the impulse isn't already there. But I am all too aware that, in her present condition, Sybil is very unlikely to initiate a solo shopping spree. The visit has reaffirmed my connection to Sybil, and has generally lifted my spirits about the upcoming trip. I shudder now to think of how Sybil and I would both be feeling if I hadn't come.

* * *

I eventually join up with Molly and Neil at Queenstown, where, almost immediately, Neil declares we should make a 'family phone call' to Sybil. Tremulously, we put through the long distance call, trying to compromise between letting her know what we've been up to and not making the trip she's missing sound too wonderful. She sounds reasonably composed. Phone calls to her continue to punctuate our journey from the South to the North Island, about every three or four days. Much to our surprise, a package from Sybil arrives at Neil's brother Ian's home, where we are staying, just before Christmas Day. In it are two huge Christmas cards, one for Molly and one for Neil and me, as well as a cute smurf-like knick-knack bearing the message "This is a Santa Hug.". The loving note she writes on her card to us touches us deeply:

446

"THE THING INSIDE MY HEAD"

You're the best and most loving parents in the
world. You do so much for me. I hope you
have a lovely Christmas and a great holiday.
I'm sorry I can't be there with you but I think of
you every day lots.

The whole package implies a state of organised
competence and an upbeat mood on her part that reassures
us. On the morning after Christmas, New Zealand time, we
make a call to find out, crucially, how she's managed on
Christmas Day and to bestow holiday greetings. Much to
our relief, she sounds quite chirpy, reeling off to us a list of
the gifts she's received from her local friends and
careworkers.

Her mood continues mostly positive in the
immediate aftermath. June Keyte, Sybil's pen-pal and our
friend, has promised to keep in contact with Sybil while we
are away. She calls Sybil from Southgate the day I leave,
carries on calling her every few days (like us) and drives up
to Woodland Lodge with her husband, Christopher, for a visit
shortly after Christmas:

*Initially, I was a bit shocked, because her
hair looked as if she hadn't had it washed it in I
don't know how long. It was all greasy and she
had a scrappy-looking jumper on. I hadn't seen
her like that before because her hair always
looked pretty. She was dressed just as if we'd
called on her at 6:00 in the morning rather than
going out to lunch really. But, generally, as
always when we were with her, she was very
chatty.*

*We left the car, and we had a walk all
along the promenade. Eventually, we found*

Lois Chaber

*this fantastic little Italian restaurant which we
had lunch in, right on the sea front. And there, I
couldn't believe it—the biggest excitement for
us when we came away was when we went into
the restaurant; she was so composed, and so
confident, walking in before us. She had the
choice of the menu and ate as if she hadn't
eaten for a week. I couldn't eat any afters, as I
normally do, but she had this huge slice of
chocolate cake at the end of that as well—
which was wonderful. We were coming back,
driving along in the car, thinking, "This is some
sort of a miracle, really; when you think she at
one point didn't eat for months on end and then
ate only a little—worthy of a sparrow."*

However, her mood takes a downturn very soon
after this pleasant visit with the Keytes, perhaps
foreshadowed by the lack of personal care June has noticed.
When we phone her on what is New Year's Eve for us, she
presents quite differently, sounding timid, distant, and quite
fragile, and reverting to her old habit of suddenly dropping
the receiver every so often, repeatedly severing
communication between us. Our festive spirits somewhat
dimmed, after a while we give up trying to talk to her and say
goodbye.

At the end of our sojourn in New Zealand, during
which Neil has been more than gratified by the contact he's
had with old friends and family, we start our long, three-
stage journey home, which includes a small treat for us, a
two day stay in Fiji, on a tiny island resort called Sonasali,
before we take off for Los Angeles. Our first morning there,
we ring Sybil at Eaglehurst as soon as the time difference
permits. We are told by a careworker whom we don't know
that she is not there. We ask the man where she is. There

448

"THE THING INSIDE MY HEAD"

is a silence, and after some hesitation, he tells us she is in Colchester Hospital. We panic. "Why?" Reluctantly, again, he tells us that she has taken an overdose of paracetamol a couple of days ago. She is all right physically, but, because of her disturbing behaviour, she is going to be discharged that very day, not back to Eaglehurst, but to the Peter Bruff Ward in Clacton Hospital.

We are shocked at this terrible news and thrown into disarray. How can she have metamorphosed from the cheerful and considerate young woman of the days leading up to and including Christmas to one who would commit this seemingly unmotivated act of self-destruction? We call Colchester hospital and manage to locate Sybil there. She is crying and unable to say much, virtually incoherent. With no attempt at admonishment, we simply reiterate over and over again our love and concern for her, Neil crooning to Sybil in his special, tender voice. We call Molly at home (she has had to leave New Zealand in advance of us), urging her to make contact with Sybil just as soon as possible. Molly later tells us that they have cried together over the phone, Sybil sobbing out, "I knew it would hurt you, but I had to do it."

We are deeply disturbed, but after the initial shock, we optimistically assume that our return home and the reunion of the family will ameliorate the situation. Meanwhile, our remaining day and a half (it is too late to change our two onward flights) in a well-appointed thatched hut on this tiny island, close to the white beach and the sparkling blue water, plus the local entertainment and the sumptuous buffets, lulls us into temporarily submerging our grief and worry over Sybil.

* * *

Arriving home late on Friday afternoon, January 8th, 1999, we lose no time in visiting Sybil on Peter Bruff Ward, all three of us, the very next day. We find her hunched up in bed in a little cubicle, separated from other cubicles on the

Lois Chaber

ward only by surrounding curtains. We have not seen her look so poorly since the dark days of 1992 before she entered the Bethlem Royal Adolescent Unit. She appears drugged, listless and apathetic, and can barely respond to our questions and remarks. Her face is pallid, her mouth half-open, fish-like, and her head lolls forward and to the side on her neck, as if she has been partly decapitated. The cubicle is untidy and strewn with neglected Christmas gifts. We have brought yet another pile of gifts with us for her, from New Zealand relatives, from Lesley the dance teacher and others, hoping to cheer her, but she adamantly refuses to open any (and I can almost tangibly 'see' her self-punitive thoughts crystallising there in the room); instead, she feebly offers gifts to us, which we open with exaggerated enthusiasm.

We also bring post for her that has come to Chase Side, but, unbeknownst to us, the letters bear disturbing surprises. The first is from fifteen-year old Alice from Reading, our friends' daughter and Sybil's pen pal. Sybil reads the letter under our eyes, only to stop, horrified and puzzled, when she comes to the line, "I was quite shocked to hear about the trouble Molly's in." In fact, Molly has had some sensitive problems only known to a very few friends of ours, not meant to be divulged to anyone else—especially Sybil. It seems my confidante has incautiously told her daughters about this matter. Molly is furious, but Neil and I manage to brush the trouble under the carpet, leaving Sybil disturbed but not insistent, as she is so enfeebled.

The second letter, from Michelle, the former Latymer classmate whom Sybil has hero-worshipped for several years, I place triumphantly into Sybil's hands. Michelle has not written to Sybil for many months, presumably preoccupied with preparing for and adjusting to her first year at Cambridge University. In desperation during this past autumn, I wrote to her, explaining about Sybil's relapse and her poor condition, suggesting that it would make a significant difference if she could get back in touch. On arriving back at Southgate, the letter from Michelle,

"THE THING INSIDE MY HEAD"

addressed to Sybil care of me, was awaiting us, and I was so hyper-excited that I just grabbed the enclosed envelope and brought it along to the hospital. Sybil doesn't open the letter during this visit—presumably to savour it alone—but some time later I am to find it amongst her belongings and to realise with horror that this envelope contained two letters, one for Sybil and one for me, not meant for Sybil's eyes:

> Thank you very much for writing to let me know about Sybil. I'm very sorry about it all and feel terrible that I haven't written for so long. In my letter I've apologized for not writing for so long, and explained that I've sent the letter via you because I didn't know which address to use. I'll speak to Ivana [another classmate] as soon as possible. Please don't hesitate to let us know if there's anything else we can do—telephone calls—visits—anything; we really want to help.

Yet again my bumbling interference will have caused Sybil pain.

* * *

Meanwhile, other faithful friends from the Granta Staff are visiting her during this critical time. Tracey describes how she ministers to Sybil:

> Since she'd have been washing her hands constantly, I would get out the hand cream and sit there and massage her hands and rub them. It was quite high up where the chaffing was, and she'd say how nice that was, and how

lovely that was. By that stage, she couldn't sit very long; she was having to get up and walk around and come back to me.

Michael is due to go on annual leave during this time in January and goes to the hospital to say goodbye: "My last message to her was that we were 'here' for her. Before I left, I asked her if there was anything I could do. She said 'No', so I just said goodbye; I didn't pressure her or anything."

The three of us visiting the next weekend, by now mid-January, find to our relief that Sybil is looking and feeling considerably better, although her OCD rituals are much in evidence. She eventually consents to open the deferred presents, growing increasingly pleased and calm, and we open some held-back ones of our own alternately—just like old times under the Christmas tree. We take heart.

Nevertheless, a couple of days beforehand, Neil has had a very ominous telephone conversation with Hazel, our first one since Sybil's overdose, and so crucial that he takes extensive notes while talking, especially as he senses a withdrawal of sympathy taking place. Hazel seems to Neil quite annoyed that Sybil seems to have no view on what she wants to do at this point. Peter Bruff Ward is okay for now, but (once again) she can't stay there indefinitely; Eaglehurst doesn't want her back (Hazel says this to Neil quite bluntly). Unless Sybil improves enough to go back to Granta (she's not even sure *they* want her back), the only option left is long-term residential hospital care in an adult ward at the Bethlem Royal Hospital.

She has explained this to Sybil, and Sybil (obviously) recoils from this possibility. But, Hazel claims, Sybil is responsible for putting herself in this situation. Today, says Hazel, Sybil seems improved, but still very unclear about what to do; she is visibly frightened that she is

452

"THE THING INSIDE MY HEAD"

back in Clacton hospital. The only positive note that Hazel strikes at all, when Neil anxiously queries her about what can be done for Sybil, is to mention the possibility of long-term art therapy to get Sybil to open up. Hazel comments that Sybil tends to react against her own success.

We are extremely upset by this phone call. Rather than just focusing on Sybil's recuperation process, it seems to us, her medical team is already giving her an ultimatum. Is Sybil really being pushed to a discharge because they think she's ready for it, or is it just the usual pressure on resources, shortage of beds, etc. that has haunted her treatment by the NHS? The thought of Sybil indefinitely confined in the Bethlem asylum, totally institutionalised, strikes terror into our hearts: no more challenging Dial-a-Ride days, no more tenderly caring for cats, no more gratifying trips to the pub with her role models, no more progress in her formal education, no more pride in a growing independence.

Sybil must feel the same way—and *what* can be keeping her, we wonder, from making a clear commitment to Hazel that she will work hard at getting better so that she can return to Granta Housing and her old life? We surmise that it is probably a paralysing sense of déjà vu, of fear, of inertia. We recall earlier remarks by her Granta carers that Sybil may have progressed too far too soon. Since the time of her collapse at Jacques Hall at the beginning of 1996 and her relapse in September '98, Sybil had made such a tremendous effort, in graduated stages, to slough off her worst OCD symptoms and build up a 'life' for herself, making commitments to activities that were both therapeutic and normalising. The prospect of having to summon up the psychic stamina to begin the whole process all over again must be staggeringly prohibitive.

Diane, writing to Sybil from London in the autumn, has tried gently to cajole Sybil into facing this enormous challenge:

Lois Chaber

Try to remember that you did it once
before and then draw on all you learnt last time
and use it as hard as you can. It will be a
difficult thing to do, you will need every ounce of
strength you can muster, you will feel like giving
up because it is easier to give up, but I know
you have a lot of hidden strength and you are
more capable that [sic] people realize. You can
do it my little angel. I have a lot of faith in you.

On the phone with Hazel, Neil has kept his own
counsel and said little. There will be a major formal review
or "Care Plan Assessment" for Sybil in a few weeks, on
February 5th, and we intend fully to speak our mind there
about what *we see* as the horror and unfairness of the threat
hanging over Sybil, to plead for patience and to urge once
again, very strongly that Sybil's medication be changed.
Sybil's' team view this CPA meeting as the occasion for
Sybil to decide her future and make a decision as to whether
she "moves on" or not. In that respect, however much *we*
look forward to this opportunity, it is a black date on the
calendar for Sybil, who, in the best of circumstances over
the years, has always dreaded the formal meetings and
reviews that focus on her so intensely and force her to make
declarations.

Despite Hazel's disturbing phone call, the recent
visit, mid-January, has cheered us up, and since I have a
meeting of my Women's Studies Group on the coming
Saturday, I rationalise that I can skip seeing Sybil this
weekend. Molly, with her busy social life, makes a similar
decision not to go. Neil goes by himself on Saturday and
recounts his visit to me in the evening.

"THE THING INSIDE MY HEAD"

When I arrived, she was quite agitated and found difficulty in sitting for a long period and would have to go out of the room. The previous weekend she'd been much the same when we had arrived, but in the course of our visit she had steadily become more composed. However, on this visit, she stayed at the same level of agitation throughout. At one point, she said to me, "I'm afraid," and I said to her then, and a few other times in the course of my visit, that she must try and talk to someone—the sort of thing I'd said to her on other occasions, to encourage her not to bottle up her difficult feelings. She promised—in fact she went off at one point, to find someone, one of the staff, I think, and may have spent a few minutes with them.

I had brought with me the photographs from our New Zealand trip, but she didn't feel that she wanted to look at them. I stayed a lot longer than I had intended because of her condition, up till dinner time, and I said I was willing to stay till after she had finished and talk to her again, but she didn't want me to. Generally speaking, we had always put things to her and gone along with doing them the way she wanted.

When I left, she gave me a hug, but it was a very decidedly strong hug, quite different than hugs she'd given on visits before, not at all gentle. Before I left, when she had gone to the dining room, I spoke to one of the male nurses and asked that somebody take some time to talk things over in the evening with Sybil; I told him that Sybil had said she was "afraid", and that, to my recollection, she'd never said that to any of us before.

Lois Chaber

We decide we'll call her Sunday evening and try to have a 'good talk'. Circumstances thwart us, however. We find out that the patients' phone is not working and that we can only talk to her on the nurses' line. Sybil knows the nurses don't really like this, and with her strong concerns for others' feelings, especially their possible disapproval, she tells us we can't talk for long, and there is a note of constraint and anxiety in her voice in the very little she does say. Neil chats briefly and hands the phone to me. I can sense so strongly that Sybil wants to get off the line that I say little before bidding goodbye. I manage to squeeze in the anxious, almost pleading "I love you" that I often resort to when I don't know what else to say. She replies, very faintly, "I love you, too," but in a very flat, mechanical tone, and hangs up.

Kim, from Granta, has also been one of Sybil's regular visitors in hospital. She sees Sybil on Monday evening, the day after our disappointing phone call:

> That night Sybil was very chirpy. We watched East Enders together; Sybil made some coffee for me. Sometimes she was "elsewhere" and sometimes she did her OCD repetitions, but it was not the worst that I had ever seen. In fact, she managed to come to the door to see me out. And before that, when I said goodbye, Sybil gave me an especially big hug. I should've picked up on something, but I didn't.

* * *

Just a couple of hours earlier on this same Monday, late in January, I am on the last leg of my journey home from work, riding on a bus from Southgate Station to my house. I am musing to myself that everything has gone particularly well this day: my class, the underground and bus connections, etc. A shiver of contentment passes through me, only to be followed by a sudden breath-accelerating premonition of danger, a gut fear that by being so complacent I am tempting the gods. I immediately start worrying whether Neil or Molly has had a car accident. This is, of course, classic OCD 'magical thinking', but these apprehensive feelings are nevertheless powerful and real to me at this moment—and I am to remember them always.

After a routine evening, Neil and I retire to bed at about 10:45. Suddenly, at about 5:00 am, we hear loud noises coming from downstairs—someone pounding on the door? Or burglars? Neil goes downstairs to investigate, while I lie in bed, still half asleep but on edge. I wait about five minutes; then Neil comes slowly up the stairs, and sits down on the bed, stricken. "What's happened?" I ask, even more terrified. "Has Molly crashed the car?" (she was still out when we went to bed). "No," he answers; "The worst has happened. Sybil is dead!"

He explains, brokenly, that two policemen at the door have conveyed this bald message and given him the number of the County Coroner's office to call in the morning. Initial disbelief in both of us gives way to a torrent of grief, and we both sit there sobbing loudly and uncontrollably.

Molly, who has come home while we were sleeping, is awoken by all the noise, and when we break the news to her, joins us on our bed, all three of us howling in pain and weeping for a long time. Exactly at 9:00 Neil phones the coroner, who confirms the death: Sybil has hung herself from the curtain rail of her cubicle with an electric cord at about 11:50 in the night.

Lois Chaber

Chapter 4: Last Words

Diaries and the Chaplain—Excerpts

> Hopelessness is not simply a contrived
> psychological construct. There is evidence of
> hopelessness and unbearable psychological pain in
> over 90 per cent of suicide notes—the closest we
> get to the suicidal mind.
>
> (Rory C. O'Connor and Noel P. Sheehy, "Suicidal
> Behaviour," *The Psychologist*, vol. 14, no. 1, 21.)

The diary entries here were found, scrawled on pads and barely readable, among Sybil's belongings at the hospital where she died. Most of the entries are undated, but internal clues suggest that they date from sometime in December '98 up to late January '99, just before she took her life. The first group of entries, in particular, is an undifferentiated stream, and it is impossible to know whether it was written in one go or over several days or weeks or exactly which venue she was writing from. Sybil did not leave an 'official' suicide note, but several of these entries could serve in lieu.

* * *

Sometimes I think a thought of pushing the Holy Spirit out through my urine when I pass water. Sometimes I think I push it out through my poo. Sometimes I think a thought of pushing it out through my breath. Sometimes I think a thought of pushing it out when I let off wind. Sometimes I move my hand and for a second I move it to hurt the Holy Spirit. Sometimes I think I've told God through hand movements that what I'm throwing away represents the Holy Spirit so I avoid throwing things. Sometimes I think thoughts of linking the Holy Spirit to sexual ideas, parts of the body or acts or the same with God or Jesus. Sometimes

"THE THING INSIDE MY HEAD"

I feel or get angry with God & wish he didn't reign.
Sometimes I think that God should forgive me. Sometimes I
think or feel like joining the devil. Sometimes I try to hurt
other people through the devil. Sometimes I think thoughts
like 'the devil reigns'. After thinking the thoughts I have to be
sorry because they're bad and not for a[n]other reason.
Sometimes I don't feel sorry. I have to reason with myself
until I feel sorry. Sometimes I doubt or sometimes wish
there isn't a God. If I do this or don't feel negative, I turn to
God. I have to go through thinking and feeling "Love is
stronger than hate, the world has to have been created by
someone, & if love is stronger than hate it has to be a good
God," & this & all other evidence points to the story about
Jesus in the Bible [probably that passage about sinning
against the Holy Spirit] being true & what he preached being
true even if the chaplain said he doesn't believe God
punishes people or sends them to hell it's still sin & I want to
be good. ~~God will be so angry at me, I'll be separated from
God, I won't be in his~~... [broken off] I think bad thoughts of
rudely swallowing or trying to swallow the Holy Spirit when I
swallow. I have to try to bring some of it back up & swallow
without doing what I did before. When I eat sometimes I
think thoughts & maybe do things or try to do things that
signal me, sort of, putting, or asking God to, or saying that it
represents, the Holy Spirit in my mouth, on my food that I'm
putting in or is in my mouth & then can't chew it, and if I do,
I'm chewing the Holy Spirit which is bad, chomping on him &
I have to spit it out. I get thoughts when I'm about to
swallow a drink, that maybe [through] small actions that I'm
saying to God that what I'm about to put in my mouth, or if it
is in, swallow, is or represents the H. S. and I have to put it
back in the cup again and if I swallow it, that's bad, but
sometimes I swallow it, rudely pushing it down, or suck it in,
or putting it into my mouth, rudely, forcibly, & thinking bad
negative thoughts about it & feeling thoughts of evil & power
over God. Sometimes I get a thought/feeling that I'm
standing on It or God or Jesus so I have to move.

When I go to the toilet & I'm trying to undo my
trousers I think thoughts that I'm pointing with my finger &
signing & thinking the vague thoughts it's hard to describe

Lois Chaber

linking It [the H.S.] with my sexual parts & sexual acts. When I pull my knickers down I get feelings/ideas thoughts at the back of my mind almost all the time going 'think it, think it', after I do. When I don't they carry on & it feels so strong & I have to keep moving my head & neck this way & that or I'll think a bad thought.

I try to fight the thoughts but a lot of the time recently it's very hard because what I do to fight them in a short time becomes meaningless or bad itself, so I have to so I think something different. I try to imagine the bad thoughts blocked out. I try to imagine them behind bars. I try to imagine that I've killed them and the devil. I've tried to imagine that my thoughts go into a vacuum. I try to think other thoughts. Often I think bad thoughts about God or about [a symbol representing Jesus Christ], so I try to instead think I hate me or the thoughts.

I get thoughts that I have to go into the toilet or I'll think a bad thought. I think thoughts of joining with the devil, going with the devil selling my soul to the devil. Sometimes I get a horrible thought/feeling that if I do what I'm about to do someone will get hurt.

[These' thoughts' described above are probably the "horrible thoughts" or "bad thoughts" to which Sybil had often referred, without further explanation, for many years. They also may explain many of her actions, like stopping and starting.]

I want to get qualifications and good marks & please & impress & live up to expectations of family & friends including 2 GCSE's. I want to qualify to work with people I want to have place of my own & a boyfriend, not living in & eventually get married. No children. 1 cat & when married for a while a dog. I want to maybe be a psychiatric nurse, or an O.T. [occupational therapist].

I think the repentance is maybe partly (going back to what you said) about fear of losing control over myself or losing my soul or being evil.

"THE THING INSIDE MY HEAD"

[This last sentence seems to be addressed to someone—possibly Rev. Smith, the chaplain, although he does not recall reading this material. Perhaps Sybil was writing out in the diary entries above what she planned to show him. Perhaps it was meant to be a 'confession"?]

I think the bad thoughts maybe partly because I'm scared of God & angry at him & so rebel. I feel stuck in a dark hole of fear & anger at God. I want to get out but feel it's impossible. It's a vicious cycle. I feel scared & angry, > think bad thoughts > feel guilty scared & angry > think bad thoughts. > I make God angry > I feel scared > I feel angry & bad towards God > I think more bad thoughts > I make God angry > etc. *[half the page is torn away here].*

I think it is also to do with rebellion. Part of me really wants to rebel against God. I sometimes see him as maybe a rebellious teenager might see their parents and I think sometimes that's why I think the thoughts & do the actions. Because I've relaxed my beliefs and punishments my thoughts have changed into thoughts about actions, and actions, for example hitting at the Holy Spirit. [I] say 'get movements' because I'm not sure how much control I have over them. Sometimes it feels like a reflex, other times accidental; sometimes I feel compelled to. I don't know. I get other thoughts coming into my head & if I don't react to them correctly it's a sin. These thoughts are like I suddenly get a thought, it feels like it's not my own, telling me that God's spirit is right in front of me, so I have to stop in my tracks, even walk back and check out in my mind whether he's there or not & enforce it in my head & then carefully walk on, trying to think 'good' thoughts.

I don't want to think a bad thought/action ever again but sometimes I feel like there would be something missing without them, I don't know what.

A problem that I've got is that part of me doesn't accept and doesn't want to accept that I'm bad because of the bad thoughts and that I'm really so guilty and that I really have to do my behaviours or I'll be punished and because all that is so scarey for me I run away from it & try to deny it by continuing to think bad thoughts on purpose.

I also join the devil or make pacts with him in my heart or soul or with movements or 'sounds'. I keep on not wanting to do these things & I regret them as soon as I've done them, but I keep on doing them.

I feel I've lost normal thinking. The thought sticks in my head & blocks normal reasoning out. I then have to stop what I'm doing or go back a few steps or start again & check in my head whether the thought is true. If I don't do this I'll be guilty or punished.

* * *

On Tuesday 29th Dec I saw Hazel. I had been feeling very low and hanging on & hoping something Hazel would say would 'click' something in my mind & make things a lot better. I had a good session & she was really understanding & helpful & we had good plans for the future.

She said that OCD is caused by a problem underneath & my bad thoughts & compulsions to hurt people were probably underlying anger that needs to be addressed & worked through & let out 'cause I'm not good at crying (which is true) & I find it hard to talk about my feelings (which is only sometimes true). She suggested art therapy because of this & also because I've got such a mixture of feelings & don't know how I feel. She mentioned, slightly, convos *[conversations?]* in the past about home & stuff, but I'm not sure, I never have been sure, that that has been the cause of my problems. She was saying that I wasn't psychotic. She said that I have to channel the anger & compulsions into better behaviour. She was very supportive & understanding & said the discharge wasn't on Mon [probably her discharge from Eaglehurst back into Granta Housing, Woodland Lodge—which never took place]. It was a good session.

"THE THING INSIDE MY HEAD"

Before the session I had been building up & hoping that Hazel would make things better & I felt that God was telling me she would, through Him, so I had to do all my penances/undoings, etc. until she came. Then she arrived & came upstairs to where I was which saved me from doing the going up & down rituals I was supposed to do but I don't think I did everything I was supposed to do before I went to talk with her in my bedroom so, although I felt like I might have found some relief through her talk & God, looking back I think it might not have been from God because I didn't do all I was supposed to do beforehand.

On Tuesday eve/Wed it finally sunk in that it wasn't going to get right quickly it was going to take quite a while and I didn't know if I was strong enough. I felt depressed trapped & scared so angry at having my life ruined, from 14 [her breakdown in 1992] & again now has enough good come out of it? Am I strong enough? I feel so tired I feel ~~suicidal~~ somewhat trapped & scared.

~~I feel like a bad person. I want to be at peace with myself & God. I talked to the chaplain today. He is SO nice. He said God wasn't angry at me.~~

I feel confused ~~abou~~ about what God wants me to do when I get these bad thoughts. ~~I don't kn always know if I've just thou~~

~~I avoid shaving.~~
I feel ill

* * *

[The following entries all occur *after* Sybil's overdose at Eaglehurst, when she had been returned to Peter Bruff Ward.]

Lois Chaber

12 January 1999: I feel so alone. E H [Eaglehurst] don't want me. P.B. [Peter Bruff] don't want me. I knew E.H. didn't but I thought that the staff at P.B. genuinely cared. Karen [Sybil's keyworker on the ward] seemed so caring. They think I'm a loser, a parasite, an institutionalized waste of time. The worst thing is I feel I haven't got myself, not the Sybil I like, I was, I want, I need I don't like me now I don't recognize myself.

~~God is there but I reject Him, I feel estranged from Him I'm a sinner. My family are there but~~ I use and hurt my family. I take them for granted I do care and love them but I don't think so much as they do me so I feel very guilty. I'm scared of hurting them I feel so guilty.

~~I use my friends. WHO AM I!!!! I feel so cold, selfish, & wooden, loveless. I feel very guilty. I'm scared of hurting them. I feel so guilty I use my friends.~~

I feel a shell of my former self. How did I get like this? Why?

Even Hazel is very angry & fed up & disappointed with me she is on the verge of giving up. She was so cold today I was just thinking about it. I can't talk to her now. Who can I go to? I can't go to God.

I'm a sinner and I keep on sinning I don't know how to turn around that's why I want to kill myself. I feel so alone. I want someone to put their arms around me and comfort me and be there, always be there & not judge but love me for me not themselves (like mum, I know that sounds cruel & ungrateful but I'm not ungrateful & it isn't all for her).

What's Karen going to think

I FEEL LONELY

"THE THING INSIDE MY HEAD"

15 January: I've had a good day considering. I still feel estranged from the nurses and like they are not truly on my side. Karen is doing my head in. She really is. She keeps going on about how I'm an adult which really annoys me because its like she's saying I'm behaving like a child, like I'm being naughty. It's a criticism, which I don't take well. Also, maybe it's because the truth hurts because although I am not doing what she thinks I am doing I still feel like a teenager a minor & don't want to be treeted like an adult. I've still got that problem of wanting people to mother me.

I feel so frustrated because no client in here really likes me they pity me or laugh at me because I'm weird but I can't stop being weird yet. I'm angry at Karen because she keeps saying that they can support [me] but its me who has to do it which I take as a criticism & judgement and maybe I shouldn't but she obviously doesn't think much of me I feel so disappointed & frustrated that she is like this. She was so nice, now Dr. Smith & [Dr.] Kent have turned her against me. I don't feel like I can talk to her I'll try again, maybe it will be better.

I hope the nurses don't expect too much of me cause I've had such a good day I hope I don't have worse days until I can handle it. When I say I've had a 'good day' it's still been really hard really frightening at times and touch and go. I have to take each second at a time It's really scarey & lonely when you don't know how you are going to cope with the next day and how its going to be still hard.

Positives
Warm Fuzzies
Barbara [a nurse] – always kind
David [unclear whether he and others below are staff or patients] – speaks to me & kind
Charles – speaks to me & nice
Barbara – caring kind sweet > I give back.
Tomorrow is a fresh new day
Goodnight

Lois Chaber

[The exact order of the remaining entries in this notepad is unclear; Sybil's writing becomes increasingly chaotic]

Thoughts that are a problem

1. Bad thoughts coming into my head
2. compelled to think bad thoughts
3. compelled to do bad things
4. compelled to say bad things (bad = blasphemous/devil worship)
5. fear of thinking bad thoughts
8. compelled to hurt someone
9. Trying to hurt someone in my head
10. Wanting to hurt someone
11. Feeling that I have to do something I don't want to do (like stand up, or anything) else I'll think bad/do bad/say bad/hurt someone/feel like hurting someone etc.
12. fear of contaminating people with germs
13. fear of getting germs to contaminate with *obsession
14. feeling like/that (I don't know) I'm going to murder someone
15. Feeling that I should deny myself even when I haven't done anything wrong
16. Feeling angry & frustrated & anxious & lashing out by thinking/doing bad things

"THE THING INSIDE MY HEAD"

[Scrawled across a whole page]

I'M ANGRY THAT I HAD TO GET ILL

again why did I have to get ill in the first place when I was 14

WHY?

I feel suicidal. I feel like I can't carry on. I'm scared every day & night. I feel so alone. The nurses I can't talk to them & when I do they won't help or don't understand. There is this great block between God & I so I won't can't tell Him help me. I hate myself. I hate being like this I want to die please let me die soon.

I'M BORED!
& FED UP

God has left me that's partly why I can't get to sleep

16 January: I feel *soooo* angry at the nurses because they don't like me & Karen because she is horrible & convinced that I'm putting on an act. Then she tells me to speak to a nurse if I need to but keeps on saying I don't need to & when I do she tells me to distract myself & she is really unsympathetic because Dr. Smith & Dr. Kent have changed her, she was so lovely & kind when I first came.

I FEEL SO ANGRY AT THE NURSES & HELPLESS I NEED THEM I FEEL *[Two words are illegible]* ANXIOUS & AGITATED & FIDGETY & ANGRY & FRUSTRATED I FEEL DIRTY

I'm angry at Dr. Smith & Dr. Kent. I hate them they are so cold they don't care how I feel. They seem to think I got myself into hospital & like this on purpose but that is so wrong my life was going so well. I never wanted to go backwards I tried to kill myself because I was desperate & very unhappy I still am unhappy. I feel lonely because everyone's angry at me for trying to kill myself even Hazel. The only ones who are not angry with me are my family & they are the ones who should be. They love me so much & are so good to me. I don't deserve it & I feel so guilty. I don't give as much back. I do love them. I feel so guilty. I don't deserve all their dedication I've put them through so much pain all these years. But I haven't meant to. I've often meant the opposite.

I hope I can see the chaplain often I feel so agitated & in a cage.

Ralph [her CBT therapist] will be really disappointed with me & angry. I'm dreading seeing him. I'm worried about the CPA [Care Plan Agreement] meeting. I want to be at peace with God. I wish Hazel was here now.

I want to be at peace with God I think the chaplain was here.

I feel so fed up
I'm scared

* * *

[All that remains is a tiny notepad with a few words scrawled in pencil on each page. There is no telling how long after January 16th she scribbled these words or how close to her death.]

I AM SO FUCKING ANGRY

Fri, January: I feel hyperactive I feel like I want to tidy wash clean write & anything hyper How can [I] relax I'm talking to myself. I feel I've lost the part that cares in me; the

part that needs to serve. I'm lost I've lost my love of God.
Why did all this have to happen I don't know what to do or
where I'm going I feel like I'm floating, unsure, no base for
me (as in where I'm going) aghhh help what can I do
tomorrow laundry OH NO! I'm terrified of all the germs in
there they are going everywhere.

I don't know what's God's voice & what isn't HELP

HELP

Sat, January: I'M ANGRY

bedtime: I'm frustrated at the thoughts I'm frustrated
because of my behaviour I have to do which then is a
nuisance—makes me look strange I look strange in other
ways I feel like harming myself I want to die

HELP

I want to stand up & look pretty like a young lady I
feel so angry that my life has fallen apart so but even worse
is the thought that it's my fault. My problems are
complicated

I hope tomorrow is better. Goals for tomorrow? Too
much!

I want to

*[Sybil's writings, as far as we know, end here. We gained
access to her diaries only after her death. In the autumn of
2000, I sent these last two diaries, above, to Sybil's
'chaplain', Reverend Smith, to read and comment on.]*

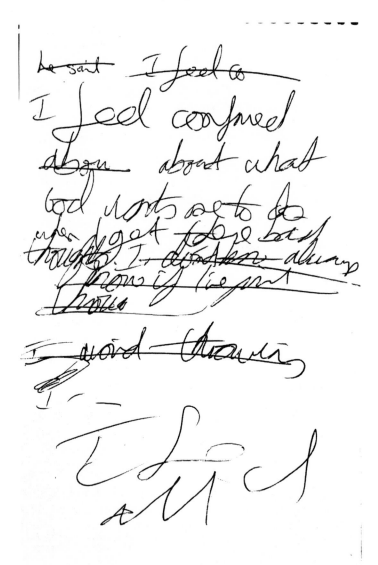

From Sybil's diary (See Dec. 29th, 'Tues eve/Wed')

"THE THING INSIDE MY HEAD"

An Informal Conversation with the Reverend Canon Richard Smith: October 2000

Rev. Canon Smith is the Senior Chaplain to the Essex Rivers Healthcare Trust, embracing Colchester, Clacton and Harwich. He holds an MA in Theology and one in Psychotherapy. Seven years ago, he kindly agreed to talk to me informally in his office about some aspects of his relationship with Sybil. His comments, recorded by me and slightly abridged below, represent his personal, off the cuff views at that time, rather than a formal written statement.

When did you first meet Sybil and how long did you have contact with her?

I met Sybil two years prior to her dying. I think, on reflection, it could have been very helpful if I could have known her longer than that. I met Sybil through Hazel making appointments for her to see me. Partly, I believe, Hazel was thinking that because I am also a qualified psychotherapist I might be able to give a psychotherapeutic input into Sybil's care. I think Sybil saw it more as wanting to see a Christian chaplain and just wanted to talk through how she saw the spiritual component to her illness. She wasn't actually on Peter Bruff Ward at the time, but she would come here to the hospital to see me in this office regularly, once a month, for a while... Very often I wouldn't see her because something had happened; something would get in the way etc. When she became really poorly, I used to see her on the ward whenever I could, and sometimes she wanted to see me and sometimes she didn't, so then it was dependent on how she was feeling at the time. But that... would be within the context of illness.

The $64,000 question is: what did you make of Sybil's 'voices' or 'thoughts' that she at times thought were the voice of God? Do you know of other cases where this has happened and what is your interpretation of the voices?

Lois Chaber

I never felt at the time that I knew Sybil, at the time I actually talked to her, that there was any time when she was psychotic. I think it is quite unusual for psychosis to be a symptom of OCD. I have to say to you that I have never met anybody so severely suffering from OCD as Sybil. In a sense it is a bit difficult for me to be able to comment on the voices from a medical perspective. This was my own interpretation—that when she talked about voices, they were more like intrusive thoughts, but I guess they can become so intrusive and so prominent that they could almost be voices in a sense. But I do want this to be put on the record, that I never ever thought of her as being psychotic.

Did I think they were voices of God? Well, the honest answer is 'probably not'. When I was reading this typed material [of extracts from the diaries] and the material there [in the last notebooks], I found it easier to reach a psychological than a spiritual understanding of what was going on for her. I think people with OCD, obsessional people, one of the problems they have early on in their lives is that they have a huge super-ego. And so they get into a state where they feel they have to severely judge themselves; it's like a big policeman in their head: everything they do is wrong, everything they think is wrong, thoughts become bad, etc.

One thing that stood out for me there was that Sybil seemed to identify her problems from about six years old; that is quite a significant age for a child, for a boy or a girl, because they would have just gone through the Oedipus complex and gone through all of that, a huge judgmental period. I don't really know what was going on with Sybil when she was six years old, but I think it was at that age that this super-ego started to attach itself to her and she started to feel guilty or bad about things. I might want to interpret that in terms of object relations rather than in terms of religion as such; I mean early relationships with parents, siblings, etc.

"THE THING INSIDE MY HEAD"

Now I thought long and hard before saying that to you because I know you have been through enough pain and turmoil, and you don't want any more thrown at you. It is not about blaming parents or scapegoating parents because I don't know any perfect parents—my parents weren't perfect... I think God is in there because I think Sybil was a religious person who genuinely had a relationship with God, but it might not always have been possible for her to see God as a loving parent, to see God as a loving father, because once the super-ego starts to get in the way, then He becomes the judge, He becomes somebody who always condemns her, He becomes somebody who is always saying you must do this and you mustn't do that.

What, then, would you say in response to Sybil's question, posed at one point in the journal, "How do you know when it's God talking to you and not yourself thinking or your illness?" Do you believe that God talks to anyone?

My own experience of God is that he usually talks to me through other people and through my prayer-life and my meditations. Sybil never actually asked me that question, or maybe she did (I can't quite remember), but I know the way I would answer that, and it would be the same to Sybil as to anyone else. If you are having thoughts that are causing you distress and hurting you, those thoughts couldn't possibly be from God because my own understanding and my own relationship with God tells me that he would not put thoughts in my head that would cause me to harm others, to harm myself or to make myself feel bad about myself... But what could well happen is this: If you have an image of God as being a judge in the sky, somebody who is quite condemning, somebody who is there to tick you off, ... to discipline you in some way all the time, you might project that onto God, and that might be projected into you, and you would feel that this is your God. It is not my God, it is not my understanding. I know there are many passages in the Bible that seem to suggest a God like that, but I would actually argue that these are more about how people were seeing God for themselves at that time...

Lois Chaber

How I used to try to be with Sybil is this: I wouldn't really engage in intellectual arguments with her. I didn't really want get taken down the line of discussing theological concepts with her. I think that actually that's not a terribly good idea with obsessional people; it distracts them from thinking about their feelings; it distracts them from trying to become who they are meant to become. I tried to create a threat-safe space for Sybil in which she could just *be*, but my frustration, and to some extent anger, is that I felt it was too late for me really to be able to do that. I think Sybil had become so severely ill even two years prior to her death that it really limited what kind of relationship I could form with her and what I could do for her... Sometimes we'd just laugh and joke. She liked talking about her animals quite a lot and the cat at home... It sounds silly but what I tried to do was this: OK, I'm the priest, I'm the minister, I'm the chaplain, so what I tried to convey, if I represented anything about God, is just the concept of a loving God. He didn't create the illness, and in that illness (it's my own theological belief coming out now), He suffers too. My feeling is that God just tried to be with her in that illness somehow...

So a lot of my ministering to Sybil was just trying to be with her without trying to be too interpretive. She used to ask me things like, did I think she was wicked, did I think this or that was the devil, and I always replied that I didn't think it was the devil, partly because I didn't want her to get obsessed with the idea of the devil and evil and so on. I certainly with all my heart tried to convey to her that I didn't in any way see her as wicked. She was a beautiful, loving person. But it was very difficult to put her in touch with her own love and her own beauty and her own self-worth. Too much had gone on, including the various treatments she had had. I am not condemning any of those treatments, but my own feeling with OCD is that the earlier you put somebody in therapy the better it is for them...

... I wonder whether she could have had a therapist with a more spiritual perspective. I think very often the

"THE THING INSIDE MY HEAD"

problem with analytical therapy or the medical model is that it doesn't acknowledge the spiritual component, or if does, it simply says, 'We'll call the chaplain, and he'll say a little prayer or something,' without really entering the therapeutic relationship. My frustration, and I have repeated it now several times, is that I didn't really feel that I was engaged soon enough...

What always stays in mind is a conversation that I had with her shortly before she died. She took part in one of our chaplain's groups that we were having on Peter Bruff Ward at the time. She came out after a while, and when the group finished, I came out. She seemed quite cheery, more cheery, strangely enough, than I had seen her for some time. We talked about the animals. I had just taken on looking after a dog for a while, and she wanted to know all about Charlie the doggy. She wanted to tell me about her cat, and she became quite hysterical, laughing-wise; she really got into a sense of humour, and we had a really nice conversation, with which, from my own selfish point of view I suppose, I was very pleased. And so my last memory of Sybil was of her laughing, which was not a very common experience, and then I was amazed just a couple of days later to hear what happened. She had been quite distressed earlier on that day, but sometimes Sybil would get a glimpse of something that gave her hope, although it didn't stay for very long, and I think she had just got one of those glimpses; she seemed lighter and just happier for a short while... When she laughed her whole faced changed, didn't it? You got a glimpse of who she could have been, what she might have been...

May I ask you specifically about the sin against the Holy Spirit that Sybil was obsessed with? She talked to me a couple of years before she died about this passage. It's Mark 3:28-29:

> *Verily I say unto you, All sins shall be forgiven unto the sons of men, and blasphemies werewith soever they shall blaspheme.*

Lois Chaber

But he that shall blaspheme against the Holy Ghost hath never forgiveness, but is in danger of eternal damnation.

I have never actually read a satisfactory explanation of what the sin against the Holy Spirit is supposed to be about, what Jesus actually meant. Lots of people have come up with explanations, but my own feeling about the sin of the Holy Spirit is that it probably means that when you have real evidence within yourself of the power of God, of the love of God, and you still deny that, then that is the sin against the Holy Spirit... I think sometimes, maybe just once in our lives, maybe never in our lives, people get a real glimpse of God. It doesn't necessarily mean that they are going to accept him, that they are going to love him; they might in actual fact look him straight in the face and say, 'So what, but I don't want to know'. That is my interpretation of the sin against the Holy Spirit.

There is a place in Sybil's diary where she refers to "that passage" with a question mark and writes the word "forgiveness" with a question mark. She must have talked to you about forgiveness.

She did talk to me about forgiveness, and what I remember saying to Sybil about forgiveness is: God could shout from the rooftops that you are forgiven and loved, but if you are not prepared to forgive yourself, then in a sense it will make very little difference because one of the things we have to do is to learn to love ourselves... It is not always easy, then, for us to see any good in ourselves, to be able to forgive ourselves... If you are looking for spiritual symptoms of OCD, that would be top of my list. OCD people are quite judgmental about others, but that is because they are quite judgmental about themselves as well. However, looking in terms of object relations and how you first relate, if a child sometimes feels that he is always having to work hard to please, that could, of course, mean that he has to work hard to please God...

"THE THING INSIDE MY HEAD"

... I think in the diary somewhere Sybil said she wanted to do well in her exams, she wanted to do well in this, that and the other, which again is typical of people with obsessional personalities; they are always looking for accolades. It doesn't matter how many accolades they get, they still need another one because they are always looking for this affirmation. In a sense, there is nothing on this earth that we could do that would be good enough for God, but then we don't have to do anything because God loves us unconditionally.

... Jung was always talking about having to unite the opposites and to bring them together, the dark and the light sides. He actually talked about the dark side of God, which I find interesting, but which, obviously, as a Christian, I find a very difficult concept to actually comprehend. But Jung also went on to talk about the 'shadow'. You, me, we present to people what we feel they want to see about us; we present what we perceive as being the good in us and everything else gets repressed, whether it is to do with our sexuality or whatever, anything in us that we feel wouldn't be acceptable out there gets repressed. And of course when you do this, you get a bigger and bigger 'shadow'.

Obsessional people very often try very hard to present a good boy or good girl image all the time, and, of course, there is a huge price to pay for that because all the stuff that you perceive as being bad about yourself just gets more and more repressed, and this is like a volcano just waiting to go off. With Sybil, I suppose there was one huge 'shadow', and it all got mixed up and may well have got so psychologically deep that it was difficult for her. There was lots of scary stuff for her that she thought was really bad, and some of it may well have been to do with sex, something I never touched on with Sybil because I wasn't able to build up a deep enough relationship to be able to do that. Very often with obsessional people there are fears about sex and about perceptions around that.

Lois Chaber

Yes, she talked very often in her diary about feeling guilty over masturbation and couldn't find anyone to talk to about it.

I am a priest saying this to you, but I don't have any problems saying masturbation is one of the most normal outlets that boys, girls, adults have, and yet it has so many bad connotations attached to it. I felt there were huge things going wrong for Sybil about sex. Spiritually, what I try to say to people as well is that God created us to be sexual beings—and I am not one of the people who feels that God just created sex for procreation; he created it as a vehicle of love and pleasure and beauty and all of those things as well. I would like to have conveyed that to Sybil but I never really had the opportunity to do that.

Did she ever talk to you about the devil?

Yes, she did, and I don't think I gave a satisfactory answer because the ploy I took with Sybil was not to really engage her in talking about the devil. Now, whether that was right or wrong is debatable, but my experience working with such people as Sybil is that blaming the devil is almost comforting, in a way. If you are saying something is the devil, you are saying it is not part of me, it's got nothing to do with me, so if I go off and masturbate, it is all the devil's work; it's got nothing to do with the fact that, if I could come to terms with it, I just enjoy masturbating... So anything good is to do with God, and anything bad is to do with the devil. I think this is what Jung's challenge was about. If we look at the 'shadow', there are a lot of potentially good things in there; sex doesn't have to be bad.

Did you read at the beginning of the turquoise notepad the litany of thoughts about the Holy Spirit—about pushing the Holy Spirit out through her nose, her urine, etc.? What do you think made her think along those lines?

"THE THING INSIDE MY HEAD"

... If she was feeling in some way that she was being taken over by bad thoughts, by the devil, then I suppose she might well logically reach the conclusion that anything to do with the Holy Spirit, to do with God, she must wash out through her urine etc.

The way I interpreted those pages was that these were the sins against the Holy Spirit that she thought she was being punished for; these were the 'bad thoughts' that constituted her 'sin' in her mind.

Yes, I think that would make sense because one explanation of the sin against the Holy Spirit is the denial of the Holy Spirit when you have evidence of the Holy Spirit being there. But I also think they are bizarre obsessional thoughts, and I think there is a tendency for obsessional people to always think the worst and always believe the worst, not about other people, interestingly, but about themselves... It was almost useless to say to Sybil things like 'God loves you' because in a sense you actual trigger off a neurosis simply by saying that because then she will get into this philosophical, argumentative mode within her mind saying 'God doesn't love me', etc., etc... In my naivety, I guess I just believed that if I sat here as the chaplain, as the priest, and if I could express some kind of love for her, then it might suggest to her that God loves her. My own experience of God has usually come through the love of other people and being in a relationship with other people, which was something Sybil found very difficult to do. My feeling is that where it started to go wrong for her is that she found it difficult to be in relationships with other people because she had such a poor self-image.

At one point in her turquoise diary she says something about seeing herself in relationship to God as similar to a rebellious teenager. Did you suggest something like this to her or do you think anyone else did?

Lois Chaber

I certainly don't ever remember having a conversation with Sybil in which I would have suggested that she was a rebellious teenager because I never actually saw her as being that. What I did see in Sybil was the child, the suffering, child and I think that the problem as I saw it was that we were never really dealing with the adult Sybil. The adult Sybil would come through some of the time, but for most of the time you were dealing with somebody in child ego-state. It was really the pain of childhood that you were dealing with. If you looked at her face, for example, she seemed very childlike—not childish—but childlike.

I guess she felt it was easier to be angry with God and project her anger onto God when really she wanted to be angry with her parents. I am uncomfortable in saying that to you, but it is probably a true psychological assessment. She found it difficult because she wanted your approval all the time... If you are feeling angry towards your parents, it's quite easy to project that anger onto God because it is easier to be angry with Him. If that goes on and on, then eventually it could be conceived in a person's mind that this God is going to answer back at some point and be angry in turn. So maybe she wanted to be the rebellious teenager to you.

Yes, I accept that. In her last weeks in Peter Bruff Ward, did she ever talk to you at all about her suicide attempt in January, the overdose, or the nurses' treatment of her, the way they were behaving to her in the last few weeks?

Yes, she did; she spoke of at least one suicide attempt. She also spoke about feeling that the nurses were not really giving her the attention she felt that she needed at that time, and she did that within a few days of the last time I saw her...

I responded by going to see the nurses and conveying my concern that Sybil seemed more distressed than I had ever seen her. They responded sympathetically to that by indicating to me that, yes, they understood what was going on, etc... I think the nurses took on board Sybil's distress. I think they were attempting some new medication at that time... I will put on record that I never felt or had any indication that the nursing staff or anyone else was being neglectful or deliberately neglecting Sybil.

I have the impression from reading her journals that the nurses were perhaps angry beneath the surface at her because of her January suicide attempt, that they somehow saw that as a betrayal of their efforts.

I don't know, but I can imagine they might be... Although you try to do all that the textbook says to you about what you should do and what you shouldn't do, if there was anger, and I couldn't actually say there was, I think it could well have been about their own frustration with her. They were really running out of ideas on how to help Sybil, and I could empathise with that because I too was. You used to have conversations with Sybil, and you used to feel that you were saying all the right things or the things that you should be saying to her, but it never seemed to make any difference, so that could be quite frustrating at times.

As a minister, what could you say about Sybil's final thoughts and her suicide? Do you consider her, from your religious perspective, as a sinner or not?

Certainly not. I never thought of Sybil as a sinner—well, no more a sinner than anyone else is—and certainly don't think of her in that context now. As far as the suicide, I am not really convinced that she ever intended to commit suicide. I think it was more an acting out of crying for help that went badly wrong. I always felt that in spite of all the pain she was experiencing and the darkness she was going through, there was always a spark of hope, something about life that she wanted to hold onto and enjoy. As to where she is now, I have no doubts in my mind that she is happy, she is at peace, and she is able to be what she wants to be with God. I wouldn't say that was God's ultimate plan for her because I don't think God wants any of us to commit suicide, but when you think about the depth of Sybil's despair and the seriousness of her illness and the problems with her thought processes, no one would be totally surprised that it happened...

My own observations of those people suffering from OCD, and from what I have read about it, is that very few OCDs actually commit suicide, which you might consider odd when you think of the amount of psychological pain that they endure. But very often with OCDs, their obsession is about staying safe, and suicide would be contrary to their thinking.

I saw her as a beautiful child; in many ways, the great sadness was that she was never able to see that for herself.

"THE THING INSIDE MY HEAD"

Endnote to 'Last Words':

My friend, Susan Teich, who has studied Jung in depth, made the following observations after reading this chapter:

I made a mental connection between Sybil's thoughts regarding God and defecation (i.e. pushing the Holy Spirit out through her "poo") and thoughts that Carl Jung had regarding God and defecation. In his autobiographical memoir, "Memories, Dreams, and Reflections," Jung recorded his torment as a child when thoughts intruded upon his mind of God sitting high above the world on a golden throne defecating upon the Cathedral at Basil. Jung's account may be of some small aid in putting Sybil's thoughts into a larger context. Jung imagined that God himself was doing the defecating, and Sybil imagined it was her own defecation that pushed out God, but in both instances the horror to the imaginer was the close association of God and faeces. It is particularly interesting that the child Jung thought, like Sybil, that he was committing the sin against the Holy Spirit, the unforgivable sin.

Jung resolved his dilemma by deciding that God had put these thoughts into his mind, and that he did so to test Jung's obedience to God. Jung, by thinking thoughts that he most passionately did not want to think, but then had to think because they were put there by God, showed his obedience to God, and, further, provided God with an opportunity to show his Divine forgiveness and grace by forgiving Jung for the thoughts. Perhaps Sybil's excremental thoughts were not entirely a manifestation of her illness. Rather, it was Sybil's illness that prevented her from choosing a meaning for them that would not torment her, as Jung was able to do.

Lois Chaber

Chapter 5: Post Mortem

> A little-known statistic reveals more suicides occur in hospitals than at home.
>
> (Gravitz, Obsessive Compulsive Disorder, p. 198.)

> About 1,300 suicides by psychiatric patients over the past five years could have been prevented by better health service care, an inquiry reported.
>
> (The Guardian Weekly, March 22-28, 2001, p. 10.)

There is a complicated aftermath to the death of any person that endows the deceased with a ghostly, lingering 'life'. Not only was Sybil still 'there' in the minds and hearts of many long after her demise, but her life and death were inevitably rehearsed and variously interpreted in the medical and state procedures that follow on from a suicidal death in an NHS hospital—the hospital's inquiry and report, the official inquest, and so on (whose intricacies we had, naïvely, never imagined before this tragedy)—as well as in the condolences, the funeral eulogies and other personal responses. Our family's post mortem 'journey' through these events was startling and harrowing.

* * *

This book as a whole attempts to understand the *multiple and various "causes"* of Sybil's tragedy, and, as part of this, it acknowledges the unfortunate role that her family (especially myself) and its experiences played in Sybil's long and severe illness. However, our family also feels that particular circumstances in the NHS care environment of Sybil's last weeks facilitated to some extent the *effectual* 'when', 'where' and 'how' of her death, and that more could have been done to prevent it happening.

"THE THING INSIDE MY HEAD"

To be sure, some people will say, "Well, she was bent on suicide and would have found another way to do it." However, this commonplace attitude has been publicly deplored by the National Schizophrenia Fellowship (now known as *Rethink*) in their 1999 report, *'One in Ten': A Report... into Unnatural Deaths of People with Schizophrenia,* whose observations and recommendations have implications for treatment of *all* the mentally ill. The report asserts: "Severe mental illness is not a hopeless cause from which people never get better, and suicide and unnatural death is an outcome that can be greatly reduced." An even more extensive report produced later the same year, *Safer Services: National Confidential Inquiry into Suicide and Homicide by People with Mental Illness,* also rejects that fatalistic cliché:

It is a commonly held view in mental health services that suicides by people with mental disorder are often impossible to prevent because of the unpredictability of suicide and the high risk that is inherent in most disorders. Our data do not support this pessimistic view.

In fact, the *Safer Services* report found that thirty per cent of in-patient suicides, in particular, were preventable. In keeping with our deep down faith in Sybil, we believe that if she had lived to attend the important Care Plan Assessment scheduled for February 5th (sadly, this became the day of her funeral), that occasion would have been an opportunity for us to suggest some important changes in her treatment, including her medication; urge that problems underlying her fear of leaving the ward be dealt with and, most of all, help mediate the vexed issue of her looming 'discharge'. This, in conjunction with the input of her team, could have made a difference to her prospects, *as had the 'case conference' for Sybil in which we participated at Clacton Hospital in the*

485

spring of 1996, and which opened the door to her behavioural therapy and so much more in Clacton. Instead, taking part in the bureaucratic procedures attendant upon her death, we were to learn of decisions concerning Sybil's care that we felt—and still feel—were misguided.

A highly illuminating four-part Channel 4 series, "Why Doctors Make Mistakes," to which I have referred earlier, provides a larger context for the errors of judgment that we feel were made in Sybil's case. This October 2000 series exposed, through the examination of sample cases from the UK and the US in which doctors, nurses, and other medical professionals "confessed" to errors of various kinds, just how common mistakes are in medical treatment. It examined the culture that fosters these mistakes and their cover-ups—especially the "myth of infallibility" that surrounds medical personnel, doctors and surgeons in particular, thwarting attempts to learn from mistakes and improve.

According to this television documentary and its accompanying booklet, one in every ten persons in the UK becomes the victim of a medical incident in which something goes wrong or is done wrongly and the patient suffers harm. At the date of the programme, there were 850,000 such "adverse events" a year in the UK and approximately 40,000 deaths as a result. The programme booklet points out that this is more than the total numbers who die from breast cancer or lung cancer each year. Similar problems exist in the US.

Take the means of Sybil's death—she hanged herself from the curtain rails of one of the ward's cubicles: It is a terrible irony that Sybil should have died in the mental health hospital ward where she was put after her overdose, *purposely* to provide the safest possible environment for a suicidally-minded individual—the very Peter Bruff Ward that she idealised and clung to as a safe haven in her diaries, a "womb" to which she could return when the stresses of trying to live a normal life with her illness overwhelmed her. The simple fact that the ward at that time had not been provided with collapsible curtain rails was a major factor in her death and is a testimony to a disinclination to change and act on the part of the NHS, which the programme booklet highlights under the heading "Preventable Suicides". According to its statistics, between 1996 and 1998, eighty-one patients on mental health wards took their lives by hanging themselves from either curtain or shower rails. In 1971, a report had warned of this tendency and recommended substituting collapsible rails, which give way under the weight of a person. But in 1999 an inquiry found that hanging was still the most common form of suicide on mental health wards. "Why," asks an article in *The Guardian* discussing this phenomenon (10 May 1999), "non-collapsible rails are still in use needs investigating."

We learned only little by little, in the painful aftermath, about the other preventable circumstances of Sybil's tragic death at age twenty.

* * *

That is not to say that we, her family, felt blameless. Guilt, justified or not, almost invariably accompanies grief. That Tuesday morning, January 26th, Molly and I bemoan aloud our failure to have gone with Neil on what was to be his last visit to Sybil. Would it have made a difference to see the whole family together, united in love and sympathy for her? We will never know. Neil berates himself for not having really 'focused' on Sybil's situation in ways he had done at earlier times—largely a result of his preoccupation with the diminished position on the Heathrow project in which he found himself upon returning from New Zealand. And I succumb to an avalanche of 'if onlys': *If only we'd known Sybil's feelings, however irrational, about the nurses; if only we had transferred Sybil to a private institution, like the Priory Hospital so very close to us in Southgate, specialising in mental health care, even if it meant re-mortgaging or selling our home; if only I had volunteered to sleep at the hospital near Sybil, to be always by her until the review, if only...*

Lois Chaber

The sympathetic middle-aged bereavement counsellor provided by Barnet Social Services tries her best to listen and to comfort, but she is not in the end particularly effective for us, and Molly impatiently drops out of the counselling process. What does enable us to hold together physically and emotionally is the preparation for Sybil's funeral, a practical focus for our grief as we determine to pay appropriate tribute to our daughter.

For me, teaching offers temporary relief. Having to concentrate intently on holding the attention of my twenty-five Composition students at the American College—there only because it is a required class—forces me to shut out the painful awareness of Sybil's death during each two hour session. In fact, my first day back, a difficult but satisfying lesson pushes thoughts of our family tragedy back into the far recesses of my mind. Only as the students file out of the classroom am I suddenly and brutally recalled to reality: "Sybil is dead!" A wave of hot then cold flashes is followed by my stomach lurching on a roller coaster descent. Our bereavement counsellor later tells me this is "shock".

Also sustaining me is Neil's support—the absence of reproaches to me about my flawed mothering. In fact, mutual tenderness sustains us both. I have been debunking some clichés, but the proverbial 'absence makes the heart...' worked for Neil and me, his Nigeria years away having increased our intimacy (ironically) and our appreciation of each other.

Neil, already unhappy in his job at Heathrow, finds returning to the workplace almost unbearable, and can only work half days for some time. In the coming weeks and months he manages and diffuses his pain by meticulously organising every single document pertaining to Sybil's illness and death in a series of thick black ring-binders. Molly is extremely torn up and totally unable to concentrate on her Art Foundation Course. She has to request an extension for a required essay and puts off choosing a university and a course for the coming year.

The process of discovering more about Sybil and her death begins when Neil, helped by his brother Ian who has thoughtfully flown over from New Zealand with his wife, musters all his stoicism to travel to Clacton to collect Sybil's belongings. As he pulls into the hospital drive his heart literally stops for a second—and then restarts with a violent jerk. Included in Sybil's personal effects are her diaries and other revelatory papers and effects, which open a window onto her mind that, sadly, we did not have earlier. Molly starts reading one of her 1997 diaries and is shocked and devastated by how many times Sybil expresses suicidal thoughts, even during a period when we thought her so well in herself. Neil, sorting out Sybil's financial estate, finds that shortly before her death she made out and sent four large cheques (£100 each—a very large amount for someone on income support) to four different charities.

Meanwhile, expressions of sympathy and grief flow in, through e-mail, post, and phone. That over two thousand, three hundred pounds are raised for the two mental health charities we nominate, 'Mind' and 'Obsessive Action' (now called OCD-Action) testifies to how many people's lives Sybil's touched on. On the phone with Barbara, the director of the local advocacy group, Tendring Mental Health Support, I blurt out, brokenly, "If only she could have known how she was so beloved"—but Barbara wisely interjects, "That was part of her illness, wasn't it, that she couldn't digest that, couldn't accept it." Many persons involved in Sybil's past care—from the Bethlem Royal, from Jacques Hall, from Peter Bruff Ward and from Granta and Eaglehurst, travel to Southgate for the funeral tribute.

The funeral becomes an opportunity for those of us close to her to proclaim the meaning for each of Sybil's life and death. As we have tried to do for so many years, we defer to Sybil by deciding at once that it must be a Christian funeral, even though Neil and I are at best agnostics, with the Reverend Richard Smith, Sybil's spiritual confidant from Clacton Hospital, to lead the service. I suggest that Molly read from Sybil's nostalgic essay, "The Beach" (see Part I, Chapter 3) to affirm Sybil's role in the family in happier times. Striving to honour her achievements, when Christopher Keyte, the husband of Sybil's pen pal June and a professional opera singer, offers to sing at the funeral, we choose "Plaisir D'Amour," the tune with which Sybil won the recorder contest so many years ago in Qatar. And we select "Morning" from the Peer Gynt Suite, which Sybil once took so much pride in playing for us on her flute, to lead our guests out from the crematorium.

Neil, with his immeasurably tender feelings for Sybil, takes this opportunity to pay unabashed homage in a eulogy he calls "Shining Star:"

> *In the many messages of support and sympathy Lois, Molly and I have received, in those from people who knew Sybil, certain qualities of her personality are brought out again and again. She is remembered as "loving" and "caring", but almost without exception all who knew her speak of her "gentleness". Yes, Sybil was intelligent and talented and we have the various certificates at home that tell us so, but gentleness and like qualities and the simple direct ability to move others with those qualities are truly her most wonderful achievement.*
>
> *To hold to such qualities through the years of anguish, of mental pain and affliction from the intrusive obsessions of her illness and in a world where aggression so often seems a norm, is truly amazing; it leaves me profoundly humble. To move so many people, whether the sixteen-year old daughter of a friend in Reading or Sybil's eighty-year old great aunt in New York, amazes me. That power of loving*

490

"THE THING INSIDE MY HEAD"

gentleness is a part of our being here now, and of why this week in other places, in churches and synagogues, prayers are being said and candles burning in memory of our Sybil.

In the messages we have received a simple phrase said more than once and from different countries seems so right and has been both painful and delightful because it is so right. These people called Sybil a "shining star". We have taken these words to our hearts: they will never leave us.

Reverend Smith echoes Neil's views of the "gentle" Sybil, but he also mentions the "darkened" forces, both without and within Sybil, that she could not come to terms with. Inevitably, moreover, he uses the occasion to proclaim the general Christian message of resurrection following death, hope in new life succeeding despair, even delicately drawing a parallel between the "angelic" Sybil and Christ, both having suffered much on earth and died before their time.

* * *

After the funeral, the period of greatest stress for us, her family, begins. An excerpt from *Levine on Coroners' Courts,* by Sir Montague Levine and James Pike, obtained from the charity Inquest, articulates our own feelings: "Families and interested parties are particularly, and understandably, aggrieved if a death occurs in a mental hospital... 'How could this have possibly happened in a mental hospital where the patient was admitted primarily because he was a suicide risk?'" Our own dismay is increased when we learn that another suicide, of a fifty-year old depressed woman, had occurred only three weeks earlier on Peter Bruff Ward.

Lois Chaber

Soon, we receive a letter from the Community Mental Health Centre in Clacton inviting us to attend an internal inquiry into Sybil's death, called a "Critical Incident Review," on February 26th. Allowing us, the victim's parents, to participate is, the letter explains, a departure from their usual practice, and we greatly appreciate this. The letter declares that the Review will not be a formal enquiry but rather a learning opportunity to avoid such incidents in the future. We are somewhat wary of this intentionally limited remit; Sybil's death, for us, warrants a formal, evaluative review, with peers from outside Clacton hospital present to guarantee objectivity and thoroughness. To be sure, the Channel 4 series on doctors' mistakes advocates going "Beyond Blame" (the title of the last programme) and establishing a "learning culture" whose main purpose would be to avoid repeating mistakes. However, the programme booklet also cites government research showing that among the things aggrieved patients or their relatives desire from the NHS are an acknowledgment that a mistake has been made and an apology (although it warns, "Nobody apologises in case this lays them open to litigation"). We are never to get such an admission or receive a *formal* apology.

On the day, the conduct of the Review, it seems to us, bears out our suspicions that it will not be thoroughgoing enough and thus limited even as a learning experience. Most of the chief persons involved in Sybil's final care programme are arranged around the edge of a large, neutrally-decorated meeting room, and we are asked not to question what the witnesses say or speak until they have all finished—a frustrating restriction.

To begin with, there is no one here representing The Eaglehurst Rehabilitation Unit and thus no one to emphasise either the fact or the implications of her overdosing in early January—the very *raison d'être* for her readmission to Peter Bruff Ward. Although Hazel, Sybil's beloved Community Psychiatric Nurse, comments that Sybil had given up on herself, she nevertheless insists that for Sybil, self-harm was only a way of coping with distress—particularly distress

492

about "moving on"—not genuinely suicidal behaviour. Dr. Smith also comments that he never considered her a suicide risk, telling the Review that she appeared to be like a normal girl at the Eaglehurst Christmas party.

Various other members of staff offer examples of Sybil's contradictory and fluctuating behaviour. Sybil's young keyworker, Karen, is still so upset about Sybil's death that she has to be taken from the room in tears; one of her colleagues tells us that Karen has previously described how Sybil had been chatting and laughing with her on a walk along the seafront on the Sunday before her death. Sybil's young cognitive behavioural therapist adds to staff members' thesis by explaining that in their sessions, Sybil had a positive long term view of herself and more than once would describe how she envisioned herself in a flat of her own, with a cat and a dog. Only Michael from Woodland Lodge points out a pattern of escalating self-harm leading up to Sybil's first re-admission to the hospital ward in September '98; it had caused concern amongst the Granta team. All the other testimony appears *to us* to have been building up to the implicit conclusion that there were insufficient grounds for anticipating Sybil's suicide and hence, understandably, no special precautions taken.

The attitude that a suicide is 'unpredictable' is repudiated as another false commonplace by the National Schizophrenia Fellowship in the "Conclusion" of their 1999 report, *'One in Ten',* already mentioned. In an earlier section, they explain, moreover, how "improved behaviour" can be misleading, emphasising the need for *both* optimistic encouragement *and* careful monitoring in such situations:

> A number of researchers have drawn attention to the pattern of suicide acts in hospital following short periods of improvement. It may well be that the person, who possibly could have been a suicide risk and on 15

> minute checks, having decided upon their course of action, becomes more at ease. This behaviour can be interpreted by hospital staff as an improvement and result in more freedom which can then lead to an opportunity for the person to carry out their chosen course of action.

By asserting the 'unpredictability' of Sybil's action, the Critical Incident Review, Neil and I feel, is not only absolving the hospital of responsibility but also failing to lay the groundwork for better risk assessment in the future.

Additionally, there are specific revelations about the circumstances surrounding Sybil's death that surprise and upset us at this Review. We only now learn that Sybil was *not* under 'close observation'—fifteen minute checks—at the time of her death, but had been changed to 'general observation'—hourly checks—about a week before her death due to what her team felt was her improving condition. In fact, the nurse Erica (about whom Sybil cared so much) reveals that on the day of the suicide, she found Sybil in the toilet cutting her arm with a broken vase she had found there. Yet it was decided *not* to put Sybil back under 'close observation'. Had Sybil been on fifteen-minute checks, she probably wouldn't have had sufficient time to leave her cubicle, set herself up in the one opposite, prepare herself for hanging, and jump off the chair. Or at least she would not have been hanging there for more than five minutes (the doctor's estimate) when the nurses found her and vainly attempted resuscitation.

Later, we are to perceive some parallels in the case of Sarah Kane, the brilliant but psychologically disturbed avant-garde playwright who commits suicide further along in 1999. *The Guardian* of September 23rd reported on Kane's death by hanging in a hospital toilet. It was ascertained at the inquest that, although she had been diagnosed as suicidal and in need of constant monitoring, she had gone unchecked for ninety minutes. We identify strongly with what Miss Kane's father has to say: "I am not seeking financial compensation for the death of my daughter. I want answers as to why she was not given proper care in order that this does not happen to somebody else's daughter." The *Safer Services* Report found that mental health teams themselves identified "closer supervision" as one of the two most important factors that would have reduced risk in the majority of suicide cases and goes on to say that the need for intensive observation is greatest in the evenings and at night, when the majority of suicides occur—as did Sybil's.

At the Critical Incident Review, we are so upset at the disclosures I have mentioned, that we don't fully register Dr. Smith's brief mention that Sybil was found with an electrical cord in her hand, trying to strangle herself, a couple of weeks before her death.

Sensing our very strong feelings, the facilitators, at the conclusion of the review, very considerately offer us an informal follow-on session with the main people responsible for Sybil. We learn that the doctor who was called in to treat the cuts on Sybil's arm discussed with the staff and the consultant whether to put Sybil back on close observation, but the team rejected this course of action because they considered the broken vase incident just a further instance of Sybil's self-harming habits, and because Sybil herself had seemed to take it very lightly. (It is worth noting what the National Schizophrenia Fellowship has to say regarding risk assessment: "[I]t is important to bear in mind that people with a mental illness are no less capable than any other members of society of hiding thoughts and emotions if they want to.")

At this juncture, we argue our strong disagreement with the team over their assumption that self-harm is entirely separate and distinct from suicidal behaviour. Neil and I view the two as just different points on a fluid continuum of self-destructive behaviour. What is "suicide" but "self-harm" taken to its logical conclusion? The *Safer Services* Report lists "self-harm" as one of three "main indicators of risk" in its Conclusion, and Table 2 of the Report shows that a "History of Self-Harm" occurred in seventy-five per cent of in-patient suicides.

In the end, however, the team members do not admit to any mistakes, and we agree to disagree.

We leave Clacton in a fog of grief and dissatisfaction. Earlier that day, distracted, I had hurriedly grabbed what I thought was a full bottle of water sitting outside Molly's room and added it to two other small water bottles. Now, on the long drive home, the others having been already emptied, I hand that final bottle to Neil, who is thirsty. He takes one large sip, recoils, choking and spitting, and says "My God, what have you given me?!!" I suddenly realise from the caustic fumes released that this clear bottle must be the white spirits that Molly uses in her hobby of glass painting! If this had been an ordinary day, I would have noticed the tiny warning label. Now, I am nearly hysterical at the prospect of having poisoned Neil. Am I to lose a husband as well as a daughter? I urge Neil to get off the highway at the next junction. Much to our relief, the pharmacist we find tells us it was probably an insufficient amount to seriously harm Neil; we should seek a hospital only if he starts foaming at the mouth. That evening, Neil's disappointment at the Review is laced with a lingering stomach ache.

* * *

The first draft of the Critical Incident Report from the Clacton Hospital comes to us on March 30th, and overall, we feel that it has not been written up as carefully as the situation warrants. There are many formal errors and some inaccuracies about Sybil's past and recent life and one glaring contradiction in particular: On the first page, it clearly states that at Eaglehurst, after Christmas, Sybil took an overdose, while nearer to the end, the Report explains that staff at the hospital were surprised by Sybil's suicide, having not considered her a risk because she had had the opportunity to obtain medicine outside the facility while at Eaglehurst but had never done so. This comment ignores the two bottles of paracetamol that Sybil had purchased and then used for her overdose there. Other references to the fact that Sybil was not considered a suicide risk abound. Hedged with such defences, the report, we feel, tends to support the view of the Channel 4 series that hospitals, fearing possible litigation, are disinclined to admit mistakes or misjudgements.

We are pleased, however, that the Trust has invited us to comment on the draft, and we throw ourselves into this task, perhaps obsessively—perhaps a way of countering the real helplessness we feel after the fact of Sybil's death—and we send back the text overlaid with corrections and a lengthy letter with our broader criticisms. Although the report makes two "Recommendations" that reflect some of our own concerns—one concerning improvements in identifying patterns of deterioration in self-harming patients, and another about adjusting the physical environment for the minimal amount of risk to patients—we suggest three more—the need for peer reviews, more training in risk assessment, and more family involvement (the last of five "Main Recommendations" on the first page of the *One in Ten'* report is: "That the role of families and friends in suicide prevention is recognized by health and local authorities by providing training and information to them and acting on the information which they provide", a recommendation that *Rethink* (the present Schizophrenia charity) is now seriously engaged in putting into practice).

When the revised final draft comes back to us in mid-May, we are chagrined to see fewer changes than we had hoped for. Some factual errors that we pointed out have been rectified, but what we see as the most glaring error of all—the discrepancy between the reference to Sybil's overdose at Eaglehurst and the later assertion that she never tried to obtain any medical substances or abuse them while there—stands uncorrected, even to the point of leaving in a typographical error we had noted. Of our three suggested additional recommendations they add a qualified version of the one relating to the involvement of family in the patient's care programme. Nevertheless, we are gratified that they have responsively strengthened the recommendations they already had. The comments we perceive as self-justifying remain; however, as the cover letter points out, the report itself acknowledges that the staff and Sybil's family view events differently.

We now feel that the upcoming inquest by the Coroner for the County of Essex, scheduled for April 28th, is probably our last chance to obtain a full and open assessment of Sybil's care leading up to her death and to draw public attention to the unacknowledged mistakes we feel were made, in the hope that they will never again be repeated, at least not on Peter Bruff Ward. Having spent an inordinate amount of our time critiquing the Critical Incident Report, we just about manage, three days before the inquest, to take advantage of our legal entitlement by faxing to the Coroner's Office a three-page "Statement to the Coroner", setting forth our concerns about the Trust's practice in the case of Sybil.

Our "concerns" in the letter are the ones we have previously raised with the Trust: the decision not to return Sybil to close observation on the day of her death when she cut herself with a broken vase, the failure to remove all potentially dangerous items from her environment (we are thinking of the electric cord, but at this point we see it merely as a general, common sense precaution to have removed it and other risky paraphernalia), the pressure put on Sybil to consider discharge when she was fragile and unwell, our disagreement over Sybil's medication, the withdrawal of therapy in 1997 by Allen Brown, the absence of peer review in the conduct of the case, the withholding of information from us, Sybil's family, and finally, the reservations we have about the Critical Incident Review and the subsequent official report.

"THE THING INSIDE MY HEAD"

Towards the end of our "Statement", Neil, writing out of his experience in industry, anticipates a major point in Channel 4's documentary on medical mishaps: "The NHS Trust has not exhibited to us a culture that places the prevention of deaths by unnatural causes among its highest priorities. We would contrast their approach with companies in high risk industries such as oil and gas where the investigation of accidental death is in depth and automatically the personal responsibility of the most senior executives and must be placed ahead of all other business at hand." He also suggests the larger significance of Sybil's case: "In the report [of the National Schizophrenic Fellowship into suicides, '*One in Ten*'] we have found so many parallels to our daughter's death that we can only begin to think that our tragedy is part of a wider national pattern."

A day later, we receive a phone call from the Coroner's Officer: the inquest is to be postponed till later in the year and it may be heard before a jury. We are gratified that our concerns have been taken seriously by the Coroner's Office; nevertheless, this indefinite postponement leaves our feelings about Sybil's death in a state of uncomfortable suspension for the next few months.

* * *

In late October a letter informs us that the new inquest date is November 25th and that it *will* be before a jury. In a phone call a few days later, we ascertain that we will be permitted to ask questions and to raise the points in our "Statement." Upon our request, copies of other people's official statements in the case file are sent to us. Some years later, we obtain access to two documents from 2002 that are related to a new government initiative to reform the Coroners' Service, *Certifying and Investigating Deaths in England, Wales and Northern Ireland, An Invitation for Views*, an interim government report, and *How the Inquest System Fails Bereaved People: INQUEST'S Response to the Fundamental Review of Coroner Services*, a report by the charity INQUEST, and we realise that many, many families have far less cooperation and help from a coroner's office than we received in 1999.

First among the items in Sybil's case file that arrest our attention is a letter to the Coroner for Essex from the Director of Acute Services for the North East Essex Mental Health Trust, complying with the Coroner's request to the Trust for a response to our "Statement to the Coroner" back in April. I transcribe most of this letter here as it represents the Trust's point of view and its main defence against our criticisms:

> ... Ms Macindoe was transferred from Colchester General Hospital and admitted to Peter Bruff Ward on 7 January 1999. She was actively engaged by staff during 15 minute observational intervals from admission. The following day after admission, she made an attempt to hang herself and was placed on one-to-one (continuous) observations and observed through the night. She remained on close observations until 12 January when she saw her consultant and the observations were reduced to 15 minutes with active engagements. Her observation levels were reduced to general observation on 20 January 1999.

> On 25 January, Ms Macindoe was discovered making superficial cuts to her arms. There was no change to her observations at this time, but this incident was discussed at length with medical staff.

> Her consultant, Dr. [Smith], believes that Ms Macindoe's self-harm attempts were a

coping mechanism, rather than an attempt to take her own life...

... Risks due to [a] patient's behaviour which may be affected by the environment form part of the risk management plan for that patient. Ms Macindoe was an informal patient who was admitted to an open ward environment. Every effort is made to minimize the risks but this must be a balanced approach between being over-intrusive and preserving a patient's civil rights within "informal status".

The Trust has conducted a detailed audit of the environment since her death and actions have been taken to reduce risks the physical environment may present to patients with self-harming behaviour.

For many patients with mental health problems discharge from an environment where they may have felt safe such as an in-patient unit is stress-provoking, therefore every effort is made to minimize this problem. Staff were constantly reassessing the pace of Ms Macindoe's care to minimize the stress that the prospect of discharge may bring. Meetings had been re-scheduled to allow Ms. Macindoe more time.

It is factually incorrect that Eaglehurst did not want her back. When deciding upon when and where a patient should be discharged to, a patient's needs are paramount. [Comment: Hazel had told Neil otherwise].

Mr. Macindoe spoke at length with Dr. [Smith] after the review in relation to research, drug therapy and other treatments for Obsessive Compulsive Disorder (OCD). It was agreed that the research does state that drugs for this illness should be changed if they do not work but this relates to simplistic cases where OCD is the only factor being considered... Ms Macindoe was on a mixture of drugs, including Lithium and therefore any changes to her medication or dosage had to be carefully considered. Her consultant also explained that there was a psychotic and behavioural dimension to Ms Macindoe's illness and therefore drug therapies were not the only treatment she was receiving, her care also included cognitive behavioural therapy.

There appears to be some confusion by Mr. Macindoe about Cognitive Behavioural Therapy and Behavioural Therapy. Her behavioural therapy was discontinued [in 1997 by Allen Brown—Cf. Part II, Chapter 6] due to the clinical judgment of the therapist who felt she needed a more structured environment to progress further. This was sought from the Maudsley Behavioural Unit, however, upon assessment it was their opinion that Ms Macindoe's commitment may have not been sufficient for her to complete the treatment programme offered. However, she was undertaking a Cognitive Behavioural Therapy programme locally up to her death.

There is acknowledgment that there were difficulties relating to family involvement in Ms Macindoe's care and this is covered comprehensively in the [Critical Incident] report... Mental health care presents staff with constant challenging patient behaviours which are often unpredictable and staff need to balance risks as part of their everyday work... The issues which Mr. Macindoe has raised in his letter represent the dilemmas which all staff

"THE THING INSIDE MY HEAD"

*who work in the mental health field have to face
on a daily basis. The Trust recognizes that Ms.
Macindoe's death has caused a great deal of
pain and suffering and learn[s] from events like
these to prevent further tragedies in the future...*

Over and above our ongoing disagreements with the
Trust, what leaps off the page for us in reading the Director's
letter now is the stark sentence, *"The following day after
admission, she made an attempt to hang herself..."* We had
not been informed about this incident last January, nor was it
discussed at any length at the Critical Incident Review. We
learn more about this disturbing event when going on to read
the summary of Sybil's case by Dr. Smith and his assistant,
Dr. Kent: It records that Sybil tried to hang herself on the
night of January 9th with an electric cable-cord attached to a
curtain rail, and that witnesses described Sybil as extremely
disturbed. This differs from Dr. Smith's brief reference at the
Review to an attempt by Sybil to 'strangle' herself; it means
that her earlier attempt anticipated her final suicide in every
way. "My God," we exclaim to each other, "she must have
used her stereo cable then as well, and they didn't even
remove it from her room!" We determine to draw the
Coroner's attention to this fact at the inquest. Learning of
this 'dress rehearsal' for Sybil's suicide and the precautions
never taken adds a new dimension to our grieving.

Part of the summary is Dr. Smith's final psychiatric
assessment of Sybil—yet another interpretation of her life,
this time from a clinical viewpoint—and what a contrast to
the funeral orations! According to him, OCD was not the
primary diagnosis in Sybil's complex case, albeit she was
very distressed by its symptoms. Rather, he decides, hers
was a case of Borderline Personality Disorder (on the
borderline between neurosis and psychosis) as well as a
general anhedonia—an inability to enjoy life ("What would
Diane, her exuberant and plain-dealing former keyworker,
make of that last?" we think). Further, in what seems *to us*

503

to be 'blaming the victim', his report claims that Sybil's intermittent manipulative tendencies made it difficult for those trying to manage her case. How this bleak and unflattering final assessment squares with the view of Sybil conveyed by her own words and those of others in this book, is for the reader to decide.

* * *

Neil feels emotionally and morally impelled to conduct our 'case' at the upcoming inquest, even though we are allowed to hire a barrister. The day before the inquest, Neil, beginning to get panicky, decides he will seek help from Citizen's Advice. He arrives at their North London office, after a day's work at Heathrow, just at closing time, but he desperately talks his way in. They refer him to the charity INQUEST, and he is lucky to find a member of staff willing, that evening, to fax helpful advice and information to us. An evening of hectic activity follows, and we go to bed late, bristling with tension.

Molly has, very loyally, insisted on coming to the inquest with us to present a united front under the ordeal and to give us moral support, but, typically, she rises late from bed the next morning and holds up our departure, ratcheting up our anxiety. Sure enough, when we arrive at Shire Hall, the Coroner's Court in Chelmsford, the other participants are already there. We exchange stiff and uncomfortable greetings with all those witnesses affiliated with the Trust. The Peter Bruff Ward Manager sits down next to me, and, meaning well, tries to start a conversation, but I am so distraught on the day that her name slips completely from my mind when I want to introduce her to Molly. One of the criticisms in the 2002 report, *INQUEST'S Response* (also made in *Certifying and Investigating Death*), is that the majority of inquest venues fail to provide a private space for the bereaved family to wait or meet with their own legal team: "This has been particularly distressing for families where the death has occurred within an institution and they have had to wait or discuss their case next to people who they believe may have been responsible for the death."

After an excruciating wait, we are finally told to file into the courtroom, where we are hit by the stuffy, sour smell of an enclosed space that has witnessed the presence of many unhappy and anxious people in the course of the week. We are directed to sit at a table facing the coroner across the room, with the other witnesses ranged on wooden benches behind us. At right angles to where we are sitting, on the left side of the room, are the double row of jurors, a mixture of ages and sexes, with, as I note, only one man wearing a suit, and to our right and central in the room is the witness box. While the Deputy Coroner for the County of Essex presides today, it is the Coroner's Officer, with whom we've had several contacts, who stage manages, so to speak, the comings and goings of witnesses and instructs us, the participants, when to rise or sit, as in a church service.

The Coroner's opening remarks set the scene: the inquest has a limited scope—just to find out the "who, how, when and where" of this suicide—with no apportioning of blame. The Officer announces that the cause of death was "hanging" and proceeds to read out the post-mortem report, which, to us, Sybil's family, seems distressingly to deal with Sybil like a hunk of dead meat. Among other things, the report confirms the presence of external lacerations on Sybil's body, evidence of her "self-harming".

From here on in, Neil takes it upon himself to cross-examine each witness, controlling his emotions with great difficulty. He does go overboard a few times, holding forth at length rather than just questioning, but the Coroner, with a couple of exceptions, is very tolerant. Neil begins by questioning the Officer as to whether Sybil's last two diary notepads, which had been seized and retained by the police, have revealed anything significant. He replies that there was nothing relevant, no mention of suicidal intent *[but see previous chapter!!]*, and at this time we ourselves are in no position to contradict him. Had we had access to these diaries at the time, the inquest verdict might have gone differently.

The two nurses from Peter Bruff Ward who found Sybil on the night she hanged herself give cut and dried testimony which more or less repeats their written statements in the file, except there is one new detail—another distressing 'if only' for us. The female nurse explains that when she first discovered Sybil out of her bed, she looked at once, but only quickly, into the empty cubicle opposite and did not see Sybil because she was in a corner not immediately visible. Only later, when they did a more thorough search of the ward, did they find Sybil in that same cubicle, dead. Had the nurse seen her *the first time*, even if Sybil were already hanging, that resuscitation attempts would probably have been successful.

In Neil's questioning, he focuses on the issue of the stereo electric cord, trying to get the nurses to admit openly before the jury and the Coroner that it is the same one with which Sybil had previously attempted to hang herself, but they both profess ignorance, and the male nurse remarks dryly that it is not really hospital policy to take away personal belongs.

Dr. Smith next takes the witness stand, introduced by the Officer, who *seems to us* to recite with a grand flourish the psychiatrist's long string of professional titles and qualifications. (In this case and in that of the Director of Acute Services, we agree to *some* extent with INQUEST'S observation in their "Response": "[T]he common experience in all cases involving institutions [hospitals, care homes etc.] is that there is a perception of a professional closing of ranks and institutional bias from Coroners in favour of professionals.") Dr. Smith's emphasis once again is on Sybil's complex diagnosis, which included a psychotic depression. He tells the court she had a personality disorder and a fear of leaving the institutional network that made treatment difficult. By December of '98, he insists, she appeared to have completely recovered.

"THE THING INSIDE MY HEAD"

At this point the Coroner interrupts to query Dr. Smith about the implications of Sybil's "self-harming". He replies with the party line, that it was just an expression of distress, and that there was no manifestation of a serious suicide attempt (thus ignoring the previous 'hanging' incident). The Coroner asks him pointedly whether he "addressed his mind to it [her self-harming]", and he defends his position by explaining how the observation levels for Sybil were only gradually reduced over a few weeks following her overdose in early January.

As Neil begins his cross-examination, I become flushed and tense, worrying that he will make a fool of himself in trying to tackle this suave, confident professional. Among other things, Neil brings up the comment by Dr. Smith's colleague in September '98 when Neil had his 'showdown' with Dr. Smith in Peter Bruff Ward, that Sybil was not psychotic. "Why the contradiction now?" Dr. Smith responds by stating his belief that Sybil's was a case of 'Borderline Personality Disorder', between neurosis and psychosis. At this point, I interrupt and try to explain that Sybil's apparently bizarre religious beliefs are a recognised feature of OCD called "scrupulosity", but Dr. Smith insists that her beliefs went beyond OCD. Unfortunately, I cannot respond further as I have not yet read *OCD: A Guide,* which points out (as cited in Part II, Ch. 2) that *"[b]ecause obsessions can be so strange (even bizarre) they are sometimes mistaken as hallucinatory or delusional symptoms of psychosis."*

When Neil questions Dr. Smith about Sybil's suicidal tendencies, the psychiatrist responds with a "yes, but" answer, which causes the Coroner to interrupt him and point out that he has given a flat "no" earlier. Neil now has the opportunity to publicly challenge Dr. Smith's prescription of the drug Venlafaxine, but the psychiatrist rebuts him by repeating his previous diagnosis of Sybil. Neil's attempts to extend the argument over drug therapy by explaining his own understanding of "best practice" are thwarted when the coroner politely but firmly cuts him short. All in all, despite our efforts, despite his backing down on a couple of minor points, Dr. Smith's testimony has appeared to greatly impress the lay jury.

The Coroner calls a one-hour recess for lunch. The three of us go off alone, feeling grim and strung out, to find something to eat, but we have no appetites and converse little before returning to the courtroom.

The first witness after the recess is the Director of Acute Services, whose letter I have cited earlier, representing the Trust, and the Coroner's Officer again *appears to us* to give vocal emphasis to his impressive qualifications. The Coroner puts to him each point of our "Statement to the Coroner," but his answers are very fluent, very assuaging, virtually a repetition of his points in the letter. His only concession is that it was a mistake not to use collapsible rails in the ward, but that has now been implemented, he explains. As to family involvement, he insists that Sybil herself wanted clear boundaries and that the staff respected her decision. (Indeed, this has been a tricky ethical dilemma for us, but potentially resolvable, we feel, though we don't dwell on this at the inquest.)

The most contentious issue—the Director's moment of greatest vulnerability—concerns the non-removal of Sybil's stereo cord. By this time in the trial, it has been so well highlighted thanks to Neil's persistence that the Coroner herself brings it up to the witness. Very composed, he answers that taking it away would have lowered the morale of the patient. Neil counters, "You could have given her a shorter cord, or substituted batteries for her stereo," but the *best* answer (which unfortunately doesn't come to our minds, brittle with tension and anger at the time) is that all other 'patient's rights' issues should have been outweighed by the patient's right to life!

Michael Grey from Granta is the last official witness. He points out, mildly, that Sybil's instances of "self-harm" had been escalating and had included an attempt to cut her wrists at Eaglehurst, not mentioned at all up to now. The Deputy Coroner asks, "Did Sybil ever discuss suicide with you?" Michael answers "No", but states that on one occasion, when Dr. Roberts asked Sybil whether she was feeling suicidal, Sybil had answered, "Yes". He also brings up that especially big hug Sybil gave to Kim, the Granta care worker, on the night of her death. Michael's testimony aids our contention that there were more than sufficient indications of Sybil's suicidal tendencies, but, conveyed in his typically low key manner, it doesn't come across powerfully.

Speaking for us both, Neil then asks if Hazel, Sybil's CPN, not on the witness list, can be allowed to come to the stand for questioning. The Coroner gives her permission, but this proves to be a dubious move on our part. We are well aware that Hazel had been very supportive of Sybil in the past, but we want, here, to challenge her views on self-harming and her pressuring of Sybil over discharge plans. Hazel disputes the idea, presented several times by Neil in the course of the inquest, that Sybil herself wanted Cognitive Behavioural Therapy during the period when she wasn't getting any. She is very well-spoken and wins over the Coroner and the jury by her confident self-presentation, insisting that she knew Sybil better than anyone else did and was even allowed to read from her diaries.

Sybil, she argues, wanted confidentiality in order to *protect* her family. Sybil experienced stress from family pressure, she charges, bringing in again the controversial New Zealand trip, thus turning the tables on us. But, to our minds, under Neil's questioning, she fudges the issue of why she was pressing discharge plans upon Sybil so soon after her overdose. She tells the jury that Sybil was in despair in January, because, after all her struggles, she was back in hospital again and it was almost exactly three years to the day since she had first come to the Peter Bruff Ward from Jacques Hall. Nevertheless—and no one thinks to bring up the inconsistency—Hazel emphatically reiterates her theory that Sybil "self-harmed" only to relieve pressure; even her death, she claims, was just an attempt at "self-harm" that went wrong.

Molly is very upset by Hazel's testimony. She has already (before any of us) read through one of Sybil's earlier diaries, and she reminds us of the many references to suicide she found there. Neil obtains permission for Molly to speak, and after the break, she gets to her feet hesitantly and timidly speaks her piece about what she has seen in Sybil's diary, citing some graphic examples. This hard-won little speech of hers, however, seems to have little impact in light of what the Officer has declared (misleadingly) about the final hospital diaries.

The Coroner sums up, reiterating that this is only a "fact-finding inquiry" and briefly summarises the various testimonies—stressing Dr. Smith's insistence on the complexity of Sybil's case. Hazel, she says, knew Sybil in depth and has told us she believes Sybil did not intend to kill herself. She gives the jury the three short form verdict options: suicide, accidental death, and open verdict, and appears *to us* to emphasise by tone and volume of voice what she is legally required to state: that if the jury is not *one hundred percent sure that suicide was intended,* they should reach a verdict of "accident".

The jury, apparently affected by Hazel's climactic testimony and the Deputy Coroner's summing up, returns from its consultative break with a verdict of "accidental death". From our point of view, even this unsatisfactory verdict implicates the Trust for its failure to prevent such an accident. Nevertheless, it weakens our main contention, a justified one we feel, that Sybil should have been taken more seriously as a suicide risk. We are dismayed.

* * *

It is more than a matter of our personal disappointment. This misleading verdict of "accidental death" as well as the

"THE THING INSIDE MY HEAD"

Deputy Coroner's later failure to make recommendations in her report (which she has the legal power to do) is a setback, too, for other NHS patients. The Schizophrenia report, *'One in Ten',* concludes that coroners have an important role to play in the monitoring of good and bad practice in the state system:

> 8.1 NSF believes that when an 'open', 'accidental' or 'misadventure' verdict is returned instead of 'suicide', the chance of useful feedback to service providers is lost. When an accident is recorded as 'suicide' there is a greater chance that purchasers and providers will review their policies and procedures because a deliberate act (involving choice) has taken place which could have been prevented.

> 8.2 These 'non-suicide' verdicts give the impression that the victim and the illness are responsible and that their professional carers were powerless and not responsible.

Besides the misleading verdict, our frustration with the outcome relates to an issue of greater scope: is the whole approach and structure of the coroner's court procedure really satisfactory? Certainly both the initial inquiry of the government-appointed committee reviewing coroners' services in 2002, *Certifying and Investigating Death,* and *INQUEST'S Response* think they are not. *Certifying* articulates what we feel on this day:

> We are... clear that in some respects the customary verdict structure for England and

Wales needs amendment, if any verdict structure is retained. Many families have said to us that some 'verdicts' of 'natural death', 'accidental death' or 'misadventure'—not a word with much natural meaning to the general public—are in some circumstances meaningless and can be offensive. If an inquest is held into the complex circumstances of a hospital death—a category of death that has in recent years increasingly occupied coroner's [sic] attention—and there are serious issues about the suitability of the treatment given, it is inadequate to summarise the outcome as an accidental or a natural death...

INQUEST'S Response comments similarly: "For many families it is hard to understand the narrow remit of the inquest... They are shocked to discover the limits to the issues that will be discussed as many see systemic failings as responsible for their relative's death and want the court to look more deeply at the underlying events."

As a result of the many reactions like our own that the inquiry uncovered, the government committee in its final report some months later (June 2003) *Death Certification and Investigation in England, Wales and Northern Ireland: The Report of the Fundamental Review 2003,* suggested that the scope of an inquest should have more flexibility and lead to fuller conclusions, recommends scrapping the short form verdicts, and specifically suggests replacing the "suicide" classification with "death from a deliberate act of self-harm or injury"—far more appropriate in our opinion. In the case of institutional deaths, the report suggests that the inquest's conclusion should provide an assessment of the institution's relevant regulatory or safety systems and whether or not they were followed. Moreover, the report opines that it should be mandatory to send the court's findings to the relevant body.

"THE THING INSIDE MY HEAD"

Following this final committee report, in March 2004, a government position paper, *Reforming the Coroner and Death Certification Service*, which appeared to a large extent to have taken on board the recommendations of the committee's previous reports (qualified, as ever, by the concern for "affordability") was presented to Parliament. Although the reform of the coroners' service was then delayed by the transfer of responsibility from the Home Office to the Department of Constitutional Affairs after the 2005 election, a Draft Bill was drawn up and circulated for discussion in June 2006. Our family especially welcomed two features of the Draft Bill: the assertion of the right of bereaved parties to legally appeal the outcome or 'verdict' of an inquest or make a complaint, and the inclusion of a lengthy "Draft Charter for Bereaved People" with an unprecedented new emphasis on their other rights and needs—for example, the right of the bereaved to a private room on the day of the inquest, whenever possible.

However, to our mind, the Draft Bill fails to fully live up to the promise of the earlier committee reports. For one thing, it retains the old short form verdicts—particularly the ambiguous "suicide" one—and although it allows for "narrative verdicts" this option, to our mind, would most likely be waived when a jury is involved or when individual coroners find themselves too busy.

Following a three-month's consultation period with stakeholders and with the general public, the portion of the Draft Bill relating to coroners' recommendations and thus to public safety has been strengthened, we have learned. It now makes it mandatory for institutions to respond in writing to a coroner's report, and the Chief Coroner each year will have to summarise for Parliament the recommendations made and the responses given nationally. This, we personally hope, will galvanise the government to take action when dangerous patterns emerge, which, in turn, should have some positive outcomes for mental health sufferers, along with other victims.

Lois Chaber

But in the Draft Bill as it now stands it is still *optional* for coroners to send a report suggesting changes in the case of institutional deaths, and equally optional for the institutions to implement such changes, although they must explain their decision in writing. The Coroners' Reform Bill unfortunately was not able to be included in the most recent Queen's speech. It is still being refined as I write [February 2008] and will be introduced to Parliament when time allows. Some of the proposed measures, such as the mandatory responses from institutions, may be introduced in Parliament before the full bill is passed. We can only hope for the best.

* * *

On the day of Sybil's inquest, several people come up to us afterwards to pay their respects. Both the Deputy Coroner herself and The Coroner's Officer explain to us that she and the Coroner for Essex had consulted and agreed to allow us a broader scope than was usual for questioning. We are very grateful for this; it has at least enabled us to achieve our goal of having a full and open inquiry into Sybil's case. Two local reporters (for the *East Anglian Daily Times* and the *Clacton Evening Gazette*) who have been sitting through the inquest also come up to us with some questions. We are expansive with them, believing that Sybil's case deserves public attention. Two articles on Sybil's death and inquest duly come out the next day headlined, respectively, "Parents of hanged woman hit out at her care" and "Parents believe daughter's suicide was avoidable."

I have made some criticisms of the conduct of the inquest, but, compared with many of the respondents to INQUEST'S 2002 survey, we have been treated quite well. Nevertheless we can attest to "the additional grief and stress that [the inquest process] causes to bereaved people" (*INQUEST'S Response*). Despite the sympathy of the journalists, and some kindly-meant small talk about New Zealand from the inquest officials, we return home depressed and shaken, a state of mind that lingers

"THE THING INSIDE MY HEAD"

insidiously for many months. Similar reactions, many times over, are what led to the suggestion of a charter for the bereaved in the reform committee's final report and to this charter's prominent place in the intended legislation.

Beyond these dismal proceedings in the coroner's court, "sudden death bereavement" itself, as *INQUEST'S Response* points out, can have consequences similar to post traumatic stress disorder for the bereaved family members: medium to long term negative effects on their health and personal lives. Neil is to suffer for quite some time with mysterious bodily symptoms and a generalised feeling of being unwell that never really receives an adequate diagnosis. He never *entirely* regains his personal and professional confidence, as far as I can see, or his constitutional optimism. Molly, despite support from a large network of friends, begins to suffer an array of tension symptoms, various nervous tics and the beginnings of muscular pains that will eventually become a serious back problem and ongoing disability, diagnosed as having no clear physical cause. She eventually has to take up benefits and see a psychotherapist, who terms Molly's bodily symptoms "a classic case of trauma". For me, in order to cope, the trauma means seriously backtracking on the programme I had begun to reduce my psychotropic medication. It is to be almost seven years before I venture again to reduce my anti-depressants.

Our disagreements with the Trust, of course, need to be balanced against our appreciation of the many kind and sympathetic efforts made by particular individuals on Peter Bruff Ward and by others under the Trust's umbrella to help Sybil during her times in hospital. The errors we feel were made are to some extent systemic ones, largely a result of the endemic time and budget constraints of the NHS—which I witnessed myself as a patient, however briefly, in the overheated, poorly supplied, understaffed Chase Farm Mental Health Ward of the early 1990s. We make a firm decision after the inquest not to pursue the issues any further legally. We feel it would not be fitting to seek any financial compensation for Sybil's death, and we do not wish to subject ourselves to possibly years more of anxiety and aggravation, caught up in the tentacles of the law. We are ready to re-engage in ordinary life and in the future.

"THE THING INSIDE MY HEAD"

Conclusion: Regrets and Hopes

[T]he combination of poor upbringing and bad genes produces bigger effects than the simple sum of their separate effects—their interaction can be particularly destructive.

(Richard Layard, *Happiness: Lessons From a New Science, London*: Allen Lane, 2005; p. 59.)

This weekend Professor Louis Appleby, the government's mental health czar, admitted that the standard of treatment of mental patients in hospitals was "not satisfactory". He said the Department of Health was working urgently to overhaul the system.

(Robert Winnett and Holly Watt, "Doctor Warns on Freed Mental Patients," *The Sunday Times*, Jan. 8, 2006.)

Lessons can be gleaned from Sybil's brief life and from our family's harrowing experience. By attempting to trace the sources of the extreme form Sybil's disorders took and the factors involved in her final tragedy, I hope I have called attention to the complex interplay of nature and nurture, the personal and the public in mental health issues.

* * *

A genetic role in the emergence of OCD now seems more than probable according to recent research, and it is likely that Sybil inherited her disorder and its related depressive component from me. Tendencies to anxiety and depression, to neurosis in general, seem to run in the female line of my paternal family (my father, by all accounts, was a stable, sanguine individual). My grandmother on my father's side was to a significant extent mentally unbalanced, suffering increasingly from paranoia as she aged, and similar instabilities afflicted my paternal aunt and my oldest

517

Lois Chaber

cousin, her daughter. My cousin and I have needed the support of psychotropic medication, but no one in the family has required the extensive hospitalisation that Sybil needed.

I suggest that without our cumulative family experiences—her 'nurture'—Sybil's problems would not have become so acute and destructive. What a child inherits is a *predisposition* to OCD or other anxiety disorders. The disorder can then remain relatively dormant or mild, or, alternatively, it can be triggered by stressful life experiences into overdrive. Sue Gerhardt, in *Why Love Matters*, explains that the precise manner in which genes are "expressed", that is, manifested in any individual, is ultimately a result of environmental stimuli, and the child's earliest 'environment' consists of its parents. She presents a convincing case for the damaging effect of inadequate care-giving on a baby's not-fully-developed brain. My equivocal feelings about motherhood, exacerbated by postnatal depression, and my consequent erratic behaviour were thus major factors in getting Sybil off to a bad start in life.

Unlike Sybil, despite my own demons and disorders, I am a survivor, and I now believe I owe that to the strong bond forged between me and my mother in my early years, despite our later drifting apart. This primal connection, I believe, has enabled me to form close attachments with both men (as lovers) and with women (as friends), which have sustained me through difficult circumstances and through my own mistakes and failures. Sybil's is a different 'story', one which certainly supports the contention in a leaflet from the Anna Freud Centre Parent-Infant Project in North London, a therapeutic centre for new parents and their babies, that "Problems in the parent-infant bond can... cause serious difficulties which affect people throughout their lives." Sybil's adolescence and early adulthood can, in fact, be seen as an unsuccessful quest for maternal surrogates, a yearning for the *unconditional* and *unlimited* nurturing that I wasn't able to give her in infancy. Moreover, forming and maintaining relationships with her peers was all too often a dispiriting struggle for Sybil throughout her life.

"THE THING INSIDE MY HEAD"

Surely, then, there is a need for more programmes like the Parent-Infant Project and the Organization for Post-Natal Disorder, and they should be publicly funded and well-publicised to help new mothers who have difficulty coping with childrearing in a complex world. As Sue Gerhardt points out, "There is a growing recognition that finding ways to improve the relationship between parents and their babies is a much more cost effective (and less painful) way of improving mental health than any number of adult therapeutic treatments." Lord Layard, in *Happiness,* also emphasises the crucial influence of parental behaviour on the mental well being of the developing individual and similarly recommends innovations in public health policy. The government, he advises, should institute compulsory parenting classes in secondary schools as well as voluntary but strongly encouraged parenting classes when a woman becomes pregnant, alongside ante-natal classes. The "cost-effectiveness"—to use Gerhardt's term—of all such suggestions is apparent when we consider that working days lost through mental illness (more than 91 million a year) cost UK industry approximately £11.8 billion annually ("Mental Health in the Media," *OCD Action Newsletter*).

While acknowledging these very important parenting issues and shouldering my hefty share of the responsibility for Sybil's tragedy, as an ongoing if chastened feminist I am hesitant about contributing to the already prevalent tendency to stigmatise mothers. One reader of my original typescript perceived me as torn between acknowledging the complex factors that led to Sybil's defeat and constructing *a direct line* between my maternal failures and her death. Perhaps my memoir dramatises an ambivalence that, though different in degree, is surely not different in kind from what *all* mothers must feel when weighing themselves in the balance. At its most extreme, the cultural warp of 'mother-blame' has been evident in those several notorious convictions of UK women for supposedly murdering their babies, which were eventually overturned in recent years.

Lois Chaber

A portion of the blame for instances of inadequate mothering, Gerhardt believes, falls on our modern Western European culture, in which the separation of the private and the public, of home and work, have led to the unhealthy seclusion of mothers: "Considering how to reduce the twin stresses of isolation and inexperience that plague parenting in advanced economies [and their expatriate extensions, I would add] will involve some radical rethinking of the conditions in which it takes place"—in other words, more work flexibility, more shared parenting, more community facilities. My conflicted motherhood was, *in part*, akin to that of many women who contend with the at times insurmountable practical *and psychological* difficulties of 'juggling' family and career. It is a dilemma that *I* never succeeded in resolving for myself and it is one with which society at large is only just beginning to deal through more generous and just maternity *and* paternity leave provisions. In any case, I hope that troubled mothers—or fathers—will seek help, but also spare some compassion for themselves.

* * *

Though the issue of mothering looms large in this account of Sybil's tragic case, I think it fair to say that other children have survived worse parenting than my own unsteady efforts. Sybil's extraordinary sensitivity and her inherited pathology made her more vulnerable, not only to my ambivalence but also to the several other unusually adverse environmental factors that impinged on her. The infant Sybil was plunged at once into crisis by her traumatic premature birth, by her separation from me and by poor hospital care, all in the midst of the turbulent Iranian Revolution. Spending her childhood in the Middle East, moreover, and having to make substantial psychological and cultural adjustments both there and afterwards in England seems to have damaged Sybil's sense of identity. Pollock and Van Reken suggest that "Third Culture Kids" *may* end up lacking "a sense of stability, deep security, and belonging."

"THE THING INSIDE MY HEAD"

Successive family traumas throughout her life exacerbated these uncongenial beginnings. Neil's employment crises, largely a result of social forces beyond his control, were devastating for Sybil as she grew up. Neil's unfortunate involvement with the devious Qatari company that entangled him in the Sharia court system, the unjust seizure of his passport, and the intense anxiety these difficulties and dangers caused Sybil were consequences of working within an alien culture that played by different rules. In London, with Neil's inability to find a position in the deteriorating economy of New Zealand, we were prevented from emigrating to a country where their would have been the emotional safety net of Neil's extended family as well as a less frenetic, more child-friendly culture, both of which would have greatly benefited Sybil.

Then, the economic forces of severe recession in 1990s England catapulted Neil into joblessness; our resulting financial struggles, so much a contrast to our comfortable life style in the Gulf, were a terrible shock to both the girls, but Sybil was already unwell, and our consequent family tensions, particularly Molly's truculent adolescent rebelliousness, poorly handled by us, and my own neurotic lapses, further unhinged Sybil. We were caught up in an ever-worsening spiral of what Gravitz has called "family illness"—*each* member of the family interchanging psychological harm with the others. The coup de grâce was Neil's desperate attempt to resolve our financial dilemma by working in Africa. Sybil felt she had been abandoned, in different ways and at different times, by both her mother and her father.

* * *

Nevertheless, in our capacity as parents, we did our earnest best in England to obtain treatment within the National Health System for this damaged child. Unfortunately, the NHS is a bureaucracy that delivers uneven care, and we cannot help feeling that it ultimately let

Lois Chaber

us down, despite dedicated efforts at various points on the part of particular individuals.

Part of the problem was timing. As with other aspects of culture, medical knowledge and practice evolve over time. Had Sybil been born ten years later—say in 1988—her childhood symptoms might have been caught early and treated in good time due to the rapidly expanding awareness of OCD and the evolution of therapies, like CBT, appropriate to it, from about 1992 onwards.

Despite this concession, however, our family believes that the institutions that touched on Sybil's fate could and should have done more for her The Child Guidance Clinic in Barnet, though extremely well-meaning, was too limited in its resources and too hidebound in its overall philosophy, we feel, to predict and prevent Sybil's breakdown in 1992. The Hill End Adolescent Unit to which the Clinic referred us was an inappropriate venue for Sybil with its punitive philosophy aimed at substance abusers and delinquents. Sybil's treatment at the Bethlem Royal Adolescent Unit was very mixed in its helpfulness. Despite a lot of theorising, the consultants, in our opinion, did not have much of a beneficial impact on Sybil, mostly because they had little hands-on contact with her. It was the informal, day-to-day intimacy with caring nurses, and the influence of her peer group there—Sybil's one great social success— that eventually brought our daughter out of her paralysis. We feel that at that point, when Sybil finally became treatable, the Adolescent Unit, with its specialist resources, should have dealt with her severe OCD. However, thanks to the perennial concern about availability of beds and the pressures to *move patients on*, the Bethlem, it seems *to us,* manoeuvred her into a therapeutic community that turned out to cater specifically for abused and abusing adolescents with whom Sybil had little in common, and where she received no treatment for her specific disorder.

The bewildering, multiple manifestations of Sybil's worsening mental illness, the scarcity of information and of

522

"THE THING INSIDE MY HEAD"

specialists during her earlier years, our own relative ignorance, the inappropriate placements and the funding issues—all these contributed to the belatedness of Sybil's treatment and thus to the severity of her OCD when she finally did receive appropriate care in 1996 in Clacton. The staff at Clacton Hospital and Dr. Smith, under the then North East Essex Mental Health Trust, were instrumental in putting Sybil on the effective SSRI drug Prozac, in initiating helpful behavioural therapy and in plugging her in to the community mental health support network. Eventually, in the therapeutic halfway house provided by Granta Housing at Woodland Lodge, she was able to make remarkable progress for a time. It must be said that Sybil herself contributed to her difficulties by her fainthearted reluctance to participate in the Maudsley's intensive OCD behavioural programme. Nevertheless, from the very beginning, the North East Essex Trust had been reluctant to take her on and was, *from our point of view*, all too often more concerned with the issue of 'discharge' than with treatment, never more so than near the time of Sybil's death.

A recent *Sunday Times* article, cited in my "Acknowledgments," profiled the mental health campaigner Marjorie Wallace and discussed the "shocking inadequacy" of UK mental health care. Its author, Minette Marrin, claims "Another driver for this lack of inpatient care is the government's target to prevent extended inpatient stay. A recently leaked report suggests the Department of Health is actually planning to fine hospitals for every day a patient remains there who could and should have been discharged" ("Broken Promises"). Always, always, the concern with financial 'targets' rather than with healing and wellness hampers the efficacy of the NHS, looming over the patient like the Damoclean sword.

The case of Roz Durham, another young mentally ill suicide victim in an NHS hospital, discussed on the Radio 4 programme "You and Yours," Feb 13th, 2003, suggests that the inadequacies and errors we perceived in Sybil's later treatment *were not isolated instances*. Roz, who (like Sybil) was thought of as a difficult patient, was streamed into the adult system at eighteen after having earlier benefited from treatment in a specialist adolescent centre. After several years in and out of hospital, Roz was reluctantly admitted to a psychiatric ward in West Suffolk Hospital in January 2002 and evaluated, due to staff miscommunication, as a "low suicide risk" despite a previous attempt to hang herself. She went missing for three days, and was eventually found hanging in a cupboard. The hospital's in-house inquiry, although it made future recommendations, concluded that the staff had acted properly "within existing policy and procedures".

The NHS mental health service up to now, we believe, has particularly failed young persons like Sybil, Roz Durham, and Sarah Kane.

On the Radio 4 programme, Peter Wilson, from "YoungMinds", argued that adolescent services strive for an overall view and keep in mind the family context, while adult services are less holistic, with a focus on diagnosis and medication (and getting the patient 'discharged' as quickly as possible, I should add!). Dr. Paul Robinson, an eating disorder specialist, commented that the patient's right to exclude his or her parents in eighteen-plus cases is "tricky" and can create problems (certainly we found it so!). Dr. Robinson concluded by calling for a "young person's service" covering those from fourteen to twenty-five, and calling for an improvement in the transition between adolescent and adult care. My husband and I could not agree more fully. Our views were confirmed on hearing, during a Parliamentary briefing on the Mental Health Bill by the Mental Health Alliance, on March 15th 2007, the painfully eloquent testimony of three young persons who had been damaged by their assignment to adult mental health wards when they were under eighteen.

* * *

"THE THING INSIDE MY HEAD"

After so many participants have spoken, what do I have to say, finally, about Sybil, my dear, tragic daughter? My own 'Sybil', based on twenty year's experience of her as well as the study of her diaries, is neither the exalted and pure 'Sybil' of my husband's eulogy nor the joyless pathological 'Sybil' of Dr. Smith's clinical assessment.

I see her as inevitably *human*—affected at times by jealousy, anger, sexual frustration, petty rivalry, stubbornness and cowardice, and afflicted by anxiety, insecurity, paranoia, depression and absurdly low self-esteem as well as by her OCD. At the same time, I acknowledge the genuine existence of idealistic principles in her keen mind and sensitive heart, despite her being pulled in other directions by more ordinary impulses or by clinical obsessions. She was by nature and on principle ardently non-violent and generous, a flawed and damaged 'innocent' trying to live simply in a very complex world. Her refusal to take the true measure of her own self-worth was at once a devastating illness and a genuine Christian humility. When not overwhelmed by the symptoms of her illness, she set a standard for everyday thoughtfulness and charitable behaviour. Whenever I am tempted to push my way into an Underground carriage in rush hour, before all the passengers have exited, when I am nearly ready to ignore scraps of paper that have fallen out of my pocket onto the ground, rather than stoop to pick them up, when I am about to rush past a man or woman selling *The Big Issue* or toss into the rubbish bin an appeal from one of the dozens of charities that assault us through the post, I pause and say to myself, "What would Sybil do?"

Impaired victim or unworldly child, she will always remain, to some extent, elusive and mysterious to me and to many who knew her. During our period of intense mourning, a poem by the Italian author, Cesar Pavese (1908-1950), was sent to us in memory of Sybil. It still seems to capture the eerie quality of her being and to encapsulate our family's feelings about her:

Lois Chaber

The hill is part of night, the sky is clear.
They frame your head, which scarcely moves,
moving with that sky. You are like a cloud
glimpsed between the branches. In your eyes there
shines
the strangeness of a sky which isn't yours.

. . . .

But you live somewhere else.
Your tender blood was made in some other place.
The words you speak have no echo here
in the harsh desolation of this sky.
You are just a wandering cloud, white and very sweet,
tangled one night among these ancient branches.

(From "Nocturne" in *Hard Labor: Poems by Cesar Pavese,* Trans. William Arrowsmith, Johns Hopkins Press, 1979.)

* * *

Coda

The pseudonym I have used for Sybil's old neighbourhood friend—'Asha'—means 'Hope' in the Bangladeshi language. It is appropriate, then, that Asha's voice is the last to resonate in this book:

> *The weird thing was that at university I met*
> *a boy who shared and reflected a lot of*
> *characteristics that Sybil had, in that he was*
> *proactively nice and very innocent about his*
> *environment. That was fine, but the odd thing*
> *about him was that he would show the same*
> *glazed-eye-look as hers, where he'd just stare*
> *out into space, not at anything specific; it's quite*
> *disarming to look at someone like that because*
> *you can't understand it. I saw this happen quite*

"THE THING INSIDE MY HEAD"

a few times and I let it pass because I didn't
know how to handle that kind of thing.

Then it happened more, and I think he was
getting quieter and not so vibrant; I felt that this
was just going to turn into another Sybil case. I
went up to him directly and I said, 'Why are you
doing that look?' He wouldn't tell me, and I had
to force it out of him until he finally said, 'Oh, I
think about killing myself'. Then I said, 'You
have to see someone about this because it's
not fair on you to feel like that'. In the end, my
friend and I persuaded him to go to counselling.
They put him on an anti-depressant, but it
shook up his system; after he was on it for a
few days, the side effects were making him
nauseous and dizzy and he didn't want to
continue. However, we said, 'Go back!' and
they gave him Prozac and that seemed much
better.

They said, 'You have to take exercise and
wake up early', and he felt these were silly
things and they wouldn't help, but I felt it was
worth doing if there might be a chance that he'd
avoid the kind of life that Sybil entered into
during the last stages. My loyalty to him arose
from what I didn't do for Sybil when I was
younger, how I couldn't help her, and so I said
to him, 'I'll wake up at seven with you and we'll
go for a walk in the park'; this, as a student,
was a big thing because we don't wake up till at
least twelve o'clock each day. He improved
from there on in.

Asha and this young man were married in 2001.

Lois Chaber

"THE THING INSIDE MY HEAD"

Lois Chaber